I0037384

Environmental Health Criteria 234

ELEMENTAL SPECIATION IN HUMAN HEALTH RISK ASSESSMENT

First draft prepared by Professor P. Apostoli, University of Brescia,
Brescia, Italy; Professor R. Cornelis, University of Ghent, Ghent,
Belgium; Dr J. Duffus, Edinburgh, Scotland; Professor P. Hoet and
Professor D. Lison, Université Catholique de Louvain, Brussels,
Belgium; and Professor D. Templeton, University of Toronto, Toronto,
Canada

Published under the joint sponsorship of the United Nations
Environment Programme, the International Labour Organization
and the World Health Organization, and produced within the
framework of the Inter-Organization Programme for the Sound
Management of Chemicals.

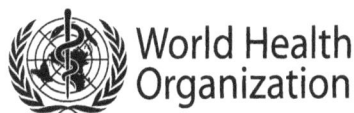

World Health
Organization

The **International Programme on Chemical Safety (IPCS)**, established in 1980, is a joint venture of the United Nations Environment Programme (UNEP), the International Labour Organization (ILO) and the World Health Organization (WHO). The overall objectives of the IPCS are to establish the scientific basis for assessment of the risk to human health and the environment from exposure to chemicals, through international peer review processes, as a prerequisite for the promotion of chemical safety, and to provide technical assistance in strengthening national capacities for the sound management of chemicals.

The **Inter-Organization Programme for the Sound Management of Chemicals (IOMC)** was established in 1995 by UNEP, ILO, the Food and Agriculture Organization of the United Nations, WHO, the United Nations Industrial Development Organization, the United Nations Institute for Training and Research and the Organisation for Economic Co-operation and Development (Participating Organizations), following recommendations made by the 1992 UN Conference on Environment and Development to strengthen cooperation and increase coordination in the field of chemical safety. The purpose of the IOMC is to promote coordination of the policies and activities pursued by the Participating Organizations, jointly or separately, to achieve the sound management of chemicals in relation to human health and the environment.

WHO Library Cataloguing-in-Publication Data

Elemental speciation in human health risk assessment / authors, P. Apostoli ... [et al.].

(Environmental health criteria ; 234)

1.Metals – analysis. 2.Organometallic compounds – analysis. 3.Metals – adverse effects. 4.Organometallic compounds – adverse effects. 5.Metals – toxicity. 6.Organometallic compounds – toxicity. 7.Risk assessment. 8.Environmental exposure. I.Apostoli, P. II.World Health Organization. III.International Programme on Chemical Safety. IV.Series

ISBN 92 4 157234 5   (NLM classification: QV 600)
ISBN 978 92 4 157234 7
ISSN 0250-863X

This document was technically and linguistically edited by Marla Sheffer, Ottawa, Canada, and printed by Wissenchaftliche Verlagsgesellschaft mbH, Stuttgart, Germany.

CONTENTS

ENVIRONMENTAL HEALTH CRITERIA FOR ELEMENTAL SPECIATION IN HUMAN HEALTH RISK ASSESSMENT

PREAMBLE   ix

ACRONYMS AND ABBREVIATIONS   xvii

1. SUMMARY   1

    1.1   Scope and purpose of the document   1
    1.2   Definitions   1
    1.3   Structural aspects of speciation   1
    1.4   Analytical techniques and methodology   2
    1.5   Bioaccessibility and bioavailability   3
    1.6   Toxicokinetics and biomonitoring   4
          1.6.1 Toxicokinetics   4
          1.6.2 Biomonitoring   5
    1.7   Molecular and cellular mechanisms of metal
          toxicity   6
    1.8   Health effects   7

2. DEFINITIONS OF SPECIES AND SPECIATION   8

3. STRUCTURAL ASPECTS OF SPECIATION   11

    3.1   Isotopic composition   11
    3.2   Electronic and oxidation states   12
    3.3   Inorganic and organic compounds and complexes   15
    3.4   Organometallic species   18
    3.5   Macromolecular compounds and complexes   21

4. ANALYTICAL TECHNIQUES AND
    METHODOLOGY   22

    4.1   Introduction   22
    4.2   Sample collection and storage   24
    4.3   Sample preparation   28
          4.3.1 Preliminary treatment of biological fluids   28

| | | 4.3.2 | Preliminary treatment of tissues and plants | 30 |

4.3.2 Preliminary treatment of tissues and plants — 30
4.3.3 Choice between low molecular mass and high molecular mass compounds — 32
4.3.4 Desalting — 32
4.3.5 Sample cleanup — 33
4.3.6 Extraction procedures — 33
4.3.7 Preconcentration of the species — 34
4.3.8 Derivatization — 34
4.4 Separation techniques — 35
4.4.1 Liquid chromatography — 35
4.4.2 Gas chromatography — 36
4.4.3 Capillary electrophoresis — 37
4.4.4 Gel electrophoresis — 37
4.5 Sequential extraction schemes for the fractionation of sediments, soils, aerosols, and fly ash — 38
4.6 Detection: elemental and molecular — 39
4.6.1 Atomic absorption spectrometry — 39
4.6.2 Atomic fluorescence spectrometry — 41
4.6.3 Atomic emission spectrometry — 41
4.6.4 Inductively coupled plasma mass spectrometry — 41
4.6.5 Plasma source time-of-flight mass spectrometry — 42
4.6.6 Glow discharge plasmas as tunable sources for elemental speciation — 42
4.6.7 Electrospray mass spectrometry — 43
4.6.8 Electrochemical methods — 43
4.7 Calibration in elemental speciation analysis — 44
4.8 Reference materials — 45
4.9 Direct speciation analysis of elements and particles — 45
4.10 State of the art — 46

5. BIOACCESSIBILITY AND BIOAVAILABILITY — 48

5.1 Introduction — 48
5.2 Bioaccessibility of elements in soils and sediments — 48
5.2.1 Factors affecting the mobility and accessibility of elements in terrestrial (soil) environments — 48
5.2.2 Factors affecting the mobility and accessibility of elements in sediment

		environments	50
5.3		Determinants of bioavailability	52
	5.3.1	Uptake by carriers	55
	5.3.2	Uptake and physical form	59
	5.3.3	Uptake and complexation	60
	5.3.4	Selective uptake according to charge and size	62
	5.3.5	Selective uptake according to binding affinity for different cationic centres	63
	5.3.6	Selective uptake involving kinetic binding traps, with or without accompanying redox reactions	63
	5.3.7	Uptake of organometallic compounds	65
	5.3.8	Exposure concentration and uptake	65
	5.3.9	Competition in the uptake and toxicity of non-nutrient elements	66
5.4		Incorporation of bioaccessibility and bioavailability considerations in risk assessment	67
	5.4.1	Bioaccessibility and bioavailability in current approaches to environmental and human risk assessment	68
	5.4.2	The biotic ligand model	68
6.		TOXICOKINETICS AND BIOLOGICAL MONITORING	70
6.1		Introduction	70
6.2		Absorption	72
	6.2.1	Chromium	73
	6.2.2	Manganese	74
	6.2.3	Iron	76
	6.2.4	Cobalt	76
	6.2.5	Nickel	77
	6.2.6	Copper	78
	6.2.7	Arsenic	78
	6.2.8	Selenium	80
	6.2.9	Cadmium	81
	6.2.10	Mercury	81
	6.2.11	Lead	83
6.3		Disposition, excretion, and protein binding	85
	6.3.1	Chromium	86

		6.3.2	Manganese	88
		6.3.3	Copper	89
		6.3.4	Zinc	90
		6.3.5	Arsenic	90
		6.3.6	Selenium	91
		6.3.7	Silver	91
		6.3.8	Cadmium	92
		6.3.9	Mercury	93
		6.3.10	Lead	96
	6.4	Biotransformation		97
		6.4.1	Chromium	98
		6.4.2	Manganese	98
		6.4.3	Arsenic	98
		6.4.4	Selenium	102
		6.4.5	Mercury	102
	6.5	Exposure assessment and biological monitoring		104
		6.5.1	Exposure assessment	104
		6.5.2	Speciation in biological monitoring	105
7.	MOLECULAR AND CELLULAR MECHANISMS OF METAL TOXICITY			111
	7.1	Introduction		111
	7.2	Mechanisms of DNA damage and repair		111
	7.3	Metal–protein interactions		114
	7.4	Generation of reactive oxygen species		119
	7.5	Effects on the immune system		120
		7.5.1	Mechanisms of sensitization	120
		7.5.2	Immunosuppression	121
8.	HEALTH EFFECTS			122
	8.1	Introduction		122
	8.2	Acute toxicity		122
		8.2.1	Chromium	122
		8.2.2	Nickel	123
		8.2.3	Arsenic	124
		8.2.4	Tin	126
		8.2.5	Barium	127
		8.2.6	Mercury	128
		8.2.7	Lead	129
	8.3	Sensitization and irritation		130

8.3.1 Chromium   131
8.3.2 Nickel   132
8.3.3 Palladium   132
8.3.4 Platinum   133
8.4 Lung toxicity   134
8.4.1 Cobalt   134
8.5 Neurotoxicity   136
8.5.1 Manganese   136
8.5.2 Tin   137
8.5.3 Mercury   138
8.5.4 Thallium   141
8.5.5 Lead   142
8.6 Nephrotoxicity   144
8.6.1 Cadmium   144
8.7 Reproductive toxicity   145
8.7.1 Nickel   145
8.7.2 Mercury   146
8.8 Genotoxicity   148
8.8.1 Chromium   148
8.8.2 Cobalt   150
8.9 Carcinogenicity   153
8.9.1 Chromium   153
8.9.2 Cobalt   154
8.9.3 Nickel   156
8.9.4 Arsenic   158

9. CONCLUSIONS AND RECOMMENDATIONS   162

REFERENCES   164

RESUME   220

RESUMEN   228

INDEX OF ELEMENTS   236

NOTE TO READERS OF THE CRITERIA MONOGRAPHS

Every effort has been made to present information in the criteria monographs as accurately as possible without unduly delaying their publication. In the interest of all users of the Environmental Health Criteria monographs, readers are requested to communicate any errors that may have occurred to the Director of the International Programme on Chemical Safety, World Health Organization, Geneva, Switzerland, in order that they may be included in corrigenda.

Environmental Health Criteria

PREAMBLE

Objectives

In 1973, the WHO Environmental Health Criteria Programme was initiated with the following objectives:

(i)   to assess information on the relationship between exposure to environmental pollutants and human health, and to provide guidelines for setting exposure limits;
(ii)   to identify new or potential pollutants;
(iii)   to identify gaps in knowledge concerning the health effects of pollutants;
(iv)   to promote the harmonization of toxicological and epidemiological methods in order to have internationally comparable results.

The first Environmental Health Criteria (EHC) monograph, on mercury, was published in 1976, and since that time an ever-increasing number of assessments of chemicals and of physical effects have been produced. In addition, many EHC monographs have been devoted to evaluating toxicological methodology, e.g. for genetic, neurotoxic, teratogenic, and nephrotoxic effects. Other publications have been concerned with epidemiological guidelines, evaluation of short-term tests for carcinogens, biomarkers, effects on the elderly, and so forth.

Since its inauguration, the EHC Programme has widened its scope, and the importance of environmental effects, in addition to health effects, has been increasingly emphasized in the total evaluation of chemicals.

The original impetus for the Programme came from World Health Assembly resolutions and the recommendations of the 1972 UN Conference on the Human Environment. Subsequently, the work became an integral part of the International Programme on Chemical Safety (IPCS), a cooperative programme of WHO, ILO, and UNEP. In this manner, with the strong support of the new partners, the importance of occupational health and environmental effects was fully recognized. The EHC monographs have become widely established, used, and recognized throughout the world.

The recommendations of the 1992 UN Conference on Environment and Development and the subsequent establishment of the Intergovernmental Forum on Chemical Safety with the priorities for action in the six programme areas of Chapter 19, Agenda 21, all lend further weight to the need for EHC assessments of the risks of chemicals.

Scope

Two different types of EHC documents are available: 1) on specific chemicals or groups of related chemicals; and 2) on risk assessment methodologies. The criteria monographs are intended to provide critical reviews on the effect on human health and the environment of chemicals and of combinations of chemicals and physical and biological agents and risk assessment methodologies. As such, they include and review studies that are of direct relevance for evaluations. However, they do not describe *every* study carried out. Worldwide data are used and are quoted from original studies, not from abstracts or reviews. Both published and unpublished reports are considered, and it is incumbent on the authors to assess all the articles cited in the references. Preference is always given to published data. Unpublished data are used only when relevant published data are absent or when they are pivotal to the risk assessment. A detailed policy statement is available that describes the procedures used for unpublished proprietary data so that this information can be used in the evaluation without compromising its confidential nature (WHO (1990) Revised Guidelines for the Preparation of Environmental Health Criteria Monographs. PCS/90.69, Geneva, World Health Organization).

In the evaluation of human health risks, sound human data, whenever available, are preferred to animal data. Animal and in vitro studies provide support and are used mainly to supply evidence missing from human studies. It is mandatory that research on human subjects is conducted in full accord with ethical principles, including the provisions of the Helsinki Declaration.

The EHC monographs are intended to assist national and international authorities in making risk assessments and subsequent risk management decisions and to update national and international authorities on risk assessment methodology.

Procedures

The order of procedures that result in the publication of an EHC monograph is shown in the flow chart on p. xii. A designated staff member of IPCS, responsible for the scientific quality of the document, serves as Responsible Officer (RO). The IPCS Editor is responsible for layout and language. The first draft, prepared by consultants or, more usually, staff from an IPCS Participating Institution, is based on extensive literature searches from reference databases such as Medline and Toxline.

The draft document, when received by the RO, may require an initial review by a small panel of experts to determine its scientific quality and objectivity. Once the RO finds the document acceptable as a first draft, it is distributed, in its unedited form, to well over 100 EHC contact points throughout the world who are asked to comment on its completeness and accuracy and, where necessary, provide additional material. The contact points, usually designated by governments, may be Participating Institutions, IPCS Focal Points, or individual scientists known for their particular expertise. Generally, some four months are allowed before the comments are considered by the RO and author(s). A second draft incorporating comments received and approved by the Coordinator, IPCS, is then distributed to Task Group members, who carry out the peer review, at least six weeks before their meeting.

The Task Group members serve as individual scientists, not as representatives of any organization, government, or industry. Their function is to evaluate the accuracy, significance, and relevance of the information in the document and to assess the health and environmental risks from exposure to the chemical or chemicals in question. A summary and recommendations for further research and improved safety aspects are also required. The composition of the Task Group is dictated by the range of expertise required for the subject of the meeting and by the need for a balanced geographical distribution.

EHC PREPARATION FLOW CHART

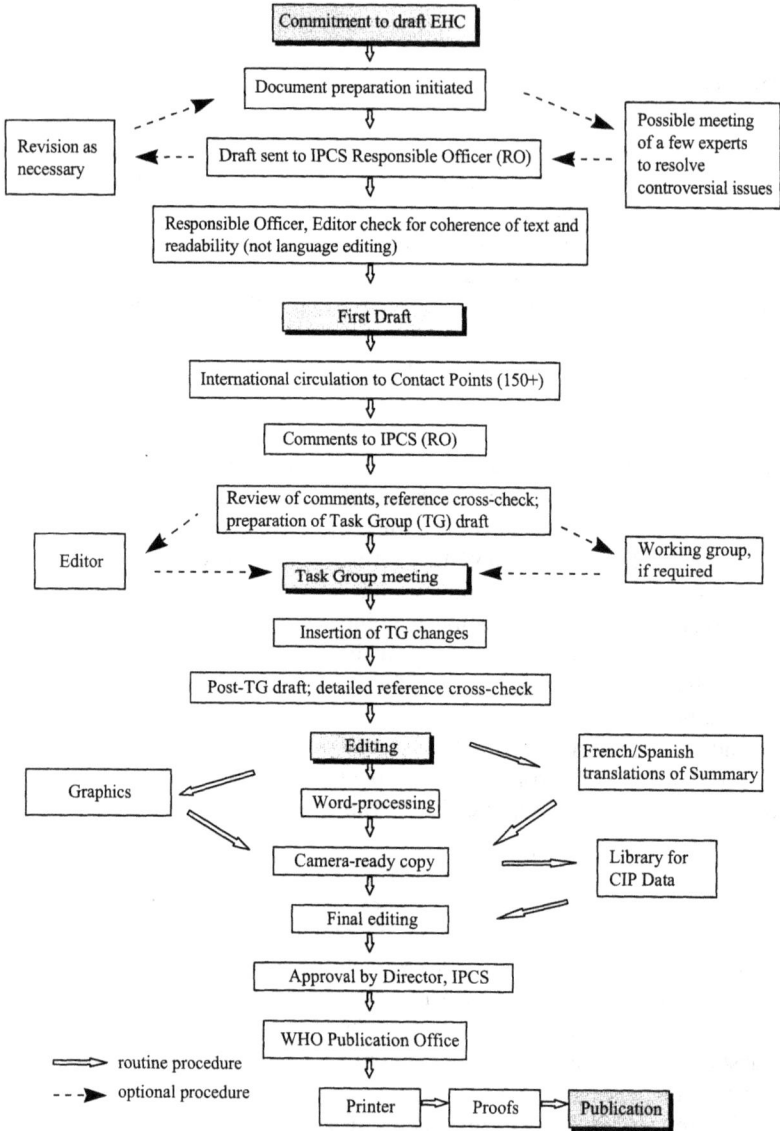

The three cooperating organizations of the IPCS recognize the important role played by nongovernmental organizations. Representatives from relevant national and international associations may be invited to join the Task Group as observers. Although observers may provide a valuable contribution to the process, they can speak only at the invitation of the Chairperson. Observers do not participate in the final evaluation of the chemicals; this is the sole responsibility of the Task Group members. When the Task Group considers it to be appropriate, it may meet in camera.

All individuals who as authors, consultants, or advisers participate in the preparation of the EHC monograph must, in addition to serving in their personal capacity as scientists, inform the RO if at any time a conflict of interest, whether actual or potential, could be perceived in their work. They are required to sign a conflict of interest statement. Such a procedure ensures the transparency and probity of the process.

When the Task Group has completed its review and the RO is satisfied as to the scientific correctness and completeness of the document, it then goes for language editing, reference checking, and preparation of camera-ready copy. After approval by the Coordinator, IPCS, the monograph is submitted for printing.

It is accepted that the following criteria should initiate the updating of an EHC monograph: new data are available that would substantially change the evaluation; there is public concern for health or environmental effects of the agent because of greater exposure; an appreciable time period has elapsed since the last evaluation.

All Participating Institutions are informed, through the EHC progress report, of the authors and institutions proposed for the drafting of the documents. A comprehensive file of all comments received on drafts of each EHC monograph is maintained and is available on request. The Chairpersons of Task Groups are briefed before each meeting on their role and responsibility in ensuring that these rules are followed.

WHO TASK GROUP ON ENVIRONMENTAL HEALTH CRITERIA FOR ELEMENTAL SPECIATION IN HUMAN HEALTH RISK ASSESSMENT

A WHO Task Group on Environmental Health Criteria for Elemental Speciation in Human Health Risk Assessment met at the Fraunhofer Institute of Toxicology and Experimental Medicine in Hanover, Germany, from 15 to 18 November 2005. The meeting was opened by Dr Inge Mangelsdorf on behalf of the Fraunhofer Institute and Dr A. Aitio, Programme for the Promotion of Chemical Safety, WHO, on behalf of the IPCS and its three cooperative organizations (UNEP/ILO/WHO). The Task Group reviewed, revised, and approved the draft monograph.

The first draft was prepared, under the coordination of Dr Janet Kielhorn, Fraunhofer Institute of Toxicology and Experimental Medicine, Hanover, Germany, by Professor Pietro Apostoli from the Institute of Occupational Medicine and Industrial Hygiene, University of Brescia, Brescia, Italy; Professor Rita Cornelis from the Laboratory for Analytical Chemistry, University of Ghent, Ghent, Belgium; Dr John Duffus from Edinburgh, Scotland; Professor Perrine Hoet and Professor Dominique Lison from the Université Catholique de Louvain, Brussels, Belgium; and Professor Douglas Templeton from the Department of Laboratory Medicine and Pathobiology, University of Toronto, Toronto, Canada.

The second draft was prepared by the same authors in collaboration with Dr J. Kielhorn and the Secretariat, which incorporated comments received following the circulation of the first draft to a group of 20 scientists identified as experts in elemental speciation and risk assessment.

Dr A. Aitio was responsible for the overall scientific content of the monograph.

The efforts of all who helped in the preparation and finalization of the monograph are gratefully acknowledged.

* * *

Risk assessment activities of IPCS are supported financially by the Department of Health and Department for Environment, Food & Rural Affairs, United Kingdom; Environmental Protection Agency, Food and Drug Administration, and National Institute of Environmental Health Sciences, USA; European Commission; German Federal Ministry of Environment, Nature Conservation and Nuclear Safety; Health Canada; Japanese Ministry of Health, Labour and Welfare; and Swiss Agency for Environment, Forests and Landscape.

* * *

Task Group Members

Professor Pietro Apostoli, Institute of Occupational Medicine and Industrial Hygiene, University of Brescia, Brescia, Italy

Professor Rita Cornelis, Laboratory for Analytical Chemistry, University of Ghent, Ghent, Belgium

Dr John Duffus, Edinburgh, Scotland, United Kingdom

Dr Stefan Hahn (*Co-rapporteur*), Fraunhofer Institute of Toxicology and Experimental Medicine, Hanover, Germany

Dr Janet Kielhorn (*Co-rapporteur*), Fraunhofer Institute of Toxicology and Experimental Medicine, Hanover, Germany

Professor Dominique Lison, Université Catholique de Louvain, Brussels, Belgium

Professor Monica Nordberg (*Chair*), Institute of Environmental Medicine, Karolinska Institutet, Stockholm, Sweden

Dr Vesa Riihimäki, Finnish Institute of Occupational Health, Helsinki, Finland

Professor Douglas M. Templeton, Department of Laboratory Medicine and Pathobiology, University of Toronto, Toronto, Canada

Secretariat

Dr Antero Aitio, International Programme on Chemical Safety, World Health Organization, Geneva, Switzerland

ACRONYMS AND ABBREVIATIONS

AAS	atomic absorption spectrometry
ADP	adenosine diphosphate
ATP	adenosine 5'-triphosphate
CE	capillary electrophoresis
DMA	dimethylarsinic acid
DMT	divalent metal transporter
DNA	deoxyribonucleic acid
EDTA	ethylenediaminetetraacetic acid
EHC	Environmental Health Criteria
ES-MS	electrospray mass spectrometry
GC	gas chromatography
GE	gel electrophoresis
HLA	human leukocyte antigen
HPLC	high-performance liquid chromatography
IARC	International Agency for Research on Cancer
ICP-AES	inductively coupled plasma atomic emission spectrometry
ICP-MS	inductively coupled plasma mass spectrometry
ICP-OES	inductively coupled plasma optical emission spectrometry
ILO	International Labour Organization
IPCS	International Programme on Chemical Safety
IUPAC	International Union of Pure and Applied Chemistry
K_{ow}	octanol–water partition coefficient
LC	liquid chromatography
MET	minimum elicitation threshold
MMA	methylarsonic acid
MMT	2-methylcyclopentadienyl manganese tricarbonyl

MS	mass spectrometry
MT	metallothionein
NIST	National Institute of Standards and Technology
NTA	nitrilotriacetate
OES	optical emission spectrometry
RNA	ribonucleic acid
RO	Responsible Officer
SD	standard deviation
SRM	standard reference material
UN	United Nations
UNEP	United Nations Environment Programme
UV	ultraviolet
WHO	World Health Organization
ZIP	ZRT and IRT-like protein

1. SUMMARY

1.1 Scope and purpose of the document

The purpose of this document is to assess, evaluate, and give guidance on the role of elemental speciation and speciation analysis in hazard and risk assessment, rather than to present a review of each element and its speciation. The effects on the environment are not considered in this document, as this has been the topic of a recent conference and associated documentation (SGOMSEC, 2003). However, exposure of the human population through environmental routes is considered.

This document is directed at risk assessors and regulators, to emphasize the importance of consideration of speciation in their deliberations. Until now, this issue has not been a part of most hazard and risk assessments. Further, one of the aims of the document is to encourage the analysis of speciation of elements to increase knowledge on the effect of speciation on mode of action and understanding of health effects.

The emphasis is not on nutritional requirements, but on the toxicity of elements to humans. Consideration is made not only of consumer/general exposure but also of occupational exposure.

1.2 Definitions

A chemical "species" is the "specific form of an element defined as to isotopic composition, electronic or oxidation state, and/or complex or molecular structure". "Speciation" can be defined as the distribution of an element among defined chemical species in a system, and "speciation analysis" as the analytical activities of identifying and/or measuring the quantities of one or more individual chemical species in a sample.

1.3 Structural aspects of speciation

The definitions of species and speciation of elements are based on several different levels of atomic and molecular structure where species differences are manifest. Here, we consider differences at the levels of 1) isotopic composition, 2) electronic or oxidation state, 3) inorganic and organic compounds and complexes, 4) organometallic species, and 5) macromolecular compounds and complexes. Some of these structural levels are more important for risk assessment than others. Thus, stable isotope composition, while important both from a theoretical point of view and in physical and environmental chemistry, is generally of minimal importance in risk assessment concerning human health. Likewise, elemental speciation at the macromolecular level has biological significance in physiology, biochemistry, and nutrition, but its importance in occupational or environmental toxicity is less well understood. Organic complexation is of intermediate importance; as most chelates are labile relative to covalent complexes, they influence bioavailability and cellular uptake. However, they form and exchange in relation to the availability of ligands in the local milieu, and their trafficking to cellular targets is somewhat unpredictable. On the other hand, valence state and inorganic and covalent organometallic speciation are of great importance in determining the toxicity of metals and semi-metals.

1.4 Analytical techniques and methodology

Remarkable advances in the performance of elemental speciation analysis have been made during the past 20 years. Speciation analysis can now be performed for nearly every element, but not for every species of every element. Insight has been acquired into sample collection and storage so as to avoid contamination and to preserve the species intact. Available knowledge allows for sample preparation in order to identify and quantify species in biological fluids, tissues, water, and airborne dust. Sample preparation may include an additional cleanup step, extraction procedures, or preconcentration and derivatization of the species, prior to their separation. The most widely used separation techniques are liquid chromatography, gas chromatography, capillary electrophoresis, and gel electrophoresis. If the species are too complex, groups of species can be isolated by applying sequential extraction schemes. This is most used in the fractionation of sediments, soils, aerosols, and fly ash. The detection is usually that of the element, although molecular detection is gaining ground, especially in clinical and food analysis. Commonly used elemental detection methods are atomic absorption spectrometry, atomic fluorescence spectrometry, atomic emission spectrometry, and inductively coupled plasma mass spectrometry. Additionally, plasma source time-of-flight mass spectrometry and glow discharge plasmas can be used as tunable sources for elemental speciation. Electrospray mass spectrometry and matrix-assisted laser desorption ionization mass spectrometry are ideal to obtain structural information about the molecular species. Electrochemical methods are further powerful tools for speciation analysis.

Calibration in elemental speciation analysis still remains challenging, especially so in the case of unknown species. There exists a limited choice of reference materials for elemental speciation. A growing number of them are certified.

Direct speciation analysis of elements in particles is of great interest in assessing environmental health hazards. It provides valuable information on the elemental species in the superficial layers of the particles, allowing deductions about the origin, formation, transport, and chemical reactions. In most cases, it necessitates highly sophisticated apparatus.

1.5   Bioaccessibility and bioavailability

Substances must be bioaccessible before they can become bioavailable to human beings. A substance is defined as bioaccessible if it is possible for it to come in contact with a living organism, which may then absorb it. Bioaccessibility is a major consideration in relation to particulates, where species internal to the particles may never become bioaccessible. Elemental species that are accessible on the surface of particles or in solution may be bioavailable if mechanisms exist for their uptake by living cells. The rate of this uptake into cells is usually related to the external concentration of either free ions with appropriate properties or kinetically labile inorganic species (free ions plus inorganic complexes). Organic complexation and particulate binding often decrease elemental uptake rates by decreasing the concentrations of free ions and labile inorganic complexes. However, in certain circumstances, organic complexes of an element may facilitate its uptake. In addition, the site at which particulates have prolonged contact with tissues, such as lung alveolar epithelia, may become a focus of chronic exposure and toxicity. Uptake systems are never entirely specific for a single element, and these systems often show competition between similar chemical species of different elements, resulting in inhibition of uptake of essential elements and uptake of competing potentially toxic elements. Because of these competitive interactions, ion ratios often control the cellular uptake of toxic and nutrient elements. Such interactions also result in inherent interrelationships between toxicity and nutrition. It is important to define chemical species interactions clearly before carrying out risk assessment because of such profound effects on availability and toxicity.

1.6 Toxicokinetics and biomonitoring

1.6.1 Toxicokinetics

Various aspects of speciation of the elements (e.g. the unchanged forms, the biological mechanisms changing species, the different valence states, and the metal–ligand complexes) must be considered when evaluating absorption, mechanisms of binding to proteins, distribution, storage, metabolism, excretion, reactivity, and toxic activity of the metallic elements themselves.

Absorption through the respiratory tract is conditioned by size, solubility, and chemical reactivity of elemental species inhaled as particles. The absorption of elemental species in the gastrointestinal tract varies depending on their solubility in water and gastrointestinal fluids, their chemical and physical characteristics, the presence of other reacting compounds, and the period of ingestion (fasting, for instance). The skin may also be an important absorption route for some elemental species.

After absorption, the elemental species can form complexes with proteins, including enzymes, such as the essential elements associated with ferritin (iron, copper, zinc), α-amylase (copper), alcohol dehydrogenase (zinc), and carbonic anhydrase (copper, zinc).

In general, the removal of electrons from or addition of electrons to the atom influences the chemical activity and therefore the ability of metallic elements to interact with tissue targets (ligands). Examples of charge relevance in crossing lipid barriers are represented by chromate/dichromate, Fe^{2+}/Fe^{3+}, and Hg^+/Hg^0 passages.

Among the other metabolic transformations, the most important is bioalkylation, which, for example, mercury, tin, and lead undergo in microorganisms, whereas arsenic and selenium are additionally bioalkylated as part of their metabolic pathways in higher organisms. Alkylation produces species at a higher hydrophobic level, leading to an increased bioavailability, cell penetration, and accumulation in fatty tissues. Bioalkylation is important for some metals, since the alkylated metal species also interact with DNA. Alkylated metal species penetrate the blood–brain barrier more readily, and it is for this reason that such alkylated species are important neurotoxicants.

Metallic elements may be stored in tissues/organs as both inorganic species or salts and species chelated or sequestered to proteins and other organic compounds.

Excretion depends on the speciation, the route of absorption, and other toxicokinetic phases. The excreted species are either inorganic or organic and frequently at the lowest oxidation state. The elements ingested with food or water are excreted through the bile and faeces; minor routes of excretion include breath, milk, sweat, hair, and nails. The excretion of essential elements is under the constant control of efficient homeostatic mechanisms, depending on the element.

1.6.2 Biomonitoring

The main purpose of biological monitoring is to measure the internal dose — i.e. the amount of the chemical that is systemically absorbed. Speciation in biological monitoring may be approached on three different levels: 1) analysis of specific elemental species (e.g. arsenic), 2) fractionation by chemical analytical means to organic and inorganic species (e.g. mercury, lead), or 3) application to the analysis of information on the differences in the distribution of different species of an element (mercury in plasma, blood cells, urine; chromium in erythrocytes/plasma).

Biological monitoring is of particular value, because the method integrates the exposure from all sources and by all routes of entry. Measurement of the internal body burden is of special importance for species of metals because of their tendency to accumulate. The ratio of the concentration of toxicologically important species at the target site to the total elemental concentration measured in bio-monitoring is different for different species.

1.7 Molecular and cellular mechanisms of metal toxicity

Metals and semi-metals have multiple effects on biological processes, and these can to a large degree be rationalized after describing interactions with the various classes of biomolecules. Such interactions show strong species dependence. The effects of individual elements on biological systems are best understood through the effects of elements on biochemical structures and processes, described at the cellular and molecular levels. Particularly in this realm, a combination of effects characteristic of an individual species is manifest. Traditionally, one has looked at interactions of metallic elements with the major classes of biomolecules — i.e. proteins, lipids, carbohydrates, and nucleic acids. This approach still has some merit, but gains significance when put into context.

Catalytic generation of reactive oxygen species by metals can damage all biomolecules: speciation determines the reactivity — catalytic or otherwise — with oxygen. Direct binding of ions, such as Hg^{2+} and Cd^{2+}, to proteins can inhibit enzymatic activities, structural assemblies, and many other functions of proteins. Here, the valence state and/or associated ligands dictate availability for binding, and hence the pattern of toxicity. Lipid peroxidation catalysed by metallic elements in their ionic form and in redox-active complexes destroys protective barriers in cells and subcellular organelles. Binding of metal ions to carbohydrates is complicated in terms of both the structural chemistry and the biological consequences, but clearly the binding affects such processes as the assembly of glycoproteins into functional extracellular matrix. Ligand exchange reactions with sugar moieties are species dependent. Binding to nucleic acids interferes with regulation of the genome on many levels. This includes both facilitating DNA damage and inhibiting its repair.

A further dimension to metal toxicity is the impact of individual elements on the immune system. While many elements are capable of producing immunosuppression, little is known of the role of individual elemental species. Some elemental species, such as those of nickel, cobalt, and chromium, are sensitizers for the skin and respiratory system. To some extent, the role of speciation is known, with therapeutic gold salts, cadmium species, and nickel species serving as interesting examples that begin to shed light on mechanisms.

1.8 Health effects

Toxicity may vary significantly according to the oxidation state of the element, the formation of complexes, and the biotransformation of the elemental species. In the chapter on health effects, a selection is given of the most significant examples (in order of atomic number) where the relevance of speciation to health effects in humans has been demonstrated, including acute toxicity (chromium, nickel, arsenic, tin, barium, mercury, lead), allergy (chromium, nickel, palladium, platinum), lung toxicity (cobalt), neurotoxicity (manganese, tin, mercury, thallium, lead), nephrotoxicity (cadmium), reproductive toxicity (nickel, mercury), genotoxicity (chromium, cobalt), and carcinogenicity (chromium, cobalt, nickel, arsenic). An overall evaluation of the data indicates that, when possible, the consideration of speciation allows a better understanding of the mechanisms of toxicity of an element and a refinement of risk assessment by focusing evaluation of the consequences of exposure upon the most relevant species.

2. DEFINITIONS OF SPECIES AND SPECIATION

The terms "species" and "speciation", in a chemical sense, have become widely used in the literature, and it is now well established that the occurrence of an element in different compounds and forms is often crucial to understanding the environmental and occupational toxicity of that element (Nieboer et al., 1999; Thier & Bolt, 2001; Ravera, 2004; Cornelis et al., 2005). A number of definitions of speciation can be found in the literature. In the past, the term "speciation" has been used to refer to "reaction specificity" (rarely); in geochemistry and environmental chemistry, to changes taking place during natural cycles of an element (species transformation); to the analytical activity of measuring the distribution of an element among species in a sample (speciation analysis); and to the distribution itself of an element among different species in a sample (species distribution).

The Oxford Dictionary of Chemistry (Daintith, 2004) defines species as "a chemical entity, such as a particular atom, ion, or molecule". A widely used glossary of terms in toxicology gives a less common definition of "chemical species" as a "set of chemically identical atomic or molecular structural units in a solid array or of chemically identical molecular entities that can explore the same set of molecular energy levels on the time scale of the experiment" and defines "speciation" as "determination of the exact chemical form or compound in which an element occurs in a sample" (Duffus, 1993). After a series of three International Symposia on Speciation of Elements in Toxicology and in Environmental and Biological Sciences, the organizers formulated the definition "Speciation is the occurrence of an element in separate, identifiable forms (i.e., chemical, physical or morphological state)" (Nieboer et al., 1999). The aim of Nieboer et al. (1999) was to include determinants of reactivity, and they produced a definition that goes well beyond speciation in a chemical sense and would include different phases of a pure substance, and even different-sized particles of a single compound.

This selection of definitions illustrates the circularity in defining a species in terms of an entity, form, or compound and indicates the lack of consensus in use of the term speciation. To attempt to harmonize the field and offer at least partial solutions to the ambiguities present in some of the earlier definitions, the International Union of Pure and Applied Chemistry (IUPAC) published guidelines for the use of terms relating to chemical species in 2000 (Templeton et al., 2000). We will use the IUPAC guidelines in this document.

Fundamental to these concepts is the meaning of the term (chemical) "species". According to the IUPAC recommendation (Templeton et al., 2000), "chemical species" is a "specific form of an element defined as to isotopic composition, electronic or oxidation state, and/or complex or molecular structure". Then "speciation" can be defined as the distribution of an element among defined chemical species in a system, and "speciation analysis" as the analytical activities of identifying and/or measuring the quantities of one or more individual chemical species in a sample.

There is necessarily some arbitrariness in our choice of levels of structure upon which to distinguish species. These will be dealt with in turn in the next chapter, and it will be seen that in terms of human health and risk assessment, some structural aspects of speciation are more important than others. Stable isotopic composition does seem useful to include in the definition, as it may influence transport properties and contribute to analytical tracer methodologies. Macromolecular species are excluded from the definition unless a macromolecular ligand is specifically defined. For example, a metal ion bound to two isoforms of a protein with defined amino acid sequences could be considered two species, but an ion bound to a polyelectrolyte such as humic acid or heparin would not be defined in terms of multiple species representing individual molecules in the heterogeneous and polydisperse population. In this case, it is advisable to refer to a fraction. "Fractionation" has been defined as the process of classification of an analyte or group of analytes from a certain sample according to physical (e.g. size, solubility) or chemical (e.g. bonding, reactivity) properties (Templeton et al., 2000).

Strictly speaking, whenever an element is present in different states according to isotopic composition, electronic or oxidation state, and/or complex or molecular structure, it must be regarded as occurring in different species. In practice, however, usage will depend on the relevance of the species differences for our understanding of the system under study. One would not generally describe a living organism or define an organic reaction mechanism by carbon speciation. Nevertheless, a pair of stereoisomers are certainly distinct species, and if each formed a chelation complex with a metal ion, these would be referred to as distinct species of the metal. Further, while the definition of species is general, in practice it is used mainly in the context of metallic and metalloid elements. Usage of speciation terminology also depends on our ability to distinguish the various species analytically. This practical analytical consideration governs whether different species should be grouped together or measured separately. Separate measurement implies minimum lifetimes and thermodynamic stabilities for detection, the values of which may change with developments in instrumentation.

The above IUPAC definition of speciation analysis deserves comment. A distinction is drawn between identification and measurement. It may be possible to identify the presence of a species without making a quantitative measurement of its concentration, and this provides some information on speciation. The definition also refers to quantities of one or more species. It is recognized that samples usually contain complex mixtures of species, perhaps with minor components, and a complete speciation analysis may seldom be achieved.

3. STRUCTURAL ASPECTS OF SPECIATION

The foregoing definitions of species and speciation imply an organizational framework to understand the concept of species at various structural levels. Various conformations, excited states, and transient forms of an elemental complex qualify as unique species under a strict application of the definition. However, both practical considerations and available analytical methodology set limits on what we can consider unique species. In practice, speciation analysis of a system should yield a set of species differing sufficiently from one another to describe the system to the required level of detail. In terms of risk assessment, this might be limited to forms of an element that have distinguishable properties of toxicity. Thus, all levels of structure are not equally important in risk assessment. Nevertheless, in this chapter we will describe the various structural levels that contribute to speciation. Specifically, we will consider nuclear isotopic composition, electronic and oxidation states, inorganic and organic compounds and complexes, organometallic species, and macromolecular compounds and complexes.

3.1 Isotopic composition

The isotopic abundances of an element can differ between samples if one or more arises from radioactive decay of another element (radiogenic) or if physical separation occurs (anthropogenic or environmental). Lead serves as an example of a radiogenic composition; of its four stable isotopes (^{204}Pb, ^{206}Pb, ^{207}Pb, and ^{208}Pb), three are radiogenic. Thus, ^{206}Pb and ^{207}Pb arise as decay products of uranium, and ^{208}Pb derives from thorium. Depending on the time of mixing of lead, uranium, and thorium in a given geological formation, the lead isotope ratios can be expected to differ (Kersten et al., 1993). This provides an isotopic signature of lead that can be used to track the movement and deposition of atmospheric lead (Maring et al., 1987; Rosman et al., 1993; Hong et al., 1994) and also to help identify sources of exposure (Rabinowitz, 1987; Reinhard & Ghazi, 1992; Kersten et al., 1993).

Elements without radiogenic precursors can also undergo isotopic separation in the environment. Differences in mass can lead to both chemical and inertial separation (Galimov, 1981). When oxygen partitions between two phases where it is bound in different species, differential enrichment of ^{16}O and ^{18}O can arise. This temperature-dependent process has been used to assess long-term trends in climate (Remenda et al., 1994). Biological separations can also occur. Disproportionation of sulfur by sulfur-metabolizing bacteria results in a different ^{34}S content of sulfates and sulfides (Canfield & Thamdrup, 1994). Anthropogenic differences in isotopic composition may also become important. Lithium, used in the treatment of bipolar disorder, has stable isotopes ^{6}Li and ^{7}Li. These have different biological properties, in part because they are transported differently across cell membranes (Renshaw, 1987; Hughes & Birch, 1992). Surprisingly, the isotopes ^{238}Pu and ^{239}Pu show differential rates of clearance from lung in dogs given aerosols of nitrates of both isotopes (Dagle et al., 1983). In general, though, only the lightest elements have mass differences that significantly affect bond strengths and primary kinetic isotope effects; apart from tracing sources of exposure, the isotopic composition is a structural aspect of speciation that is not prominent in toxicology or risk assessment. For instance, replacement of 30–40% of body water with D_2O is lethal in rodents, but replacement of 60% of body water with $H_2{}^{18}O$ is without effect (Jones & Leatherdale, 1991).

3.2 Electronic and oxidation states

This is one of the most important aspects of speciation affecting human toxicity and risk assessment. Oxidation state can affect absorption, membrane transport, and excretion, as well as toxicity at the cellular or molecular target. Examples of elements with more than one biologically important valence are given in Table 1.

Chromium serves as a good example of the importance of oxidation state. Cr^{III} is considered as an essential element (WHO, 1988), but Cr^{VI} is genotoxic and carcinogenic (Katz & Salem, 1994). Cr^{VI} does not appear to bind strongly to DNA, but is reduced inside the cell to Cr^{III}, which does. The binding of Cr^{III} alone is insufficient to damage DNA. However, the electrons released from intermediate oxidation states during the reduction of Cr^{VI} to Cr^{III} may do so (Wetterhahn & Hamilton, 1989; Aiyar et al., 1991; Standeven & Wetterhahn, 1991). Bioavailability also depends on oxidation state. Cr^{VI} is better absorbed than Cr^{III} following both dermal and oral exposure (Rowbotham et al., 2000). Cr^{VI} is taken up by some cells as chromate (CrO_4^{2-}) via anion transporters, whereas Cr^{III} ions permeate the lipid membrane with difficulty (Katz & Salem, 1994). Sulfate transporters are also involved in chromate transport through sulfate mimicry (Clarkson, 1993; Ballatori, 2002).

Table 1. Some elements with more than one biologically relevant valence
(in order of atomic number)

Atomic number	Name[a]	Symbol	Speciation
23	Vanadium*	V	IV/V
24	Chromium*	Cr	III/VI
25	Manganese*	Mn	II/III/IV
26	Iron*	Fe	0/II/III
27	Cobalt*	Co	II/III
28	Nickel*	Ni	II/IV
29	Copper*	Cu	0/I/II
30	Zinc*	Zn	0/II
33	Arsenic*	As	III/V
34	Selenium*	Se	II/IV/VI
42	Molybdenum*	Mo	II/III/IV/VI
46	Palladium	Pd	II/IV
47	Silver*	Ag	0/I/II
50	Tin*	Sn	II/IV
51	Antimony*	Sb	III/V
52	Tellurium*	Te	0/II/IV/VI
78	Platinum	Pt	II/IV
80	Mercury*	Hg	0/I/II
81	Thallium*	Tl	I/III
82	Lead	Pb	II/IV
92	Uranium*	U	III/VI
94	Plutonium*	Pu	III/IV/V/VI

[a] Elements marked with an asterisk are taken from Yokel et al. (2006).

At present, there is no general means of predicting how the oxidation state of a particular element will affect toxicity. Thus, inorganic Mn^{III} species are more toxic than other oxidation states — e.g. manganese(II) chloride $(MnCl_2)$ and manganese(IV) oxide

(MnO_2) are both less toxic in vitro than manganese(III) pyro-phosphate (Archibald & Tyree, 1987) — and the generally greater toxicity of Mn^{III} compared with Mn^{II} has been confirmed by others (Chen et al., 2001; Reaney et al., 2002). One mechanism of manganese toxicity is by disruption of iron–sulfur clusters in mito-chondrial enzymes, such as Complex I and mitochondrial aconitase. The higher oxidative behaviour of Mn^{III} and its similarity of ionic radius to that of Fe^{III} have been suggested as reasons for its greater ability to inhibit iron–sulfur enzymes (Chen et al., 2001). Greater complexation with and oxidation of catecholamines by Mn^{III} have also been noted (Archibald & Tyree, 1987).

In contrast to chromium, more reduced species of inorganic arsenic are more toxic, in general following the order arsine (arsenic(III) hydride; AsH_3) > arsenites (As^{III}) > arsenates (As^V) (Hindmarsh & McCurdy, 1986). Also in contrast to chromium species, oxidation state does not appear to be very important in determining arsenic bioavailability, as tri- and pentavalent com-pounds have similar rates of uptake, at least in mice (Vahter & Norin, 1980). However, phosphate transporters in renal epithelia and anion exchangers in erythrocytes can transport As^V species as a phosphate mimic (Clarkson, 1993). The same is true of V^V (Clarkson, 1993), which is more toxic than V^{IV}. One of the important determinants of the greater toxicity of arsenites is the increased propensity of As^{III} to combine with thiol groups. For example, inhibition of the tricarboxylic acid cycle results in part from combination of As^{III} with the dithiol group of lipoic acid, a cofactor in the decarboxylation of pyruvate and α-ketoglutarate (Hindmarsh & McCurdy, 1986). Short-lived methylated species of As^{III} are toxic, whereas methylated As^V species are detoxification products (for details, see section 3.4 below).

Oxidation state is critical for ion transport, which is exemplified by the different classes of transporters for Fe^{II} and Fe^{III}. The divalent metal transporter DMT-1 is important in uptake of iron in the gut, and also in intracellular iron trafficking following endocytosis of transferrin-bound iron (Gunshin & Hediger, 2002). DMT-1 trans-ports the divalent Fe^{II} (but not the trivalent Fe^{III}), as well as a number of other metals in their divalent state, including Mn^{II}, Co^{II}, Zn^{II}, Cu^{II}, Ni^{II}, Cd^{II}, and Pb^{II} (Gunshin et al., 1997). Fe^{II} is soluble under physiological conditions and can also diffuse across membranes. In contrast, Fe^{III} is prone to hydrolysis in aqueous environments, producing poorly soluble products [e.g. iron(III) hydroxide, $Fe(OH)_3$] (Schneider & Schwyn, 1987; Schneider, 1988; Harris, 2002). While uptake of Fe^{III} from a number of organic chelates probably involves dissociation and reduction to Fe^{II} (Templeton, 1995), there is also evidence of non-transferrin-mediated Fe^{III} transport in liver (Parkes & Templeton, 2002). Whereas generation of Fe^{II} generally facilitates its cellular uptake, oxidation of mercury vapour to Hg^{II} causes it to become trapped within cells. Some bacteria possess a mercuric reductase system that reduces Hg^{II} to volatile Hg^0, which then diffuses from the cell (Walsh et al., 1988; Misra, 1992). A similar activity has been reported to be inducible in human liver (Dunn et al., 1981).

3.3 Inorganic and organic compounds and complexes

Organic and inorganic ligands affect the properties of metal species and thus can have profound effects on toxicity. Available inorganic ligands affect properties such as charge, solubility, and diffusion coefficient and so determine transport and bioavailability.

Occupational exposure to nickel and its inorganic compounds illustrates the wide range of biological effects that can arise from a single element. Nickel salts such as chloride and sulfate are water soluble and of low oral toxicity, although when inhaled chronically in aerosols they may cause an increased risk of cancer in the respiratory system (IARC, 1990). On the other hand, in animals, α-trinickel disulfide (nickel(II) subsulfide, Ni_3S_2) is a potent carcinogen. Sunderman (1984) has established an order of carcinogenicity in rats of Ni_3S_2 ~ β-nickel(II) sulfide (NiS) > nickel(II) oxide (NiO) >> Ni^0 >>> amorphous NiS, for nickel particles injected intramuscularly. Nickel sulfides and oxides are quite insoluble in water, but may become biologically available by interaction with biological ligands. Occupational exposures to nickel usually involve multiple species. For instance, workers may be exposed to Ni_3S_2, nickel(II) sulfate ($NiSO_4$), nickel(II) chloride ($NiCl_2$), NiO, nickel(II) carbonate ($NiCO_3$), Ni^0, nickel–iron oxides, and nickel–copper oxides in various smelting and refining operations (IARC, 1990; WHO, 1991a). Inorganic ligands also affect particle size and surface chemistry of nickel, and this in turn contributes to properties such as protein adsorption. Protein adsorption correlates well with a bioassay of human erythrocyte hydrolysis, as can be seen in Table 2.

Table 2. Rank order of protein adsorption capacity and erythrocyte
haemolytic activity for a series of industrial inorganic compounds of nickel[a,b]

Nickel compound	Protein adsorption (rank)	Haemolysis (rank)
$Ni(OH)_2$ (colloid)	1	1
NiS (amorphous)	2	–
NiO	3	2
Ni^0 (1-μm powder)	4	4
β-NiS	5[c]	3
α-NiS (source 1)	5[c]	5
$Ni(OH)_2$ (dried)	7	8
α-Ni_3S_2	8	7
α-NiS (source 2)	9	6
Ni^0 (5-μm powder)	10	9

[a] Adapted from Nieboer et al. (1999).
[b] Ranking is in descending order of protein adsorption, 1 being highest.
[c] Not significantly different from each other.

A complex set of events underlies cellular transformation.
Landolph and co-workers (Landolph et al., 1996) have distinguished
true neoplastic transformation in cultured cells from morphological
changes and anchorage independence. Nickel compounds again
show the diversity of response to different inorganic species tested
in cultured mouse embryo cells (Table 3).

Table 3. Cell transformation induced by nickel compounds[a]

Compound	Morphological transformation	Anchorage independence	Neoplastic transformation
Ni_3S_2	+	–	–
NiS	+	+	–
NiO	+	+	+
$NiSO_4$	–	–	–
$NiCl_2$	–	–	–

[a] The results of in vitro studies with mouse embryo cells are adapted from
Landolph et al. (1996).

Speciation is a major determinant of the bioavailability of
aluminium. The form of aluminium in drinking-water depends on the
pH and whether the water is fluoridated. In unfluoridated water

above pH 6.5, $Al(OH)_4^-$ is the predominant species, while in fluoridated water below pH 6.5, AlF_2^+ and aluminium(III) fluoride (AlF_3) are major species (Martin, 1986). At higher pH, mixed HO^-/F^- species can occur. These inorganic forms are poorly absorbed in the gastrointestinal tract. Nevertheless, some aluminium is absorbed from inorganic forms such as aluminium(III) hydroxide [$Al(OH)_3$] and aluminium(III) carbonate [$Al_2(CO_3)_3$] and from dihydroxy aluminium(III) aminoacetate, with phosphate suppressing absorption (Alfrey, 1985). Complexation with organic acids greatly increases absorption. Administration of citrate with $Al(OH)_3$ rapidly increased serum levels in human volunteers (Taylor et al., 1992), and aluminium was available from a diet supplemented with aluminium(III) lactate (Greger & Baier, 1983). Maltol enhances the gastrointestinal absorption of aluminium (Kruck & McLachlan, 1989) and allows it to cross the blood–brain barrier (Hewitt et al., 1991).

Hydrolysis is an important part of the aqueous chemistry of metals. In aerobic aqueous environments at neutral pH, hydrolysis is a key determinant of the solubility and therefore bioavailability of many metals. The reaction $M^{n+} + nH_2O \rightarrow M(OH)_n\downarrow + nH^+$ frequently produces neutral metal hydroxides with very low solubility. With the exception of alkali and alkaline earth elements, most metals form one or more hydroxo-complexes under natural conditions. These include kinetically very stable complexes, such as $Al_{13}O_4(OH)_{24}^{7+}$ (Baes & Mesmer, 1986).

Small organic molecules can affect cellular uptake in unpredictable ways. For instance, binding of Cd^{II} to albumin renders it unavailable for uptake by cells (Templeton, 1990), and removal of cadmium from albumin by small molecules facilitates its uptake. On the other hand, the bioavailability of Ni^{II} is decreased by some ligands, such as histidine and cysteine (Abbracchio et al., 1982). In some cases, organic complexes are of sufficient stability that they can be isolated intact. An example is ferrioxamine, the complex of Fe^{III} with the hexadentate hydroxamate chelating agent, deferoxamine. In other cases, for example with bidentate iron chelators, the metal may exist in a complex equilibrium of partially coordinated forms (Templeton, 1995). If some of these species can redox cycle, the toxicity of iron may actually be enhanced through Fenton catalysis (Graf et al., 1984). Concentration-based stability constants take into account protonation of the ligand: $\beta_\lambda = [MH_\nu L_\lambda] /$

$[M][H^+]^v[L]^\lambda$, where M, H, and L refer to metal, hydrogen, and ligand, respectively, and v and λ are stoichiometric coefficients. Inclusion of HO^- in the ligand set can be taken into account by letting the stoichiometric coefficient of hydrogen, v, take negative values. It is usual for the proportion of different metal–ligand species to change with pH, and the set of β values is used to plot the distribution of species of metal in the presence of ligand as a function of pH (Martell & Motekaitis, 1992). Toxicity may then differ among body compartments, dependent on pH.

3.4 Organometallic species

This level of structural consideration in speciation is very important in human health and risk assessment. When a metallic element forms a bond with carbon that has strong covalent character, a so-called organometallic compound is formed that takes on particular biological properties. Such organification of an element may arise in the environment (e.g. environmental alkylation by microorganisms, as occurs in the formation of CH_3Hg^+), may be of anthropogenic origin (e.g. tetraalkyl lead compounds), or may occur within the body itself as part of the metabolic process (as in the example of arsenic discussed below). Organification of an element affects its solubility, lipophilicity, and volatility; all impact upon its biological availability and dissemination.

At the environmental level, an important distinction can be made between the addition of a methyl group to a metallic or semi-metallic element and the addition of a longer alkyl chain. The involvement of the methyl donors *S*-adenosyl methionine and methylcobalamin (Thayer, 1993) in eukaryotic cell metabolism distinguishes methylation reactions from other metallo-alkylations. In general, metals undergo only biomethylations, important examples being the formation of methyl derivatives of tin, antimony, mercury, lead, and germanium (Thayer, 1993). Cobalt is methylated to form methylcobalamin (vitamin B_{12}) in the gastrointestinal tract of ruminants, but otherwise biomethylation of metals is mostly restricted to activities of microorganisms in soils and sediments. On the other hand, alkylation (including methylation) of the semi-metals arsenic and selenium is a part of their metabolism in many organisms, including humans.

Methylation of metals generally increases their toxicity by rendering them more lipid soluble and facilitating their crossing of lipid barriers such as the cell membrane or blood–tissue (e.g. blood–brain) barriers. The membrane of a eukaryotic cell generally consists of a lipid bilayer through which a charged elemental species will not readily diffuse. Masking the charge by alkylation, or enhancing the hydrophobicity, will increase the access of a toxic metal to its intracellular target. An organ such as the brain has an additional mode of protection at the supracellular level. The blood–brain barrier refers to a functional barrier formed by the blood vessel endothelium and supporting tissues of the brain that prevents some substances from entering the brain from the blood. Other such barriers protect the fetus (the blood–placenta barrier) and testes (the blood–testis barrier), and the permeability of these barriers is highly dependent on the chemical species involved.

For the metalloids arsenic and selenium, methylation can serve as a means of detoxification (Hindmarsh & McCurdy, 1986; Karlson & Frankenberger, 1993). The major methyl donors in biomethylation reactions are methylcobalamin and *S*-adenosyl methionine (Thayer, 1993). *S*-Adenosyl methionine is a sulfonium ion that transfers its methyl group as a carbocation to a nucleophilic acceptor in a reaction known as the Challenger mechanism (Bentley & Chasteen, 2002). In the case of selenium, *S*-adenosyl methionine–dependent methylamine detoxifies the element by producing the more soluble trimethylselenonium ion $[(CH_3)_3Se^+]$ or the more volatile dimethylselenide $[(CH_3)_2Se]$ species (Karlson & Frankenberger, 1993).

The detoxification of arsenic is less straightforward. It was mentioned above that methylation of arsenic species is dependent on oxidation state. Arsenate reductase reduces arsenate to arsenite in human liver (Radabaugh & Aposhian, 2000). An earlier view was that methylation of As^V to methylarsonic acid (MMA) and dimethylarsinic acid (DMA) initiated a detoxification pathway (Hindmarsh & McCurdy, 1986; Aposhian et al., 2003). It is now known that As^{III} species can be methylated: mono- and dimethyl As^{III} species (methylarsonous acid and dimethylarsinous acid) apparently arise in mammalian cells from direct methylation of As^{III} species, and they may then be oxidized to MMA and DMA (Aposhian et al., 2003). Significantly, whereas the MMA and DMA species are detoxification products, methylarsonous acid and dimethylarsinous acid are more toxic than their inorganic As^{III} parent compounds (Cohen et al., 2002; Hughes, 2002).

Further complexity in arsenic metabolism is introduced by the ability of *S*-adenosyl methionine to donate either its aminobutyryl group or its deoxyadenosyl moiety instead of the methyl group (Hindmarsh & McCurdy, 1986). Reactions of cacodylate $[(CH_3)_2AsO_2^-]$ with the nucleoside function lead to arsenosugars that are metabolized further to arsenobetaine $[(CH_3)_3As^+CH_2COO^-]$ and arsenocholine $[(CH_3)_3As^+CH_2CH_2OH]$. These are non-toxic products that serve as a classic example of the fallacy of measuring only the total amount of an element in a diet and attempting to predict toxicity; ingestion of arsenobetaine and arsenocholine in seafood is without consequence.

The other class of biomethylation reactions is those that rely on methylcobalamin as the methyl donor. Here, in contrast to *S*-adenosyl methionine, the methyl group is transferred to an electrophilic metal substrate as the carbanion. Further, in contrast to the organification of selenium and arsenic, mercury and lead are two important toxic elements that are organified by this route. Organification of mercury is a clear example of the consequences of the increased lipophilicity of a toxic metal. Inorganic mercury salts are toxic to the kidney and peripheral nervous system and are corrosive at sites of mucosal contact (Campbell et al., 1992). However, they are poorly absorbed from the gut. On the other hand, organomercurials are nearly completely absorbed in the gastrointestinal tract and are highly absorbed following dermal exposure. Because of their lipophilic nature, they distribute widely throughout the body. Mono- and dimethylmercury are potent neurotoxicants that, unlike inorganic species, readily cross the blood–brain barrier. They also cross the placenta and are teratogenic (Clarkson, 1991; Klaassen, 2001).

In addition to products of bioalkylation reactions, either in the body or in the environment, manufactured organometallics have taken a prominent role in human toxicology. Elements with important organic derivatives include arsenic, tin, mercury, and lead. In some cases, introduction of the organometallic compound into the environment has been deliberate. Organomercurials have been used to treat seed grains. Triphenyltin $[(C_6H_5)_3Sn-X$, where X is an anion or an anionic group, such as chloride, hydroxide, or acetate] is a fungicide, and disodium methanearsonate [$CH_3AsO(ONa)_2$] is a herbicide. Incidental but environmentally harmful emissions include lead-based antiknock compounds such as tetramethyl lead [$(CH_3)_4Pb$] and tetraethyl lead [$(C_2H_5)_4Pb$] from gasoline combustion and leaching of organotin stabilizers [e.g. dioctyltin ($C_8H_{17})_2Sn$-X] from polyvinyl chlorides. Alkyl derivatives of lead, tin, and mercury are of major concern in human toxicology; potent central nervous system toxicants include tetraethyl lead, trimethyltin, and the mono- and dimethylmercury species.

3.5 Macromolecular compounds and complexes

The macromolecular level of speciation is structurally the least defined. For instance, it is not possible to document the state of protonation of every amino acid in metal-binding protein or in general to account for conformations representing local energy minima. The IUPAC definition of speciation considers the complex of a metal with a given protein of unique amino acid sequence and a globally averaged tertiary structure to be a single species, even though the sample will contain an ensemble of proteins in different states of protonation and local conformations (Templeton et al., 2000).

Sequestration of elements by proteins is important for toxicity. For example, Cd^{II} loosely bound to a high molecular mass protein such as albumin in the blood will be taken up by the liver. However, in the liver, cadmium induces and binds to the small protein, metallothionein (Nordberg et al., 1972). This sequesters the cadmium (Templeton & Cherian, 1991). However, if the cadmium–metallothionein complex is subsequently released from the liver and reaches the kidney, it causes more damage to the kidney than do cadmium salts (Nordberg et al., 1975; Templeton & Cherian, 1991). The Fe^{III}-binding sites of transferrin compete successfully with citrate for Al^{III} (Martin et al., 1987). However, rather than detoxifying aluminium by sequestration, transferrin probably increases its toxicity by keeping it in the circulation and delivering it around the body. Proteins provide sets of ligands to accommodate the coordination requirements of elemental ions, but it is hard to predict a priori how a given element will distribute among proteins present in plasma or cells or whether protein binding will increase or decrease the element's toxicity.

4. ANALYTICAL TECHNIQUES AND METHODOLOGY

4.1 Introduction

In order to assess the risk to human health from exposure to elemental species, analytical laboratories are being challenged to develop techniques for a widening variety of species. First comes the identification of the species. This requires reliable procedures for sampling of the material and isolation of the species without changing their composition. The detection can be based on measurement of either the element in the species or the molecule in which the element is incorporated. Generally speaking, the methods for elemental detection are more sensitive than those for molecules. Very low detection limits are needed because of the very low concentrations of species that can be expected. Individual species may represent only a minute fraction of the total, already ultra-trace element concentration.

Next come the questions as to how to calibrate the species, many of these not being available as commercial products, and last but not least how to validate the methods of elemental speciation analysis. There has been a steady improvement in detection limits of both elemental and molecular mass spectrometry over the past decades. Added to this is the progress made in the sampling procedures and separation of the species by hyphenated techniques to the point that sufficient analytical methodology seems to be at hand to analyse an ever larger array of elemental species and so improve knowledge of their role in health matters (Ebdon et al., 2001). An important group are the relatively low molecular mass molecules, such as metallothioneins (Dabrio et al., 2002).

A first group of compounds to be studied is those of anthropogenic origin and their metabolites. They have the advantage that the target species is known. Most of these elemental species do not exist in nature, and so their background level originally was zero. The organotin compounds belong to this category. They proved to be very effective as anti-fouling agents, fungicides, bacteriostats, polyvinyl chloride stabilizing agents, etc. Neither their disastrous effect on living systems as major endocrine disruptors nor their seemingly decades-long stability in the environment were ever anticipated until the time they created havoc in the reproductive system of bivalves. Analytical methodologies are available to detect these substances in a variety of matrices. Their applications are, however, still restricted because of insufficient detection limits.

Much more difficult to study are those elemental species that developed in living systems along with evolution. Where the total element concentrations are well documented, the species may be highly dynamic. Only a minority of species in living cells are present as stable covalent compounds, such as those where the element forms the core of the molecule (e.g. cobalt in vitamin B_{12}). Unfortunately, most elemental species exhibit a labile bond with their ligands, with low stability constants. These compounds may be very mobile, switching ligands and chemical form until they reach their target organ. A reliable speciation procedure will have to include stability criteria for the species during sampling and sample handling and awareness of possible species transformation. The development of reliable analytical methodology is expensive and difficult, but it is worth the investment, as it will further knowledge on the complex mechanisms of elemental species in the human body — the only way to unravel their beneficial or harmful effects to humans.

Besides the danger of displacement of the trace element that is non-covalently bound to molecules, there is also the opposite effect of capturing random trace element impurities by the ligands of matrix molecules during sample handling. These ligands may act as scavengers for trace element impurities in reagents, in column fillings, on inner walls of the apparatus, and on anything else with which they come in contact. In this respect, albumin, the main protein in human serum, is the most feared scavenger of trace element impurities. When possible, the balance must be made between, on the one hand, the total trace element concentration in a given sample and, on the other hand, the sum of all the trace element species. It is evident that the latter should never exceed the former. However, as it may be difficult to identify all the species of a specific element in a sample, this type of validation may not always be applicable.

The above paragraph made a distinction between species according to their anthropogenic or natural occurrence. From an analytical point of view, it is more relevant to know if one is looking for, for example:

- different oxidation states, e.g. Cr^{III}/Cr^{VI}, Fe^{II}/Fe^{III};
- low molecular mass organometallic molecules that are covalent in nature (e.g. MMA or DMA), or the opposite, labile low molecular mass organometallic molecules, such as aluminium bound to citrate;
- high molecular mass compounds that are covalent, such as copper in caeruloplasmin, or that form a labile bond, such as aluminium bound to transferrin.

All these possibilities have to be considered and certain options chosen when designing speciation procedures (Cornelis et al., 1996, 1998).

Most attention is focused on those elemental species that occur in low concentrations in the human body and food and those that are of importance in occupational exposure. The state of the art in analytical performance for elemental speciation has been the subject of two comprehensive handbooks (Cornelis et al., 2003, 2005).

4.2 Sample collection and storage

There are existing guidelines for sampling and storage with the aim of total element determinations (Versieck & Cornelis, 1989; Cornelis et al., 1996). Additional information about species sampling procedures is given in Brereton et al. (2003), Emons (2003), and De Cremer (2003). The main issue is to keep the elemental species unaffected by the procedure both in composition and in concentration. This remark can be simply put as: avoid contamination and keep the species unchanged. Of the two threats, contamination hazards may be the easier to master. Suppose we are interested in methylmercury in serum, urine, or hair. In this case, any fortuitous contamination with inorganic mercury goes unnoticed, as only methylmercury will be specifically isolated from the matrix, and there is no danger that methylmercury will be formed during the procedure. The same reasoning is valid when analysing organolead compounds. Although Pb^{II} contaminations are ubiquitous, those by organolead species are not that widespread. There still remains the possibility of fortuitous binding of trace element impurities with ligands in the sample. In principle, good analytical practice under well controlled, clean conditions can avoid such problems.

As mentioned previously, the integrity of the elemental species throughout the analysis is highly dependent upon the nature of the species. A first, general guideline is to store biological specimens at below 7 °C when it is only for a few days, but to deep-freeze them for longer periods. This may be insufficient. It is important to be aware that elemental species in powders may also suffer from lack of stability due to residual humidity. This was documented in the case of arsenic species in rice powder, kept at +20 °C, + 4 °C, and −20 °C. The results are shown in Table 4. At the start of the study, the rice contained As^V, As^{III}, MMA, and DMA. It was observed that MMA demethylated completely to As^{III} and also that all of the As^V was gradually reduced to As^{III} at the end of a 2-month period. The freezing temperature did little to preserve MMA and As^V in their original form. The arsenic content in rice originates from the water in which it is grown. It is thought that grinding the rice and storing it with about 18% humidity may have led to this unwelcome conversion of species, possibly induced by anaerobic activity. The arsenic species in the rice powder standard reference material (SRM) with very low residual humidity, issued by the National Institute of Standards and Technology (NIST SRM 1568a), was found to be stable.

Long-term freezing of samples is generally acceptable, although some exceptions have been reported. Arsenobetaine in sample extracts stored at 4 °C for 9 months was found to decompose to trimethylarsine oxide and two other species (Le et al., 1994). Deep-freezing samples will generally minimize any bacterial or enzyme degradation or loss from volatility. Poorly sealed sample containers let in oxygen, so that the species are oxidized, or loss of species occurs if the compounds are volatile. Bacterial degradation of the sample should be avoided. Bacteria can convert inorganic arsenic to methylated forms, and steps should be taken to preserve the original samples. Sample cleanup from a biological or complicated matrix can present problems. Ultimately, a stability study using samples spiked with known arsenic species is necessary to validate a sample storage and treatment procedure (B'Hymer & Caruso, 2004).

Table 4. Stability study of rice powder sample with 18% residual humidity during 2 months of storage at room temperature, 4 °C, and −20 °C[a]

Arsenic species	T (°C)	X ± SD (μg/kg)		
		t = 0	Month 1	Month 2
As[III]	20		88.3 ± 4.9	94.9 ± 2.2
	4		81.9 ± 7.4	92.9 ± 2.3
	−20	46.99 ± 0.75	82.2 ± 7.4	93.2 ± 1.9
DMA	20		29.7 ± 3.6	27.5 ± 2.5
	4		27.0 ± 1.6	24.9 ± 0.8
	−20	28.33 ± 1.11	26.0 ± 2.3	23.9 ± 0.6
MMA	20		nd	nd
	4		nd	nd
	−20	18.10 ± 1.7	nd	nd
As[V]	20		10.7 ± 3.9	nd
	4		10.5 ± 4.7	nd
	−20	24.45 ± 1.09	11.0 ± 5.7	nd

nd = not detected; SD = standard deviation
[a] Adapted from Brereton et al. (2003).

It appears that for biological samples, long-term preservation of species can be guaranteed only when they are kept in the dark and at very low temperatures. To prevent microbiological activity over many years, the specimens should be kept at below −130 °C. The other approach is to remove all the residual water, when temperatures of only −20 °C may be acceptable. Anyway, it is absolutely necessary to do a stability study for each individual elemental species in its particular matrix (Emons, 2003).

An interesting study was published on the stability during storage of arsenic, selenium, antimony, and tellurium species in, among others, urine and fish. The species studied were As[III], As[V], arsenobetaine, MMA, DMA, phenylarsonic acid, Se[IV], Se[VI], selenomethionine, Sb[III], Sb[V], and Te[VI] (Lindemann et al., 2000). Best storage conditions for aqueous mixtures of these species were achieved at 3 °C; at −20 °C, species transformation, especially of selenomethionine and Sb[V], took place, and a new selenium species appeared within a period of 30 days.

Special attention is needed for sampling techniques and storage of airborne metal species in the workplace (Dabek-Zlotorzynska & Keppel-Jones, 2003). The filter media must be chosen carefully. General criteria that must be considered when selecting them are 1) representative sampling for particulates of 0.3 μm and greater in size, 2) low hygroscopicity, since hygroscopicity exceeding 1 mg per piece leads to serious errors in mass concentration measurements, and hence to the improper estimate of the environmental concentration, and 3) absence of impurities that might interfere with the analysis. As an example of the latter, glass fibre or Teflon filters were found to be unsuitable for the sampling of airborne dust with low platinum content (Alt et al., 1993). Only polycarbonate and cellulose gave blank values as low as 5 pg of platinum per total filter.

Moreover, filters should be mechanically and thermally stable and should not interact with the deposit, even when subject to a strong extraction solvent (Dabek-Zlotorzynska & Keppel-Jones, 2003). This is particularly relevant in the case of the analysis of Cr^{III}/Cr^{VI} in air particulate matter. Spini et al. (1994) reported the reduction of Cr^{VI} to Cr^{III} when cellulose filters were extracted with an alkaline solution containing a known amount of Cr^{VI}. The same results were obtained by an acid (sulfuric acid) dissolution of the filters, which can be explained by cellulose's well documented reducing properties. Therefore, cellulose filters cannot be used for chromium speciation in airborne particulates. Polycarbonate membrane filters (Scancar & Milaćić, 2002) and borosilicate microfibre glass discs (Christensen et al., 1999) are suitable for this type of analysis.

Sample integrity during storage of particulate matter is another important issue. Some changes can be anticipated — for example, reduction of Cr^{VI} due to interaction not only with the collection substrate during sample storage but also with the air. Erroneous results may occur due to redox reactions. The enrichment of particles on the filter gives rise to enhanced contact of the chromium species with gaseous species (e.g. sulfur dioxide, nitrogen oxides, oxygen, ozone) and/or with material collected on the filter (e.g. Fe^{II} [iron oxide, or magnetite] and As^{III}-containing components) (Dabek-Zlotorzynska & Keppel-Jones, 2003). Such changes may be minimized by storing the samples in closed polypropylene vessels under an inert atmosphere (nitrogen or argon) (Dyg et al., 1994; Christensen et al., 1999). The shorter the time between collection and analysis, the better. Anyway, the reverse — namely, the oxidation of Cr^{III} to Cr^{VI} — is most unlikely under usual conditions of storage and sample treatment.

The rule of thumb is that when no data are available from reliable studies by other research groups, the effect of sampling and storage conditions on the stability of the species in the matrix should be studied. Many species are thermodynamically unstable. The simple act of sampling and storing the species may alter them. The information is then irreversibly lost.

4.3 Sample preparation

The main origins of the samples to be handled in elemental speciation and fractionation in human health risk assessment will be clinical, food, drinking-water, and air filter samples for occupational health monitoring. The most common approach is to aim at just one element or group of similar species at a time.

One or more of the following steps will be needed prior to the separation and measurement of the species in clinical samples and food (Cornelis et al., 1998): release of the species from the cells, sample pretreatment to select a particular group of species, and desalting. The preliminary treatment of clinical and food samples is familiar to biologists and biochemists but may be less known to the inorganic trace element analyst. Therefore, a synopsis of procedures is briefly outlined in the following sections.

4.3.1 *Preliminary treatment of biological fluids*

Blood and urine are the most commonly studied samples. For speciation purposes, it is of no value to analyse total blood because of the very different nature of the constituents: serum and packed cells.

Blood is a heterogeneous fluid consisting of approximately 55% clear, slightly yellow fluid (native plasma) and three main groups of suspended cells (red blood cells or erythrocytes, which form the main portion — around 99% of the suspended cells; white blood cells or leukocytes; and blood platelets or thrombocytes). When no anticoagulant is added, normal blood withdrawn from the circulation forms a clot due to the polymerization of fibrinogen to fibrin; this process normally requires 5–15 min at room temperature. On standing, the clot retracts (packed cells expressing serum, which differs from plasma, in that it contains no fibrinogen). After centrifugation, serum may be decanted or drawn off with a pipette (Versieck & Cornelis, 1989). Centrifugation should be performed within 1 h after sampling the blood.

For speciation or fractionation purposes, it is preferable to collect the blood without anticoagulant. It is also inadvisable to add any preservative. First of all, both anticoagulant and preservative may contain impurities (e.g. a mercury compound). Secondly, both anticoagulant and preservatives may contain substances that are liable to break up the bonds between the elemental species and the serum matrix. Most anticoagulants are either polyanions (e.g. heparin) or metal chelators and therefore have a high affinity for metal species. As a rule, neither heparinized samples nor ethylene-diaminetetraacetic acid (EDTA), citrate, or any other anticoagulant-doped samples may be used.

The spontaneous clotting of the blood lasts for about 15–30 min at room temperature. As mentioned, centrifugation should be completed within 1 h. Haemolysed samples should never be considered for speciation purposes. The distribution of the trace element species between serum and packed cells is of a totally different nature and may also differ by several orders of magnitude. The concentrations in these two phases are controlled by different mechanisms.

Packed cells have to be lysed before any speciation study can be envisaged. This can be done by mixing one part of packed cells with one part of cold toluene and 40 parts of ice-cold water. The lysate is centrifuged at 15 000 × g at 40 °C and is then filtered through a 0.45-μm filter.

Urine will usually show a deposit some time after collection. Substances that are dissolved at body temperature have a tendency to precipitate at lower temperatures. It is a matter of concern to find out if the species to be studied are also present in this precipitate. Addition of preservatives or acidification (lowering of pH) cannot be considered as a general rule, because both steps are liable to alter the species. Here again, a preliminary detailed study of the influence of a possible additive on the nature of the species is essential.

4.3.2 Preliminary treatment of tissues and plants

Sampling of tissues should be done according to a strict protocol whereby contamination is excluded and species preservation guaranteed. Tools made of stainless steel are the preferred material for removal of the samples from the organism; however, with stainless steel containing 8–20% chromium, 8–12% nickel, and minor concentrations of cobalt and manganese, the risk of contaminating the samples by contact with it cannot be neglected. Much better materials for knives from the point of view of eliminating contamination are polyethylene, polypropylene, Teflon, and quartz (Versieck et al., 1982). The listing of materials is not exhaustive, and the choice will be made on the basis of experimental data proving the validity of the sampling procedure. Chemical speciation of a trace element in tissues begins with the separation of the soluble species from those bound to insoluble compounds. The tissue is commonly subjected to a very harsh ultrasonic homogenization in isotonic phosphate-buffered (pH 7.35) saline solution using short bursts (10 s) in an ice-water bath. The homogenization can be considered sufficient when the power output on the homogenizer display decreases drastically. The homogenate is then centrifuged at 4 °C at 15 300 × g for 1 h. The supernatant is removed with a pipette. Soluble compounds trapped inside the precipitate are removed by washing 3 times with an equal volume of phosphate-buffered saline solution, followed by centrifugation of the suspended precipitate. The joined supernatants are further treated according to the procedures described in section 4.4. Some tissues, such as lung and hair, show high mechanical resistance due to the presence of fibrous, insoluble, structural proteins. Speciation of elements bound to insoluble compounds cannot be pursued any further.

In the case of tissue, the distribution of the trace elements can also be approached in a cytological way. This refers to the subcellular-level distribution of the trace elements between cytosol, mitochondria, and nucleus. An overview of the overall procedure is given in Figure 1 (Cornelis et al., 1998). The total trace element concentration can be measured in each step of these separations, in order to make up the balance, as a first check of the validity of the

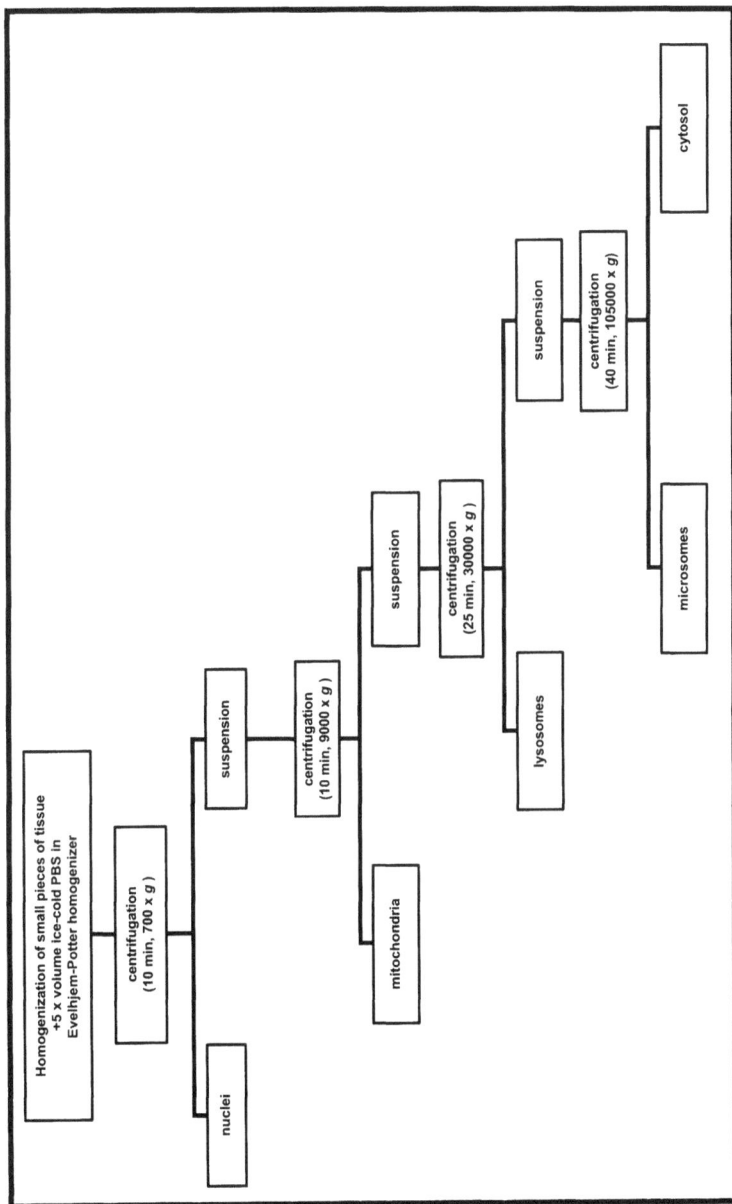

Fig. 1. Overview of the homogenization of the tissue and the separation of the soluble species from those bound to the insoluble compounds, followed by subcellular fractionation (the centrifuge is cooled at 4 °C). PBS = phosphate-buffered saline.

results. Chemical speciation of the cytosol can be done according to the procedure outlined in the following section.

4.3.3 Choice between low molecular mass and high molecular mass compounds

Once the preliminary sample preparation described in the previous paragraphs is finished, the analyst has to opt for either low molecular mass or high molecular mass compounds. This is because a good separation within the low molecular mass group can be achieved only in the absence of high molecular mass compounds. An elegant way to do this is through centrifugal ultrafiltration. The solution is held in a semipermeable membrane cone and subjected to a centrifugal force, typically at $800 \times g$. Those compounds with an effective radius smaller than the pore size of the membrane are pushed through it, whereas the other compounds are retained on the inner side of the membrane. The separation is characterized by the cut-off of the membrane, this being the maximum molar mass of the compound able to pass through the pores. If no precipitation or adsorption takes place, the concentrations of the compounds in the ultrafiltrate will equal those in the original sample. There are some difficulties that may arise during ultrafiltration, related to the thermodynamic and kinetic stability of the chemical bond between a low molecular mass compound of a trace element and a protein. Indeed, a weak and easily dissociative chemical bond may break up during ultrafiltration, freeing more low molecular mass compounds than originally present.

The thermodynamic and kinetic aspects of centrifugal filtration have been discussed in detail by Whitlam & Brown (1981). By ultrafiltering only part of the sample (e.g. 10%), possible dissociation of the protein–low molecular mass complexes is suppressed. It is advisable to work under a nitrogen blanket to create an inert environment, preferably in a cold room or with the equipment cooled down to a fixed temperature below the ambient temperature of the workplace.

4.3.4 Desalting

Desalting of the sample is necessary whenever the ionic strength of the solution does not fit that of the chromatographic separation. Urine samples have an electrolyte composition that is very variable.

Supernatant of tissue samples may also display a salt content that is too high. Desalting of the solutions allows the analyst to work in controlled conditions. Gel filtration columns with a fractionation range of 1–5 kilodaltons are commercially available. If no over-loading of the column occurs, the sample protein fraction can be collected in the first fractions of the eluate, as low molecular mass compounds have a longer retention time. Eluents for desalting are first degassed and filtered through a Millex-HV13 filter with a pore size of 0.45 μm before use. Phosphate-buffered saline can serve as an eluent during the desalting run.

4.3.5 Sample cleanup

Most biological (clinical and food) samples have a fairly com-plex matrix due to the presence of amino acids, lipids, hydrocarbons, polysaccharides, etc. Cleanup procedures are therefore necessary to remove all those compounds that are of no interest for the purpose of the analysis and whose presence may even compromise the detection sensitivity of the analytical method (Muñoz-Olivas & Cámara, 2003).

One of the fastest methods to eliminate lipids is a mixture of chloroform and ethanol in such proportions that a miscible system is formed with the water suspension of the sample. Dilution with chloroform and water then separates the homogenate into two layers, the chloroform layer containing all the lipids and the ethanol–water layer all the non-lipids.

Some analyses require an extraction step in order to isolate and also enrich the analyte. The different types of extraction procedures will be described in the following section. It may be necessary to purify the extract. Solid-phase extraction with C18 cartridges pro-vides a very useful cleanup of the sample, ensuring the stability of the compounds. This has been illustrated in the case of selenium speciation (Wrobel et al., 2003).

4.3.6 Extraction procedures

Many species need to be purified from major matrix constituents prior to further separation and measurement. There exists a broad choice of extraction procedures, varying from simple aqueous or solvent extraction to more complex methods, such as enzymatic extraction, solid-phase extraction, solid-phase micro-extraction, steam distillation, supercritical fluid extraction, liquid–gas extraction (purge and trap), accelerated solvent extraction, and microwave-assisted extraction (Muñoz-Olivas & Cámara, 2003).

Extensive research has been done on the extraction of various species of arsenic, copper, lead, mercury, selenium, tin, and zinc in biological matrices. A synopsis of a number of examples of ana-lytical procedures, including sample pretreatment for elemental speciation purposes, has recently been published by Muñoz-Olivas & Cámara (2003).

4.3.7 Preconcentration of the species

When the concentration of the analyte is very low, it is neces-sary to include a preconcentration step. This will often be followed by chromatographic separation. There are four main strategies described in the literature whose choice is determined by the chemi-cal characteristics of the species: amalgam formation, cold trap, high-temperature trap, and active charcoal retention.

In the case of mercury compounds, amalgam formation on a gold trap is most effective and widely applied. The cold trap method is used for derivatized species — i.e. elemental species that have been transformed into volatile compounds, such as tin, lead, and mercury species (Szpunar et al., 1996). The high-temperature trap has been used for arsenic in biological material (Ceulemans et al., 1993). Active charcoal retention has been employed for trapping non-polar volatile chelates (Heisterkamp & Adams, 1999).

4.3.8 Derivatization

To derivatize means to convert a chemical compound into a derivative — i.e. a new compound derived from the original one, for the purpose of identification. Derivatization of non-volatile organometallic species into volatile compounds, which are then separated with gas chromatography (GC), is common practice (Bouyssiere et al., 2003). The volatile derivatives need to retain the original moiety and be non-polar, volatile, and thermally stable. Such derivatizations have been accomplished by hydride generation, with tetraalkyl(aryl) borates, with Grignard reagents, and even through the formation of volatile chelates, such as acetonates, tri-fluoroacetonates, and dithiocarbamates. There is also mention of the derivatization of selenoaminoacids, selenomethionine, and organic arsenicals with a variety of reagents (Bouyssiere et al., 2003). Frequently, the derivatives are concentrated by cryotrapping or extraction into an organic solvent prior to injection on a GC column.

4.4   Separation techniques

Species separation is achieved mainly by one of the following well known techniques: liquid chromatography (LC), GC, capillary electrophoresis (CE), and gel electrophoresis (GE). The choice will be determined by the chemical properties of the species, the available skills and infrastructure in the laboratory, and, last but not least, the available resources.

4.4.1   *Liquid chromatography*

The sample is introduced into a chromatographic column filled with a stationary phase while a liquid mobile phase is continuously pumped through the column. The stationary phase is usually a chemically modified silica or polymer. The analytes interfere to a different extent with the stationary phase and the mobile phase. This determines the length of time each analyte resides in the column. Usually the LC system is coupled to a specific detector. Such a setup is perhaps the most common in elemental speciation analysis. High-performance liquid chromatography (HPLC) columns form a widely used subset of LC, with small-diameter particles (3–5 µm) as the stationary phase, the mobile phase being pumped under increased pressure. A good overview on HPLC in elemental speciation can be found in Ackley & Caruso (2003). The most common types of LC are size exclusion chromatography, ion exchange chromatography, and affinity chromatography. Today, it is also possible to couple an LC system to a soft ionization system in order to obtain structural information. Examples of a soft ionization technique are electrospray mass spectrometry (ES-MS) and tunable plasma.

There are multiple procedures described in the literature for the separation of specific elemental species or groups of species. As an example, more than 100 chromatographic conditions have been listed in the literature for the separation of organotin compounds

(Harrington et al., 1996), selenium species (Montes-Bayon et al., 2000), arsenic species (Ali & Jain, 2004; B'Hymer & Caruso, 2004), mercury species (Harrington, 2000), elemental species bound to proteins (Templeton, 2005), elemental species bound to humic acids (Heumann, 2005), etc. LC will surely remain the major separation technique in the foreseeable future. Electronic databanks (e.g. Web of Science) prove to be very helpful in putting together a procedure that is ideally suited for the combination of matrix, analyte, and the available infrastructure of the laboratory.

4.4.2   Gas chromatography

Only volatile and thermally stable species qualify for separation by GC. Very few compounds fulfil these requirements, but fortunately the analyst can resort to chemical reactions that transform non-volatile compounds into volatile, thermally stable compounds. This process is referred to as "derivatization" (García Alonso & Encinar, 2003) (see section 4.3.8 above).

Naturally occurring volatile species include dimethylmercury $[(CH_3)_2Hg)]$, dimethylselenium $[(CH_3)_2Se]$, tetramethyltin $[(CH_3)_4Sn]$, trimethylantimony $[(CH_3)_3Sb]$, trimethylbismuth $[(CH_3)_3Bi]$, methylated arsines, tetraalkylated lead compounds in sewage sludge, and many more gases from municipal waste disposal sites. This list is not exhaustive. Very interesting research on these compounds has been done by Feldmann (1997), who described innovative ways to convert non-volatile species into volatile species by derivatization techniques. Various separation schemes have been developed. Most common is the cryogenic trapping and sequential thermal desorption from packed columns. This method is not very selective, but unstable compounds can be preserved for a long time before analysis. Next comes GC on packed columns, offering an improved separation of the analytes through interaction with the column, combined with separation on the basis of their volatility (Szpunar et al., 1996). GC with capillary columns offers a much improved resolution. Their very small loading capacity forms the limiting factor for their exploitation.

The most common detector for this type of speciation is inductively coupled plasma mass spectrometry (ICP-MS), followed by inductively coupled plasma atomic emission spectrometry (ICP-AES). It is also possible to do isotope dilution measurements and isotopic ratio patterns when a high-resolution ICP-MS is available as the elemental detector.

4.4.3 *Capillary electrophoresis*

The principle of separation by CE is based on differences in the electrically driven mobility of charged analytes, similar to conventional electrophoresis. A high-voltage electrical field (typically 20–30 kV) is applied along an open tube column with small internal diameter (Michalke, 2003).

This technique can be used as a primary or as a secondary separation technique, for example after HPLC, when it is referred to as a two-dimensional technique. Taking into account the very small loading capacity of CE, the two-dimensional approach will yield far more interesting results, bringing the high resolution of CE to its full potential. The system is often connected to ultraviolet (UV) detection for molecular information, but also to ICP-MS or ES-MS for either elemental or molecular information.

There exist different separation modes in CE: capillary zone electrophoresis, with separation on the basis of the charge/mass ratio; capillary isoelectric focusing, based on the isoelectric point; capillary isotachophoresis, based on analyte conductivity; and micellar electrokinetic capillary chromatography, based on hydrophobicity.

CE analysis offers high resolution and high speed, and it is easily adaptable for automation and quantitative analysis. It has been successfully used for the speciation of many compounds (Alvarez-Llamas et al., 2005), among others Cr^{III}/Cr^{VI} (Jung et al., 1997), selenium and arsenic compounds (Sun et al., 2004), selenium in human milk (Michalke, 2000), and copper, cadmium, and zinc in metallothionein (Profrock et al., 2003).

4.4.4 *Gel electrophoresis*

The field covered by GE for elemental speciation consists of charged macromolecules to which a metal or semi-metal is bound, covalently or not. These macromolecules can be proteins, humic acids, or DNA. There are practical limitations due to the small amount of material that can be brought onto the gel, and, consequently, the limit of detection of the species. For protein separation, its resolution is unsurpassable (Chéry, 2003).

The first prerequisite during the separation procedure is again the preservation of the elemental species. This is not evident, considering the nature of the many reagents needed to operate GE. For example, the contamination of the samples with platinum due to the release of platinum ions from the platinum electrodes during electrophoresis completely falsifies the results when pursuing platinum speciation. Substitution of platinum by silver solves this problem when searching for platinum species (Lustig et al., 1999). Other critical parameters are the choice of buffer and pH.

When the metal is covalently bound, such as copper in caeruloplasmin, denaturing conditions can be used during electrophoresis. This is not the case for more weakly bound elements, for which non-denaturing conditions or native electrophoresis should be applied, in order to prevent the loss of the basic structure of the complex and stripping of the metal. Another factor that may even jeopardize the stability of strongly bound elements is oxidation of residues of proteins, as has been documented for selenoproteins (Chéry et al., 2001, 2005).

The method can be hyphenated with powerful detection methods, such as laser ablation dynamic reaction cell ICP-MS for elemental detection (Chassaigne et al., 2004) or matrix-assisted laser desorption ionization MS for molecular detection. A more tedious way, but reliable for quantitative measurements, consists of cutting out zones of separated proteins in the gel and measuring the element off-line with ICP-MS, by using electrothermal vaporization as the sample introduction system (Chéry et al., 2002).

4.5 Sequential extraction schemes for the fractionation of sediments, soils, aerosols, and fly ash

It is impossible to determine the large number of individual species in matrices as complicated as sediments, soils, aerosols, and fly ash. A practical solution consists of identifying the various classes of species of an element and determining the sum of its concentrations in each fraction. Such a fractionation is based on different properties: size, solubility, affinity, charge, hydrophobicity, etc. The fractionation methods are operationally defined. Despite their limitations, sequential extraction schemes provide a valuable tool to distinguish between trace metal fractions of different particle size and solubility. They are a useful approach to reveal possible environmental implications of the presence of elemental species in, for example, land disposal of waste material, of sediments, etc. They help to describe what may be "the bioavailable fraction" of the elemental species. Notwithstanding the limitations of sequential extraction procedures, they are convenient to compare results from different studies on the condition that these operationally defined fractions are linked to a very strict analytical protocol. The results produced by different laboratories show that harmonization is very difficult to achieve. Reference materials certified for specific extraction procedures constitute the cornerstone of this type of analysis.

Sampling, subsampling, sequential extraction schemes, and the application of field flow fractionation have been summarized in Hlavay & Polyák (2003).

4.6   Detection: elemental and molecular

During the last decade, substantial progress has been made in improving the sensitivity of the detection methods of commercially available equipment. The trend is to go for on-line, also called hyphenated, systems. The most convenient method for on-line coupling is ICP-MS. It is, unfortunately, the most expensive "detector" for HPLC and other chromatographic systems, as well as for CE, especially when one considers that this multielement method will be used for the detection of only a single element. For economical reasons, it is certainly worthwhile to consider what other atomic spectrometric methods have to offer.

4.6.1   Atomic absorption spectrometry

The difficulty, if not the impossibility, of making flame atomic absorption spectrometry (AAS) and graphite furnace AAS on-line methods for measuring the elements in the fractions obtained during LC makes them less popular for elemental speciation purposes. They have, however, earned their merits in the field. Graphite furnace AAS has been used for the off-line measurement of elements in the elution fractions of LC, although insufficient detection limits proved to be a serious drawback in the case of many clinical applications, where the concentrations of the elemental species in the biological fluids and tissues are very low (Zhang & Zhang, 2003).

When species can be converted to hydrides, such as is routinely done for mercury, selenium, arsenic, and antimony, then hydride generation AAS is a very interesting and cheap detection technique. An on-line method was developed for the speciation of arsenic in human serum, including MMA, DMA, arsenobetaine, and arseno-choline. It has been applied for the speciation of arsenic in persons with abnormally high arsenic concentrations in serum, such as dialysis patients (Zhang et al., 1996, 1998). The method is based on cation exchange LC separation, UV photo-oxidation for sample digestion, and continuous hydride generation AAS for the measure-ment of arsenic in the LC eluent. By developing the technique of argon segmented flow in the post-column eluent, a substantial improvement in chromatographic resolution for the separation of these four arsenic species was obtained. The LC separation, photo-oxidation, hydride generation, and AAS measurement could be completed on-line within 10 min. The response is different for the different species. The detection limits (as arsenic) were 1.0, 1.3, 1.5, and 1.4 µg/l for MMA, DMA, arsenobetaine, and arsenocholine, respectively, in serum. The concentration of the four species was determined in serum samples of six patients with chronic renal insufficiency. Only arsenobetaine and DMA were significantly detected by this method. The main part of arsenic in human serum is arsenobetaine. No MMA, arsenocholine, or inorganic arsenic were detected in these six samples.

AAS with a quartz tube atomizer is a very sensitive, specific, rugged, and comparatively inexpensive detector for GC. GC coupled with AAS has been described as a sensitive instrumentation for mercury speciation (Emteborg et al., 1996). On-line solid-phase extraction coupled to graphite furnace AAS has also been explored.

Cold vapour AAS is the most widely used technique for mea-suring mercury. Direct coupling of solid-phase microextraction and quartz tube AAS has been used for selective and sensitive determination of methylmercury in seafood (Fragueiro et al., 2004).

4.6.2 Atomic fluorescence spectrometry

When species can be converted into hydrides, such as is routinely the case for mercury, selenium, arsenic, and antimony species, then atomic fluorescence spectrometry becomes a very economical elemental detection technique. It is, however, necessary to keep in mind that the conversion of elemental species into hydrides is not occurring to the same extent and at the same rate for all species. This has been documented, for example, in the case of arsenic. The conversion of methylated arsenic species into methylated hydrides gives a different response than the conversion of inorganic arsenite or arsenate to AsH_3 (Zhang et al., 1996).

4.6.3 Atomic emission spectrometry

ICP-AES is the most common technique for emission spectrometry. It is sometimes referred to as ICP–optical emission spectrometry (OES). This method offers in principle the advantage of being multielemental, although in the case of elemental speciation, it will usually be used as a single-element detector. It is easy to couple on-line with LC because it can accept a continuous flow of eluent. The disadvantages are the overall inefficiency of the nebulizer and the plasma's sensitivity to organic solvents. The poor tolerance of the plasma source to common mobile phases, such as ion pair reagents, limits the applicability of the technique. The fact that many ion exchange chromatography elutions are not isocratic (i.e. the elution is effected under variable, usually increasing, ionic strength) requires special protocols to circumvent the problem of varying analyte response during the elution (Zhang & Zhang, 2003).

4.6.4 Inductively coupled plasma mass spectrometry

ICP-MS is based on the measurement of m/z ratios. It offers extremely low detection limits for nearly all elements. This is due to the very high degree of atomization in the plasma at about 7000 K. This extreme temperature makes it far superior as an atomization source than the graphite furnace for AAS with temperatures at only 2000 °C. There exist problems of spectral interference. For instance, when measuring ^{52}Cr, mass 52 will experience interference from the isobars of $^{40}Ar^{12}C^+$ and $^{35}Cl^{16}OH^+$, because the resolution is limited to $\Delta m/m = 1$ (Vanhaecke & Köllensperger, 2003).

Today there exist two major tools to reduce these interferences to a negligible level. The first is the dynamic reaction cell, which allows chemical reactions in a collision cell so that the interfering isobars are neutralized or the analyte is transformed into another, heavier polyatomic compound. Another very reliable, but very expensive, tool to eliminate isobaric interferences is high-resolution ICP-MS with $\Delta m/m$ from 1/4000 to 1/10 000 (Houk, 2003).

HPLC works well on-line with ICP-MS. Similar difficulties due to the influence of the eluent on the plasma can be anticipated and need careful consideration, as mentioned in the previous section on ICP-AES.

An alternative way for sample introduction is solid sampling electrothermal vaporization, followed by ICP-MS detection. An interesting application is the direct determination of methylmercury and inorganic mercury in fish tissue with non-specific isotope dilution (Gelaude et al., 2002).

4.6.5 *Plasma source time-of-flight mass spectrometry*

Plasma source time-of-flight MS is a powerful tool for elemental speciation analysis through the use of a modulated or pulsed ionization source that provides both atomic and molecular fragmentation information (Leach et al., 2003). Its use has been documented for the analysis of, among others, organotin compounds and the oxidation states of various elements.

4.6.6 *Glow discharge plasmas as tunable sources for elemental speciation*

Glow discharge plasmas offer a number of interesting possibilities as speciation detectors for gaseous and liquid sample analysis (Marcus, 2003). The plasma works at sufficiently low temperatures (kinetic temperatures in the range of 100–500 K) so as not to induce dissociation in molecular species. Detection can be achieved by OES or MS. The technique has been successfully applied for the speciation of, for example, organotin compounds.

4.6.7 *Electrospray mass spectrometry*

ES-MS offers soft ionization of metal-containing species followed by tandem MS for the precise determination of the molecular mass of the original species and that of the individual fragments. This method is ideal for obtaining structural molecular information about the species. An extensive sample cleanup is needed in order to obtain high sensitivities (Chassaigne, 2003).

The method allows the coupling of HPLC on-line, on condition of using a suitable eluent. This method has been successfully applied for the speciation of organo-arsenicals and selenium species, identification of metallothioneins, etc.

4.6.8 *Electrochemical methods*

Electrochemical methods are based on the measurement of electrical signals associated with the molecular properties or interfacial processes of chemical species (Town et al., 2003). Owing to the direct transformation of the desired chemical information (concentration, activity) into an electrical signal (potential, current, resistance, capacity) by the methods themselves, they are easy and cheap. The two major difficulties in the application of electroanalytical techniques to complex real-world samples have been the lack of selectivity of electrochemistry and the susceptibility of the electrode surface to fouling by surface-active materials in the sample. A variety of electroanalytical techniques that differ in the mode of excitation signal–response characteristics are currently being used: potentiometry, fixed-potential methods, amperometry, various forms of voltammetry and electrochemical detection in LC, and flow-injection analysis. These methods have been applied for the quantification of various oxidation states of an element (Fe^{III}/Fe^{II}, Cr^{VI}/Cr^{III}, Tl^{III}/Tl^{I}, Sn^{IV}/Sn^{II}, Mn^{IV}/Mn^{II}, Sb^{V}/Sb^{III}, As^{V}/As^{III}, and Se^{VI}/Se^{IV}), its organometallic species, or metal complexes in equilibrium with each other (e.g. butyltin species in surface water from a harbour by adsorptive stripping voltammetry with tropolone). The ideal is to perform in situ measurements with minimal sample perturbation. Despite many difficulties, well known to specialists in the field, the sensitivity of electroanalytical methods makes them very powerful tools for many applications.

4.7 Calibration in elemental speciation analysis

Nearly all determinations of elemental species are performed in a relative manner — i.e. through comparative measurement with a set of calibration samples of known content (Heumann, 2003).

Different calibration modes are feasible. External calibration modes are where the sample and the corresponding calibrant are measured separately. They do not use measuring conditions identical to those applied in internal calibration techniques and should therefore be subject to thorough investigation to prove their validity. For internal calibration modes, there are the standard addition technique and the species-specific isotope dilution technique.

The following are a few comments about these various calibration modes.

Whereas calibrants for all the elements of the periodic table are commercially available, either in some inorganic form or even organically bound, more often than not this form is not identical to the specific elemental species under investigation. Lack of availability of the specific calibrants, problems with the stability of the elemental species standards, possible species transformation during sample treatment, the aggravating situation of incomplete separation of a particular species from a mixture of species — all these make calibration of elemental species a much more difficult undertaking than total element determinations.

Isotopically labelled calibrants for elemental species are not usually commercially available. All calibrants need to be exactly characterized and must be checked with respect to species-specific purity.

Isotope dilution MS can be used in two different ways. The first technique uses a labelled species spiked and equilibrated with the sample to undergo the same separation and measurement procedure. This is isotope dilution used to its full capacity. The second method consists of injecting the label after the separation of the species (e.g. in the eluate of HPLC) or after the GC column as an internal standard for the response of the measurement (Heumann, 2004).

The stability of the elemental species standard solutions is crucial. Adsorption on the walls of the storage vessels, composition of the solvent, evaporation of solvent, pH, oxidants, temperature, material of the storage vessel, the air above the solution — all are parameters liable to jeopardize the stability of the species in solution. This has been carefully documented for Cr^{VI} standard solutions (Dyg et al., 1994).

4.8 Reference materials

Quality assurance of the analytical procedures used for speciation analysis requires the analysis of representative reference materials, certified for the relevant species and at representative concentrations (certified reference materials) (Quevauviller, 2003). There are an interesting number of reference materials currently available, including arsenic species in fish, Cr^{III}/Cr^{VI} in a lyophilized water and a welding dust, mercury species in at least 20 materials (including fish, mussels, seaweed, hair, sediment), alkyl lead in urban dust, organotin compounds in sediment and mussel tissue, and extractable species in sewage sludge and sediment (Cornelis et al., 2001; Virtual Institute for Reference Materials, http://www.virm.net/).

In addition to stable reference materials certified for species, there may be a need for a new type of reference material for method validation of labile species.

4.9 Direct speciation analysis of elements and particles

The characterization of elemental species in particles, especially aerosol particles, is of great importance in assessing environmental health hazards. In atmospheric sciences, individual particle analysis provides valuable complementary information concerning origin, formation, transport, and chemical reactions, which may never be learned from conventional bulk techniques. In occupational health monitoring, particle characterizations are instrumental in evaluating health hazards for workers exposed to dust from foundries, calcination ovens, powder handling, milling, welding, etc. (Ortner, 2003).

The special methods for single particle characterization require advanced technology. Methods that are already routinely used are high-resolution scanning electron microscopy and electron probe microanalysis. Other techniques are selected area electron diffraction in the transmission electron microscope or energy filtering transmission electron microscopy. An appropriate combination of such techniques (multimethod approach) yields conclusive answers as to particle speciation. A high-resolution scanning electron microscopy identification combined with energy-dispersive X-ray fluorescence spectrometry allows the study of the true nature of aerosol particles collected during metallurgical processes. It is beyond the scope of this monograph to go deeper into these technologies. Ortner (2003) introduces the reader to this very specialized field.

Attention should also be drawn to X-ray absorption fine structure spectroscopy and X-ray Raman spectroscopy, two highly sophisticated techniques for species analysis in solid samples. Their theoretical principles are described by Welter (2003). They are being used in environmental analysis (e.g. the binding of actinides and fission products to humic acids and clay).

4.10 State of the art

The advances in our knowledge of elemental speciation analysis during the past 20 years are remarkable. Analytical methods for the species of 21 elements, of the actinides, and of four groups of compounds (halogens, volatile metal compounds of biogenic origin, metal complexes of humic substances, and metal complexes of proteins) are described in a recent book (Cornelis et al., 2005). The total number of original publications since 1972 exceeds 16 000. The elements that are in the limelight (in the order of atomic number) are **aluminium** (Milačič, 2005a,b,c; Valkonen & Riikimäki, 2005), **chromium** (Hoet, 2005a; Metze et al., 2005), **iron** (Hoffmann, 2005; Walczyk, 2005), **nickel** (Schaumlöffel, 2005), **copper** (Artiola, 2005; Nohr & Biesalski, 2005), **zinc** (Guenther & Kastenholz, 2005b), **arsenic** (Ali & Jain, 2004; Buchet, 2005; Prohaska & Stingeder, 2005), **selenium** (Francesconi & Pannier, 2004; Michalke, 2004; Uden, 2005), **cadmium** (Guenther & Kastenholz, 2005a; Verougstraete, 2005), **organotin**

(Rosenberg, 2005), **mercury** (Horvat & Gibičar, 2005), and **lead** (Crews, 2005; Hill, 2005; Hoet, 2005b).

For more information on speciation, the reader is referred to the literature cited in this chapter and to the European Virtual Institute for Speciation Analysis (http://www.speciation.net/).

5. BIOACCESSIBILITY AND BIOAVAILABILITY

5.1 Introduction

A substance is bioaccessible if it is possible for it to come in contact with a living organism, which may then absorb it. As an example, any substance trapped inside an insoluble particle will not be bioaccessible, although substances on the surface of the same particle will be accessible and may also be bioavailable. However, even surface-bound substances may not be accessible to organisms that require the substances to be in solution. Thus, bioaccessibility is a function of both chemical speciation and biological properties. In some cases, bioaccessibility will be the limiting factor in determining uptake. This is particularly true of elements in soils, sediments, and other particulate matter to which humans may be exposed. Hence, although bioaccessibility is an important consideration for all matrices and routes of exposure, including exposure to particulates from inhaled air, an overview of bioaccessibility only in the context of soil and related matrices is presented below.

Substances are biologically available ("bioavailable") if they can be taken up by living cells and organisms and can interact with "target" molecules. Substances that are not bioavailable may still cause physical damage or may alter the availability of other substances. Bioavailability of an element usually depends upon its chemical speciation.

5.2 Bioaccessibility of elements in soils and sediments

5.2.1 Factors affecting the mobility and accessibility of elements in terrestrial (soil) environments

Elements can occur in the soil in either the solid phase or the aqueous soil solution. In the solid phase, ions can be bound to organic and inorganic soil components in various ways, including ion exchange and surface complexation, or they can exist in minerals or be co-precipitated with other minerals in the soil. In the soil solution, the elements can exist either as free ions or as complexes with organic groups, such as amino, carboxyl, and phenolic groups, or inorganic groups, such as carbonate, chloride, hydroxide, nitrate, and sulfate. Ions in solution are generally bioaccessible, and ions in the solid phase of the soil may become accessible if environmental conditions change (National Research Council, 2003).

Because most soil solutions are not saturated with respect to their inorganic components, continuous dissolution from the solid phase tends to occur, and dissolution kinetics determine the bioaccessibility of ions derived from soil minerals. Conversely, sorption of ions, compounds, and complexes limits their bioaccessibility. Sorbed compounds can occur as surface complexes or as surface precipitates or clusters. Ion exchange occurs mainly at sites where there is a permanent electrical charge (not pH dependent) on clay minerals that have undergone isomorphic substitution. Isomorphic substitution is replacement of ions in the clay mineral lattice with other ions of lower charge. Soils with significant negative charge have a high cation exchange capacity and low cation mobility. Soils high in clay typically have the highest cation exchange capacity. Ion exchange is affected by the speciation of elements as reflected in their oxidation state, as this also affects the net charge on their ions or on other electrically charged derivatives (Table 5).

Table 5. Elemental species that may determine the accessibility of elements in the soil solution[a]

Element	Aerobic soils	Anaerobic soils
Chromium	$Cr(OH)_3$ (low to neutral pH)	$Cr(OH)_3$
Nickel	NiO, $NiCO_3$, $Ni(OH)_2$	NiS
Arsenic	$Ca_3(AsO_4)_2$, $Mg_3(AsO_4)_2$, As_2O_5	As_2S_3
Cadmium	$Cd(OH)_2$, $CdCO_3$	CdS
Mercury	$HgCl_2$, HgO, $Hg(OH)_2$	HgS
Lead	PbO, $PbCO_3$, $Pb_3(CO_3)(OH)_2$	PbS

[a] Modified from Hayes & Traina (1998).

Abundant bioaccessible amounts of essential nutrients, such as phosphate and calcium, can decrease plant uptake of non-essential but chemically similar substances, in this case arsenate and cadmium. More complex interactions are also observed. For example,

Cu^{II} toxicity may be related to low abundances of Fe^{II}, Zn^{II}, sulfate, and/or molybdate (Adriano, 1986, 1992; Chaney, 1988).

In summary, soil conditions that cause precipitation or sorption of elements reduce their soil mobility and bioaccessibility. The elements that tend to be the most mobile and bioaccessible are those that form weak bonds with organic or inorganic soil components or those that complex with ligands in solution and that are not adsorbed to soil particles.

5.2.2   Factors affecting the mobility and accessibility of elements in sediment environments

Determining the bioaccessibility of elements sorbed to sediments is key to understanding their potential to accumulate in aquatic organisms and to induce toxic effects in them and in the ultimate human consumers. It is clear from the published data that total element concentrations in sediments are poorly related to the bioaccessible fraction (Ruiz et al., 1991; De Vevey et al., 1993; Allen & Hansen, 1996). A recent document (USEPA, 2005) describes the use of equilibrium partitioning sediment benchmark procedures to derive concentrations of metallic element mixtures in sediment that are not harmful to benthic organisms. The equilibrium partitioning approach is applicable across sediments and designed to allow for the bioaccessibility of chemicals in different sediments in relation to an appropriate biological effects concentration.

A large amount of the total elemental constitution of most sediments is in a residual fraction as part of the natural minerals that make up the sediment particles (USEPA, 2005). These residual elements are not bioaccessible. The remaining elements in sediments are adsorbed to or complexed with various sediment components and may be bioaccessible. In oxidized sediments, cations may be adsorbed to clay particles, iron, manganese, and aluminium oxide coatings on clay particles, or dissolved and particulate organic matter. As the concentration of oxygen in sediment decreases, usually because of microbial degradation of organic matter, oxide coatings begin to dissolve, releasing adsorbed cations. In oxygen-deficient sediments, many cations react with sulfide produced by bacteria and fungi to form insoluble sulfides. Many chemical species may be released from sorbed or complexed phases into sediment pore water in ionic, bioavailable forms following changes in oxidation/

reduction potential. Microbial degradation of organic matter may also release adsorbed species to pore water. Certain bacteria are able to methylate some ionic species, such as those of arsenic, mercury, and lead, to produce organic derivatives that are more bioaccessible than the original inorganic species.

The dominant role of the sediment sulfides in controlling metal cation bioaccessibility seems to be clear (Di Toro et al., 1990, 1991; Ankley et al., 1991). Sulfides are common in many freshwater and marine sediments and are the predominant form of sulfur in anaerobic sediments (usually as iron(II) sulfide [FeS]). The ability of sulfide and metal cations to form insoluble precipitates with water solubilities below the toxic concentrations of the cations in solution is well established (Di Toro et al., 1990). This accounts for the lack of toxicity from sediments and sediment pore waters, even when high metal concentrations are present (Ankley et al., 1991). Ankley et al. (1991) showed that the solid-phase sediment sulfides that are soluble in weak cold acid, termed acid volatile sulfides, are a key factor in controlling the toxicity of cations of elements such as copper, cadmium, nickel, lead, and zinc. Toxicity due to the cations of these elements is not observed when they are bound to sediment and when, on a molar basis, the concentration of acid volatile sulfides is greater than the sum of the molar concentrations of metals. When the ratio of the sum of the simultaneously extracted metallic elements to the concentration of acid volatile sulfides exceeds 1.0 on a molar basis, toxic effects due to cations of the elements may be expressed, if the cations are not complexed by other ligands. Thus, the element to acid volatile sulfides ratio can be used to predict the fraction of the total metal concentration present in sediment that is bioaccessible as cations, and hence provides the basis for risk assessment.

Limitations to the metallic element to acid volatile sulfides ratio approach occur when the concentration of acid volatile sulfides is low — for example, in fully oxidized sediments. Most sediments have at least a small zone where the sediments are oxic near the sediment–water interface. The importance of this zone has been demonstrated for copper relative to acid volatile sulfides and accumulation of copper in the midge (*Chironomus tentans*) (Besser et al., 1996). In these situations, other phases (i.e. iron and manganese oxides, dissolved organic carbon, and particulate organic carbon) can play an important role in determining the bioaccessibility of potentially toxic elements.

5.3 Determinants of bioavailability

Elements in non-ionic and uncombined form are mostly not bioavailable. Mercury is a notable exception because of its volatility (see below). Elements that readily form simple ions upon solution in water are accessible to living cells but may not be available if there is no mechanism for their uptake. Thus, a knowledge of the mode of uptake applicable to humans at risk is essential for risk assessment.

It is not enough to consider simple ions, since these ions may be complexed by inorganic and organic ligands or adsorbed onto, or bound within, particles. Furthermore, any metallic elements and ions derived from them may cycle between oxidation states in which they have different bioavailability. Complexation and redox cycling are often associated with large differences in reactivity, kinetic lability, solubility, and volatility because of changes in chemical speciation.

In the simplest case, uptake may be driven by an electrochemical gradient. The concentrations of substance or charge driving uptake through the plasma membrane will be those concentrations of substance or charge immediately in contact with the membrane. Both may, in turn, be dependent upon biotransformation and/or localization within cells or cell compartments. Uptake is also affected by components of the exposure medium, such as the presence of similar chemical species that may compete for uptake sites (Hare & Tessier, 1996; Playle, 1998; Alsop & Wood, 1999).

Even if the biologically available form of an element is the free ion in solution, the free ion may be derived from other chemical species, and the thermodynamic equilibrium for production of the ion or the rate of its release may be the limiting factor for its uptake by living cells (i.e. transfer from the external medium to the interior of the cell). Knowing which chemical species determine the rate and amount of uptake of an element by living organisms is essential for risk assessment. In order to determine the relevant chemical species for risk assessment, three questions must be answered (Hudson, 1998; Sunda & Huntsman, 1998a):

1. What is the mechanism of uptake of the element of concern?
2. How do elemental species interact in the uptake process? (Interactions may occur outside the organism, where elements may interact directly or compete for transport sites, or inside, where elements may compete for binding sites that regulate transport systems.)
3. Which chemical species control the rate of elemental uptake and excretion by the cell?

Most elements are absorbed by living organisms from aqueous solution, whether it is from the sea, fresh water, soil water, aerosols, or dietary intake to the gut. Seawater has been particularly well studied and illustrates well the factors to be considered in risk assessment. For seawater, most Mn^{II}, Fe^{II}, Co^{II}, Ni^{II}, and Zn^{II} are present as "free" aqua ions. Some metallic elements, such as Cu^{I}, Cd^{II}, Ag^{I}, and Hg^{II}, are complexed by chloride ions. Others, such as Cu^{II} and Pb^{II}, are complexed with carbonate, whereas Al^{III} and Fe^{III} complex with hydroxide ions (Byrne et al., 1988). Surface seawater has a fairly constant pH and major ion composition, and the inorganic speciation of elements varies little throughout the surface water of the world's oceans. In contrast, there are large variations in chloride concentration, alkalinity, pH, and redox potential in, for example, fresh and estuarine waters and soil water. These variations lead to changes in inorganic complexation. In fresh waters, pH can vary over a range from about 5 to 9; as the pH changes, so does the hydroxide and carbonate complexation of Al^{III}, Cr^{III}, Fe^{III}, Cu^{II}, Cd^{II}, and Pb^{II}, causing great changes in their bioavailability. In estuaries, large salinity gradients strongly affect the extent of chloride complexation to Cu^{I}, Ag^{I}, Cd^{II}, and Hg^{II}. It is likely that similar changes will occur locally in the aqueous media of the human body and its cells, as pH, oxygen, carbonate, and chloride concentrations change as a result of physiological events. These changes in chemical speciation will affect local bioavailability and toxicity.

Naturally occurring organic complexation of elements in the environment has not been studied as thoroughly as inorganic complexation. Organic complexation of Cu^{II} has been the most extensively studied. More than 99% of Cu^{II} is complexed to organic ligands in almost all aquatic systems except deep oceanic water (Sunda & Hansen, 1979; van den Berg et al., 1987; Coale & Bruland, 1988; Moffett, et al., 1990; Sunda & Huntsman, 1991; Xue et al., 1996). Cu^{II} is bound by unidentified organic ligands present in low concentrations and having extremely high conditional stability constants (log K ~13 in seawater and 14–15 in lakes at pH 8) (Coale & Bruland, 1990; Moffett et al., 1990; Sunda & Huntsman, 1991; Moffett, 1995; Xue & Sunda, 1997).

Some studies indicate that Fe^{III} is also >99% complexed by unidentified organic ligands in near-surface seawater (Gledhill & van den Berg, 1994; Rue & Bruland, 1995; Wu & Luther, 1995). Zn^{II}, Cd^{II}, and Pb^{II} are also complexed organically in surface seawater. Electrochemical measurements indicate that 98–99% of zinc in surface waters is complexed to organic ligands (Bruland, 1989; Donat & Bruland, 1990), whereas 50–99% is organically bound in estuarine and fresh waters (van den Berg et al., 1987; Lewis et al., 1995; Xue et al., 1995). In contrast, Mn^{II} forms only weak coordination complexes, and there is no evidence for much organic chelation of this element (Roitz & Bruland, 1997).

In addition to its solubility, the oxidation state of an ion may be crucial. Where chromium is concerned, only Cr^{VI} as chromate is readily taken up by living cells. Even so, epidemiological studies suggest that the almost insoluble chromates are more likely to be associated with lung cancer than the soluble salts (Duffus, 1996). The same may be true of nickel compounds associated with lung cancer (Draper, 1997). Readily water-soluble $NiSO_4$ gave negative results in United States National Toxicology Program tests of carcinogenicity (NTP, 1994). Thus, bioavailability in the sense of ready uptake into living cells may be less relevant to carcinogenicity in lungs than to other types of toxicity.

Redox transformations alter the speciation and bioavailability of at least eight metallic elements — namely, chromium, manganese, iron, cobalt, copper, silver, tin, and mercury. The oxidation states usually differ markedly in regard to acid–base chemistry, ionic charge, solubility, ligand exchange kinetics, and stability of coordination complexes. The stable or metastable forms of manganese, manganese(III) and manganese(IV) oxides, are insoluble and, hence, not conventionally regarded as bioavailable. However, in the particulate form, they have been associated with "manganese pneumonia" in humans following an inflammatory reaction in the lungs (Baxter et al., 2000). Mn^{II} salts are highly soluble and readily taken up by cells, but Mn^{II} is quite susceptible to oxidation by molecular oxygen to form Mn^{III} and Mn^{IV}. Mn^{II} is released into surface waters from photochemical and chemical reduction of manganese oxides by organic matter and can persist for days to months because of its slow oxidation kinetics (Sunda & Huntsman, 1987, 1988).

Iron is quantitatively the most important micronutrient element. It occurs in oxygenated water mainly in the thermodynamically stable state, Fe^{III}, which is only sparingly soluble in the absence of organic chelation. Photochemical or biological reduction of Fe^{III} can increase the biological availability of iron, since the resulting Fe^{II} is more soluble, has much more rapid ligand exchange kinetics, and forms much weaker complexes than Fe^{III}. The Fe^{II} formed is unstable and rapidly reoxidizes to Fe^{III}, especially at high pH (Miller et al., 1995).

5.3.1 Uptake by carriers

Elemental species are often transported into cells by specialized protein carriers (Simkiss & Taylor, 1995) or by organic ligands, such as chelating agents or ionophores. Some, like elemental mercury Hg^0 or the covalently bound mercury(II) chloride ($HgCl_2$) (Gutknecht, 1981), may diffuse passively through the phospholipid layers of the cell membrane. Appropriate chemical species bind to receptor sites on proteins or ligands and then either dissociate back into the medium or are transported across the membrane and released into the cytoplasm (Figure 2). The rate of uptake equals the concentration of the elemental species bound to the transport protein multiplied by the kinetic rate constant for transport across the membrane and release into the cytoplasm.

Binding of metal cations to receptor sites depends on whether the cations are class a ("hard") or class b ("soft") cations (Frausto da Silva & Williams, 1991) (Table 6). Class a cations are of small size and low polarizability owing, for example, with uncomplexed metallic elements, to a high ratio of positive charge to ionic radius, and consequently lower deformability of the electron orbitals. More polarizable class b cations, if free in aqueous solution, tend to bind to class a anions such as hydroxide and phosphate, which are common on the outer surface of living cells. Hydroxyl derivatives of the class a cations lack this affinity and therefore have poor bioavailability. Class b cations are of larger size and greater polarizability. Class b cations, such as lead, cadmium, and mercury, bind to nitrogen or sulfur centres with a higher covalent content to the bond, and from which they therefore dissociate more slowly. This is believed to be a basis of their toxicity. Further, the class b cations compete for binding sites with "essential" cations based on atomic radius. Thallium competes with potassium, while lead and cadmium compete for zinc and calcium sites.

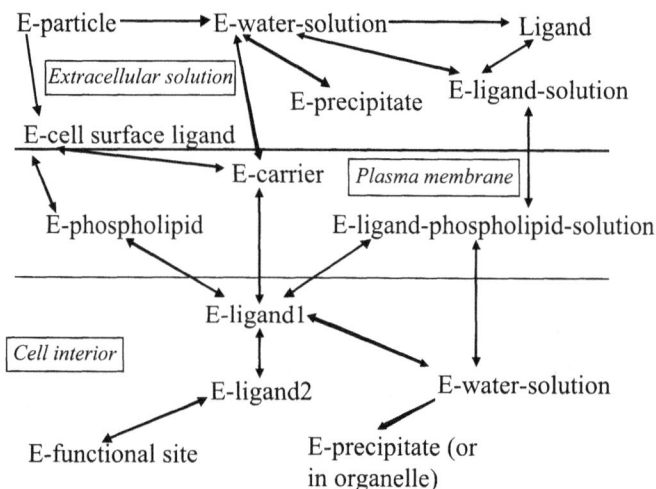

Fig. 2. Schematic representation of the relationships between the extracellular chemical species of an element E and the uptake of that element by living cells

The kinetics of uptake will vary with changes in chemical speciation (e.g. the presence of aqua ions or of hydroxide or chloride complexes). At equilibrium, the concentration of bound element, and therefore the uptake rate, is related to the external free ion concentration. Here, the uptake system is effectively under thermo-dynamic control (Sunda & Huntsman, 1998a) (Figure 3). Binding equilibration may be expected for elements with rapid ligand exchange kinetics, such as Cu^{II} and Cd^{II}. Fe^{III}, whose ligand exchange rates in seawater are only 1/500th of those for copper (Hudson & Morel, 1993), shows uptake kinetically controlled by the rate of metal binding to membrane transport sites. The rate of binding is related to the concentration of the labile dissolved inorganic Fe^{III} species [$Fe(OH)_2^+$, $Fe(OH)_3$, and $Fe(OH)_4^-$] whose exchange kinetics are rapid enough to permit appreciable rates of iron coordination to transport sites. Other elements with slow exchange kinetics, such as Al^{III}, Cr^{III}, and Ni^{II}, may also be under kinetic control, and their uptake may be determined by the concentration of kinetically labile inorganic species (Hudson & Morel, 1993).

Table 6. Class a (hard) and class b (soft) metals[a]

Class	Description/examples
Class a (hard) metals	Lewis acids (electron acceptors) of small size and low polarizability (deformability of the electron sheath or hardness)
	Li, Be, Na, Mg, Al, K, Ca, Sc, Ti, Fe^{III}, Rb, Sr, Y, Zr, Cs, Ba, La, Hf, Fr, Ra, Ac, Th
Class b (soft) metals	Lewis acids (electron acceptors) of large size and high polarizability (softness)
	Cu^{I}, Pd, Ag, Cd, Ir, Pt, Au, Hg, Tl, Pb^{II}
Borderline (intermediate) metals	V, Cr, Mn, Fe^{II}, Co, Ni, Cu^{II}, Zn, Rh, Pb^{IV}, Sn

[a] Modified from Frausto da Silva & Williams (2001).

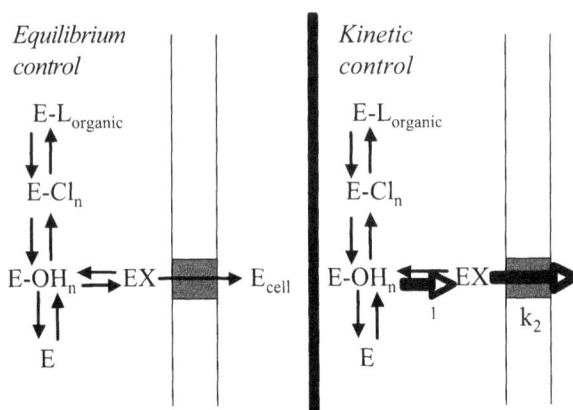

Fig. 3. Schematic diagram to show the extremes of equilibrium (thermodynamic) control and kinetic control of element E binding to cell membrane transport mechanisms. Under kinetic control, k_1 or k_2 may be the controlling rate constants. L = ligand; X = carrier into the cell membrane (after Duffus, 2001).

The iron species cited above and a number of aqueous chemical species relevant to bioavailability are the result of hydrolysis. Hydrolysis of metal ions is the process by which trivalent and more highly charged cations react with water to form hydroxo or oxo complexes, which vary in ionic charge and may be anionic and/or multinuclear (Lyman, 1995). Hydrolysis is the cause of the speciation changes with pH that affect aluminium in aqueous solution (Figure 4). The tendency to hydrolyse increases with dilution, and the hydrolysis products vary with pH. Hydrolysis decreases the availability of simple ions. This is why Be^{II}, Al^{III}, and Cr^{III} compounds in aqueous solution are poorly absorbed by cells at pHs near neutrality, where they occur as a mixture of hydroxide complexes. Clearly, any risk assessment for exposure to Be^{II}, Al^{III}, or Cr^{III} compounds should incorporate a quantitative consideration of the relative concentrations of the hydroxide complexes. Similar considerations may apply to other metallic elements, depending upon the circumstances.

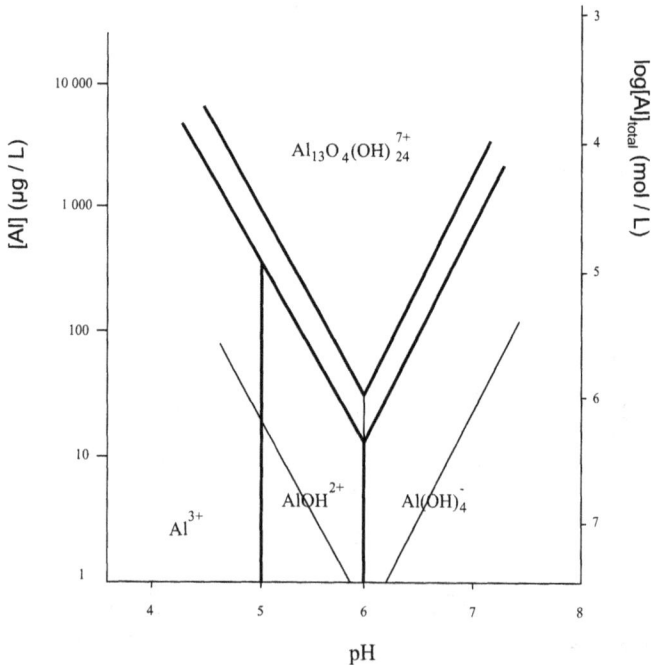

Fig. 4. Chemical speciation of aluminium in aqueous solution as a function of hydrolysis, concentration, and pH (after Nieboer et al., 1999)

Many elements, such as zinc, are taken up by more than one transport system with differing binding affinities. Each transport system may be the main one, depending upon the chemical conditions (e.g. low versus high metal ion concentrations; Sunda & Huntsman, 1992). Each system may be under differing controls (kinetic or thermodynamic), and thus it may be important to know which system predominates in order to predict effects of chemical speciation on uptake rates. Once one or more uptake-limiting species are identified, risk assessment must concentrate on determining the species concentration and the effective exposure for the bioavailable species of the element of concern.

In cases of kinetic control, elements in organic chelates and bound particulates (e.g. colloidal metal oxides) are generally assumed to be unavailable for direct uptake, since their dissociation and ligand exchange kinetics (or their diffusion rates, in the case of colloids and particulates) are too slow to permit rapid donation of free ion, or bioavailable species, to membrane transport sites (Morel et al., 1991). However, there are certain chelates, such as the crown ethers, that can bind metal ions, dissolve in the phospholipid bilayer of the cell membrane, and pass through by simple diffusion (see below). This also appears to be true for certain hydrophobic copper complexes (Ahsanullah & Ying, 1995).

Most non-metallic elements are available to biological systems as simple anions: for example, F^-, Cl^-, Br^-, I^-, or oxyanions such as $B(OH)_4^-$, $H_2PO_4^-$, HPO_4^{2-}, SO_4^{2-}, $H_2AsO_4^-$, AsO_2^-, and SeO_4^{2-}. The metallic elements chromium, molybdenum, and vanadium can also be included here as the anions CrO_4^{2-}, MoO_4^{2-}, and VO_4^{3-}, respectively, and the principles of uptake for all these elements are similar. Anions cannot cross membranes without carriers, and, once captured, they remain inside the cell unless there is a specific outward pumping system.

5.3.2 *Uptake and physical form*

Biological effects of elements depend upon physical form as well as on chemical speciation. This is relevant to the risks to human health associated with processing metal ores. Formation of aerosols during processing makes the ore or its derivatives available for inhalation. Breathing in dusts produced during ore crushing and milling may lead to localized respiratory effects, including asthma, pulmonary irritation, and oedema (Chiappino, 1994). The physical form, the aerosol produced, permits inhalation, while the relatively insoluble chemical form localizes the effects to the lungs. Metal roasting or welding leads to the production of metal fumes (oxides of beryllium, chromium, manganese, cobalt, nickel, copper, zinc, arsenic, selenium, cadmium, and lead), which can also be inhaled and which can give rise to combined local and systemic effects such as metal fume fever (Gordon & Fine, 1993; Burgess, 1995). The systemic effects are a reflection of solubility of the oxides, which in turn affects their metabolism and the related toxicokinetics. The oxides dissolve in lung fluid to release ions, which enter the blood and circulate, affecting distant organs and adding to the harmful effects of inflammatory mediators released from the lung tissue.

We have very little knowledge of what happens to particulates bound to membrane receptors (e.g. in lung tissue). Such interactions must depend on chemical speciation in the particulates and also on their surface chemistry (Nieboer et al., 1999).

5.3.3 *Uptake and complexation*

The inorganic complexation in water of many ionic species, such as those of manganese, cobalt, nickel, and zinc, is usually negligible, and the inorganic speciation is dominated by the uncomplexed aqua ions. For these elements, the distinction between thermodynamic equilibrium and kinetic control may be of little practical importance. However, for ionic species that are strongly complexed by chloride ions, such as Cu^I, Ag^I, Cd^{II}, Hg^I, and Hg^{II}, and whose complexation varies widely with sodium chloride concentration, knowledge of the type of transport control may be critical in predicting expected changes in metallic element uptake rates accompanying variations in the major ion composition of the water. Similarly, for elemental species that are highly complexed to hydroxide, such as Al^{III}, Cr^{III}, and Fe^{III}, and for ions complexed to carbonate ions, such as Cu^{II}, Cd^{II}, and Pb^{II}, changes in pH or alkalinity can lead to large differences in inorganic speciation, and therefore in metallic element transport behaviour, and related risk assessment.

As already indicated above, there are exceptions to the membrane protein carrier transport mechanism for metal uptake. Some uncharged, non-polar complexes, such as $HgCl_2$ and methylmercury(II) chloride (CH_3HgCl), can diffuse directly across phospholipid membranes owing to their lipid solubility (Gutknecht, 1981). This is true also of some organic complexes, such as Cd^{II}– xanthate complexes (Block & Glynn, 1992), Cu^{II}–oxine complexes (Croot et al., 1999), and Cu^{II}–, Cd^{II}–, and Pb^{II}–diethyldithio-carbamate complexes (Phinney & Bruland, 1994). Much detailed information about this comes from studies on diatoms, but it is likely that these observations apply to all living organisms, as we believe that all plasma membranes have similar properties for transport, dependent on lipid solubility. In experiments with a coastal diatom, the uptake and toxicity of Hg^{II} in a mercury/sodium chloride solution were related to the computed concentration of $HgCl_2$ and not to that of Hg^{2+} or of total inorganic mercury species. This implies that uptake occurred by diffusion of the lipid-soluble undissociated $HgCl_2$ complex through the cell membrane (Mason et al., 1996). Once inside the cell, the $HgCl_2$ takes part in ligand exchange reactions with biological ligands, such as sulfhydryls, providing an intracellular sink for the diffusing mercury. Other relatively lipid soluble, neutrally charged chloro-complexes, such as copper(I) chloride (CuCl) and silver(I) chloride (AgCl), may also be taken up by the same diffusion/ligand exchange mechanism. Similarly, lipo-philic chelates, such as those with 8-hydroxyquinoline and dithio-carbamate, are taken up by the same process (Stauber & Florence, 1987; Phinney & Bruland, 1994). The uptake of such chelates may be a significant uptake pathway for organisms in aquatic environ-ments receiving pollutant inputs of synthetic organic ligands that form lipophilic chelates. Similarly, drugs with chelating properties may cause significant changes in the uptake of metallic and non-metallic elemental species and in their distribution in the human body.

Other neutral molecules can also diffuse into cells. Thus, boron(III) hydroxide [$B(OH)_3$] and silicon(IV) hydroxide [$Si(OH)_4$] can carry silicon and boron to all parts of a cell by free diffusion across membranes. Compounds such as $B(OH)_3$ may be trapped by binding to *cis*-diols, probably to polysaccharides, giving moderately labile ring condensation products. $Si(OH)_4$ or any weak dibasic acid may react in the same manner. Molybdenum, in the form molybdenum(VI) hydroxide [$Mo(OH)_6$], behaves like $Si(OH)_4$.

Chelates with certain biological ligands can be transported into cells by specific membrane transport proteins. Many micro-organisms release strong iron-binding ligands (siderophores) into the surrounding medium under iron-limiting conditions. Siderophores complex and solubilize iron. The siderophore–iron chelates are then transported into the cell by specific membrane transport proteins, after which the iron is released for assimilation by metal reduction or degradation of the siderophore (Nielands, 1981). The production of siderophores is widespread in eubacteria and fungi and also occurs in many, but not all, cyanobacteria (Wilhelm & Trick, 1994). There may be many other organic ligands released by bacteria still to be discovered. Mirimanoff & Wilkinson (2000) have reported bacteria that produce a complexing ligand capable of rapidly reducing Zn^{2+} concentrations in the external medium by facilitating its bioavailability and uptake.

5.3.4 Selective uptake according to charge and size

The various anions of group VII and oxyanions of groups IV–VI show considerable variation in size, permitting separation on that basis alone (Frausto da Silva & Williams, 1991, 2001). The associated thermodynamic selectivity may be much more significant than the great differences in abundance and availability of these elements. On the basis of similar sizes, only the anions F^- and OH^- or Br^- and SH^- can show competition.

There are some differences in the nature of the binding sites for anions compared with those for cations. Anions are negatively charged, and they have a relatively lower charge density because they are large. This means that anions must bind to clustered, positively charged groups, such as the ammonium group $-NH_3^+$, the guanidinium group, and metal ions, or through very extensive hydrogen bonding. Rarely, binding may occur at hydrophobic centres or regions containing $-OCH_3$, $-SCH_3$, $-CH_2-$, phenyl, etc. These centres will take up anions only if they are surrounded by a "buried" positive charge generated by the fold of the protein.

Hydration opposes binding if the binding sites are hydrophobic, and the less hydrated anions will be bound preferentially to such sites. The so-called "lyotropic" or Hofmeister series is obtained; this is the reverse of the hydration free energy. Thus, in binding strength:

$$I^- > Br^- > Cl^- > F^-$$
$$ClO_3^- > BrO_3^- > IO_3^- > CO_3^{2-} > HPO_4^{2-}$$

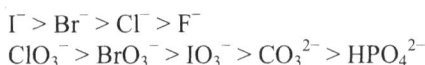

The non-polar sites in proteins that give such series often contain (buried) charged histidine residues or, sometimes, arginine and lysine residues.

5.3.5 Selective uptake according to binding affinity for different cationic centres

Binding of anions to cations or cationic centres depends upon whether they are class a or class b (Frausto da Silva & Williams, 1991, 2001). For class a (hard) cations, the order of binding by anions is $F^- > Cl^- > Br^- > I^-$, and $O^{2-} > S^{2-}$; for class b (soft) cations, the order is the reverse. The order of binding of anions to class a metal ions is overwhelmingly due to electrostatic effects, but binding to class b metal ions is driven mainly by covalence. The main cations concerned in biological systems are Mg^{2+}, Ca^{2+}, Mn^{2+}, Mn^{3+}, Fe^{2+}, Fe^{3+}, Co^{2+}, Co^{3+}, Cu^+, Cu^{2+}, Zn^{2+}, but only Cu^+ is a class b cation. Na^+ and K^+ cannot normally be considered as anion binding sites since they form only very weak complexes and are highly mobile. However, they may have a role in a few specific cases. Thus, for free aqueous ions, Cu^+ will amplify the lyotropic effect, while all other hydrated cations should oppose it to different degrees. For example, the following cations oppose the lyotropic effect in the order $Mg^{2+} > Ca^{2+} > Mn^{2+} > Zn^{2+} > Cu^{2+}$.

Simultaneous uptake of an anion and a cation is also a possibility. A common example of simultaneous uptake follows the binding of polyphosphates such as ATP and ADP with Mg^{2+}. The magnesium polyphosphates attach to very hydrophilic protein regions containing additional positive charges on basic side-chains of the proteins. This binding is very selective, since the combined requirements of the anion and the cation have to be satisfied simultaneously.

5.3.6 Selective uptake involving kinetic binding traps, with or without accompanying redox reactions

Some neutral molecules can be trapped by condensation reactions with various organic compounds, forming kinetically stable covalent bonds — for example, $B(OH)_3$, which condenses with *cis*-

diols. Other neutral molecules must be activated, reduced, or oxidized before they can bind to other compounds through kinetically stable covalent bonds (Frausto da Silva & Williams, 1991, 2001).

Phosphate anions can be retained only weakly by ionic interaction with positively charged groups (e.g. $-NH_3^+$), but they can be retained in a kinetic trap by condensing with -OH groups. In these forms, phosphate is transported (e.g. as sugar phosphate), stored (e.g. as polyphosphate and ATP), and transferred to other molecules, simple or polymerized, to give a variety of substances (e.g. RNA and DNA).

Inside cells, SO_4^{2-} is reduced and sulfur is retained in sulfide (S^{2-}), the thiol R-SH, or the disulfide -S-S- form. The same reactions occur with SeO_4^{2-}, which is bound as selenothiol, and with NO_3^-, which is incorporated as an amino group or other nitrogen-containing molecule. In the halide group, F^- and Cl^- are usually handled as such, but I^- and Br^-, once taken into a cell, can be selectively absorbed by enzymes, and the fact that they can be much more easily oxidized than Cl^- permits the reactions Br^- → Br and I^- → I in the presence of Cl^- — for example, by the action of many peroxidases. The reactive radicals so produced attack organic compounds readily (e.g. phenols), and thus bromine and iodine are inserted covalently into organic molecules. This is well seen in the biosynthesis of the thyroid hormone. In some cases, the free halogen can be formed and liberated (e.g. I_2 in some seaweeds).

There are situations in which reduction can change an anion into a cation. The uptake of vanadium and of molybdenum initially as HVO_4^{2-} and MoO_4^{2-}, respectively, is based on this principle. They are reduced to oxocations or simple cations and bound into proteins or cofactors. Oxovanadium(IV), VO^{2+}, is like nickel in its complexes with polyaminocarboxylic acids and binds quite strongly to N/O donors at pH ~7; however, with certain strong complexing agents, it can lose the oxo-group to give V^{IV} complexes. The vanadium-containing fungus, *Amanita muscaria*, contains this species, V^{IV}, bound to an *N*-hydroxy derivative of iminodiacetic acid, forming a very stable octa-coordinated complex in which the *N*-hydroxy group is ionized and binds the metal. The unusual accumulation of vanadium in tunicates as V^{III} or VO^{2+}, from the low concentrations of HVO_4^{2-} found in the environment, is probably due to this change in oxidation state, so that there is no "saturation" inside cells relative to the ionic species available outside, even when no internal ligand appears to be present and the retention of the ion (V^{3+} or VO^{2+}) is ensured by storage in vesicles.

The reactions of molybdenum are unusual, since it is the metallic element that has the most non-metallic properties. On entering a cell, the hydroxide form of the molybdate (MoO_4^{2-}) ion — i.e. $MoO_2(OH)_4^{2-}$ — can react not just with -OH groups to form MoO_2^{2+}-bound species, but also, since it is a class b (soft) metal ion, with -SH groups in the following reaction:

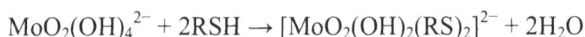

$$MoO_2(OH)_4^{2-} + 2RSH \rightarrow [MoO_2(OH)_2(RS)_2]^{2-} + 2H_2O$$

5.3.7 Uptake of organometallic compounds

In general, bioavailability of organometallic compounds reflects the lipid solubility of the organic part of the molecule. Thus, bio-availability may be determined for organic molecules from the mathematical relationship between the bioconcentration factor and the octanol–water partition coefficient (K_{ow}) (Mackay, 1982). In other words, increasing K_{ow} is reflected in increasing bioavailability up to very high values at which the molecule will tend to remain in the phospholipid of the plasma membrane and move no further into the cell or organism.

5.3.8 Exposure concentration and uptake

Uptake of bioavailable species depends upon their concentration in the extracellular medium. This may be the aqua ion concentration in solution, or it may be the total concentration of kinetically labile inorganic species (aqua ions plus labile inorganic complexes), or it may be the concentration of particulates or bioavailable complexes. In constant ionic media such as near-surface seawater equilibrated with the atmosphere (pH ~8.2), the inorganic speciation is constant, and concentrations of aqua ions and inorganic complexes are related to one another by constant ratios (Turner et al., 1981). Under these conditions, it probably does not matter whether one defines element availability in terms of concentrations of free ions or of total dissolved inorganic species, although it is important to know the concentration of the truly bioavailable species if complex interactions are suspected.

5.3.9   *Competition in the uptake and toxicity of non-nutrient elements*

Binding sites are never entirely specific for any one chemical species. Binding sites that have evolved to bind a particular species will also bind competing species with similar ionic radii and coordination geometry. Such competitive binding can occur at transport sites, active sites of metalloproteins, or feedback control sites, such as those regulating the number or activity of specific membrane transport proteins. Competition often occurs for binding to uptake sites. For example, uptake of Mn^{2+} is inhibited by the presence of ions such as Cu^{2+}, Zn^{2+}, and Cd^{2+}, which compete for binding to the relevant transport site. The inhibition of manganese ion uptake by competing ions results both from direct binding of these ions to membrane transport sites and probably also from binding to control sites regulating the maximum reaction rate of the transport system. The control site binding results in a reduction in the cell's capability for feedback regulation of intracellular manganese ion concentration. The inhibition of manganese ion uptake by other ions, such as those of cadmium, causes manganese deficiencies at low Mn^{2+} concentration. Such deficiencies can be the fundamental cause of inhibition of growth by the competing ions and emphasize the inherent linkage between toxicity and nutrition (Hart et al., 1979; Sunda & Huntsman, 1983, 1996).

Ionic species are often taken up by more than one transport system, each system being important under different sets of conditions. Although cadmium ions are taken up by the manganese system at high Zn^{2+} concentration, uptake at low Zn^{2+} concentration is dominated by a high-affinity cadmium ion transport system, which is under negative feedback control by intracellular zinc ions. Cobalt ions also appear to be taken up by this system, and their uptake also increases substantially with decreasing Zn^{2+} concentration. Because of the uptake of cadmium ions by manganese- and zinc-related systems, cadmium ion uptake by cells can be as heavily influenced by external manganese and zinc ion concentrations as it is by free cadmium ion levels. Thus, risk assessment must consider these ions as acting as a group, and not as acting independently.

Once inside the cell, competing ions may bind to nutrient ion sites such as the active sites on metalloproteins. The bound competing ion may have coordination geometry, Lewis acidity, redox behaviour, or ligand exchange kinetics that do not permit reaction of the nutrient ion with the site. There may be a loss of metabolic function and inhibition of metabolism. Damage will be made worse by high internal ratios of potentially toxic ions to nutrient ions.

Competitive interactions between nutrient and inhibitory ions and their derivatives are common. Studies on phytoplankton have provided evidence of competition between manganese and copper ions, manganese and zinc ions, manganese and cadmium ions (see above), zinc and copper ions (Rueter & Morel, 1982; Sunda & Huntsman, 1998b,c), iron and copper ions (Murphy et al., 1984), iron and cadmium ions (Harrison & Morel, 1983), cobalt and zinc ions (Sunda & Huntsman, 1995), and zinc and cadmium ions (Lee et al., 1995; Sunda & Huntsman, 1998b,c). In addition, uptake of the thermodynamically stable oxyanions, chromate ions (Riedel, 1985) and molybdate (Howarth et al., 1988), is competitively inhibited by sulfate, which is stereochemically very similar to both. The chromate/sulfate antagonism appears to be related to uptake of chromate by the sulfate transport system (Riedel, 1985). As a consequence of these interactions, variations in salinity and accompanying changes in sulfate influence both chromium toxicity and molybdenum nutrition. Chromate and molybdate should also interact antagonistically, but there appear to be no published data on this.

5.4 Incorporation of bioaccessibility and bioavailability considerations in risk assessment

The bioaccessible amount of any substance, which determines the exposure, is almost always less than the total measured amount in the environment. Oxidation state, hydrolysis, binding to dissolved compounds, adsorption onto sediment surfaces, and inclusion in organic films surrounding particles or at a water surface, among other things, may make substances unaccessible. Site-specific variations in bioaccessibility occur as a result of physicochemical and geochemical differences in natural environments. Thus, risk assessment procedures not only must allow for differing bioavailability of different chemical species of elements, but also must take into account how bioaccessibility varies from place to place and from time to time. Bioavailability can be accounted for by the selection of appropriate toxicity data in which the naturally occurring bioavailable species are considered or by the application of uncertainty factors to adjust the experimental test conditions to compare with those of the natural situation.

5.4.1 *Bioaccessibility and bioavailability in current approaches to environmental and human risk assessment*

The concentration limitation method of Aldenberg & Slob (1991) and the No Risk Area approach of Van Assche et al. (1996) acknowledge the importance and influence of bioaccessibility and bioavailability in the calculation of an environmental protection level. In the No Risk Area approach, the importance of acknowledging bioavailability in toxicity tests is emphasized. In the concentration limitation method, the calculated maximum permissible concentration can be adjusted according to the bioaccessible species of the substance in the area under study.

Bioaccessibility dependent on chemical speciation and partition between media has so far received little consideration in human risk assessment. For example, substances tightly bound to soil particles may not be accessible and may become accessible and bioavailable only when they enter the soil water or dissolve in gastric juices or inside phagosomes. In each case, the degree of accessibility and bioavailability will be different, although the original particles may be identical. If there is vaporization from solution, the substance becomes more accessible through the air and less so from the aqueous solution. There are distribution models that can describe such environmental movement quite well for carbon compounds, but they cannot be applied to most inorganic chemical species.

5.4.2 *The biotic ligand model*

Bergman & Dorward-King (1997) suggested that modelling the interactions of metal cations with biological surfaces, particularly the fish gill, might be useful as a method for predicting the acute toxicity of metallic elements in freshwater systems. The resultant models have been called biotic ligand models and are based on the gill surface interaction model for metal cation toxicity put forward by Pagenkopf (1983). Biotic ligand models link metal bioaccumulation and bioavailability with toxic impacts (Paquin et al., 2002). The biotic ligand model approach predicts toxicity by considering the chemistry of the exposure medium and the relationship between the exposure medium and the organism (the biotic ligand). The model combines factors influencing aquatic speciation and accessibility (e.g. pH, temperature, organic and inorganic anionic complexation) with other abiotic factors, specifically cationic competition (e.g. Na^+, K^+, Mg^{2+}, Ca^{2+}), affecting bioavailability and has been shown to work in practice (McGeer et al., 2000; Di Toro et al., 2001; Santore et al., 2001; de Schamphelaere et al., 2002; Heijerick et al., 2002). The model can distinguish metal species that will bioaccumulate and cause toxicity from the total pools in an organism as well as the bioaccessible pool in the exposure medium.

The biotic ligand model approach for predicting metal toxicity is being further developed for the effects of nickel, copper, zinc, silver, cadmium, and lead. Most of these developments are focusing on acute impacts, but it is hoped to extend the approach to chronic toxicity (Paquin et al., 2002). In order to develop the approach, it will be necessary to improve our understanding of geochemical speciation of metals relative to bioaccumulation and toxicity. A major area requiring further research is the role of natural and human-made dissolved organic matter. Organic compounds can facilitate or moderate toxicity, but more needs to be known about structure–activity relationships if the predictive model is to be developed further. In addition, the physiological mechanisms associated with chronic toxicity must be better characterized in order to define precisely the modelling end-point, either as accumulation of relevant chemical species or as dose of these species at a receptor. Another factor to consider with regard to chronic toxicity is that physiological acclimation changes can alter bioaccumulation at the site of toxicity, and these must be defined and incorporated into any successful model. Finally, biological species may differ considerably with regard to the uptake of different chemical species and with regard to their relative toxicities. Thus, the biotic ligand model approach has much to be said in its favour, but it has many challenges to deal with before it can be applied generally.

6. TOXICOKINETICS AND BIOLOGICAL MONITORING

6.1 Introduction

According to IUPAC, toxicokinetics is the process of the uptake of potentially toxic substances by the body, the biotransformation they undergo, the distribution of the substances and their metabolites in the tissues, and the elimination of the substances and their metabolites from the body (Nordberg et al., 2004). Exposure routes for species of inorganic elements are ingestion, inhalation, and dermal contact. Exposure by inhalation is very important, especially in occupational settings; as a consequence, the respiratory apparatus is a major route of absorption and deposition for metallic elements, both in the workplace and in the general environment. However, other routes of exposure must not be neglected in assessing risk.

Figure 5 indicates the different steps and media in which speciation must be considered when studying toxicokinetics after exposure via inhalation, ingestion, and skin absorption. Monitoring usually concentrates on urine, faeces, exhaled air, sweat, hair, nails, teeth, and blood.

In order to predict accumulation of an element in the body and assess risk, it is essential that its metabolism and kinetics are understood (Friberg & Elinder, 1993). It must be determined how much of the external exposure dose is absorbed after inhalation; how much is absorbed by the gastrointestinal tract and by the skin; whether the element is changed by biotransformation; how much is accumulated in the critical organ; and by which routes the element is excreted (e.g. expired air, urine, faeces). Consideration should also be given to the rate at which the different reactions take place, and the biological half-life of the relevant species should be determined, as this information is needed in order to predict the accumulation of elements in individual organs or in the body as a whole.

Knowledge about toxicokinetics is important for biological monitoring of an elemental species, as it influences the sampling time and the biological matrix in which the species is measured.

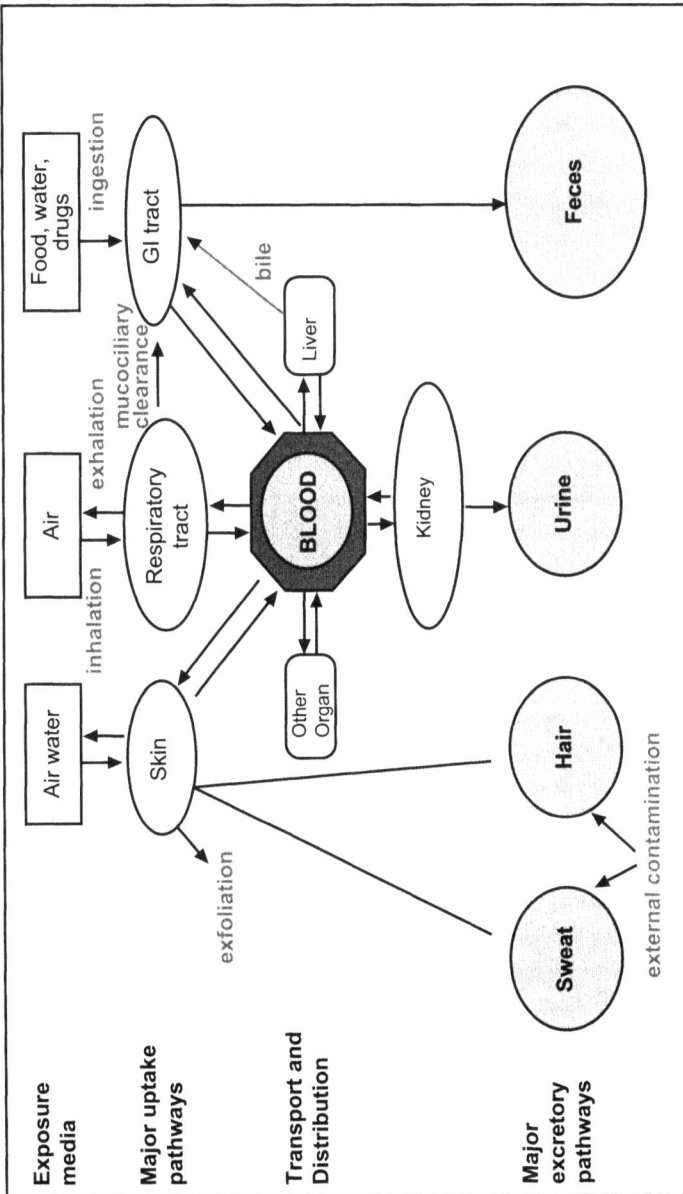

Fig. 5. Exposure and metabolic pathways for elements (from Clarkson et al., 1988). GI = gastrointestinal.

Most current methods measure the total amount of each metallic element, but the availability of methods for measuring the amounts of individual chemical species involved in toxicokinetics will make it possible to better estimate the effective dose present (acting) at different (critical) sites or levels.

6.2 Absorption

Absorption will be considered in order of importance of the exposure routes, starting with the inhalation route.

Particulates are first deposited in the upper respiratory tract (nose and pharynx). Absorption depends on both physical speciation (size, aerodynamic properties, solubility, and nature of the surface) and chemical reactivity and speciation. Particles of between 1 and 10 μm enter the trachea and bronchial tree, from which they may be removed by mucociliary action. The smallest particles (<1–2.5 μm) enter the alveolar region, where less intense airflow and system geometry may permit sedimentation, electrostatic precipitation, and diffusion–absorption of the particles. Nanoparticles (<100 nm) have properties that are now being elucidated and will not be discussed here.

Absorption of elemental species in the gastrointestinal tract varies depending on solubility in water and gastrointestinal fluids, chemical and physical characteristics, presence of other reacting compounds, and circumstances of ingestion (fasting, for instance).

For skin absorption, dose and duration of contact as well as the part of the body surface involved combine with chemical speciation and reactivity to determine whether absorption occurs and in what quantity.

Elemental species must pass through lipophilic membranes of cells in epithelial barriers or through barriers with specialized structures, such as the blood–brain, blood–testis, and blood–placenta barriers. Finally, uptake through the membranes of subcellular organelles must be considered.

Elements may undergo conversion from elemental form to cation form by the loss of one or more electrons (oxidation). The opposite process (reduction to a lower oxidation state and perhaps to an anion) may also occur in tissues, since each element has its characteristic oxidation–reduction or redox potential. Depending upon the local redox potential, a change in the oxidation state may be produced by either enzymatic or non-enzymatic reaction.

In the following sections, information relevant to the toxicokinetics of specific elements is summarized, with emphasis on species-specific behaviour.

6.2.1   *Chromium*

Because the two main oxidation states of chromium have different toxic actions, assessments of the absorption of chromium must distinguish between Cr^{VI} as chromate anion and Cr^{III} as the trivalent chromium cation. Entry of Cr^{3+} ions to cells is dependent on passive diffusion and phagocytosis (ATSDR, 2000), whereas chromate at physiological pH can enter erythrocytes, hepatocytes, and thymocytes through facilitated diffusion via the Band 3 anion exchanger, similar to sulfate and phosphate (Alexander, 1993). Chromates are structurally similar to sulfate and are believed to be transported into cells via the sulfate anion system (Ballatori, 2002; Hostynek, 2003). Absorption is faster for chromate than for trivalent chromium cations.

Respiratory absorption

Once chromium in any form is in the lung, water-insoluble compounds remain within the respiratory tract for a prolonged period of time, whereas soluble compounds readily cross the air–blood barrier (Hrudey et al., 1996).

The International Commission for Radiological Protection Task Group on Lung Dynamics has classified the chromium oxides and chromium hydroxides into a slow-clearance group and other chromium compounds into a fast-clearance group (Morrow et al., 1966). Slow clearance probably explains the much higher association of relatively insoluble chromates with lung cancer than is found with those that are readily water soluble.

Gastrointestinal absorption

Chromate anions in aqueous solution are absorbed more readily than trivalent chromium cations. However, at normal rates of intake, chromate is largely reduced to Cr^{3+} ions in the gastrointestinal tract (Hoet, 2005a), and the conversion makes it difficult to predict the absorption of chromium in food from its analysis before digestion.

Approximately 0.5–3% of chromium as trivalent chromium cations in food and water was absorbed in humans; the absorption seems to be homeostatically regulated (Anderson, 1986; Anderson et al., 1983; Bunker et al., 1984; Gargas et al., 1994; Finley et al., 1997; Kerger et al., 1997; Paustenbach et al., 1997). Absorption of trivalent chromium cations was inversely related to the dose, perhaps because of increasing chemical interactions between the aqua ions as their concentration in solution increased. For chromate in solution, absorption is dependent on water solubility and does not exceed 5% of the dose (Donaldson & Barreras, 1966; IARC, 1980).

Dermal absorption
In an in vitro gas diffusion cell study using full-thickness human abdominal skin (Gammelgaard et al., 1992), after the test duration of 190 h, when the skin barrier was still found intact, no chromium could be detected in the recipient phase after exposure to chromium(III) chloride ($CrCl_3$) or chromium(III) nitrate [$Cr(NO_3)_3$], whereas potassium dichromate ($K_2Cr_2O_7$) was found to pass through the skin. Moreover, the chromium concentrations in the skin layers were about 10 times lower after $CrCl_3$ application and about 15–30 times lower after $Cr(NO_3)_3$ application than the corresponding concentrations after application of $K_2Cr_2O_7$. Thus, Cr^{VI} permeates the skin to a larger extent than Cr^{III}.

6.2.2 Manganese

Respiratory absorption
Water-soluble manganese species are readily absorbed following inhalation. Less manganese was found in the lung after exposure to the more soluble manganese(II) sulfate ($MnSO_4$) than after exposure to the less soluble manganese(II,III) tetroxide (Mn_3O_4) or manganese(II) phosphate ($MnPO_4$), suggesting more rapid pulmonary clearance of $MnSO_4$ (Dorman et al., 2001a). The concentration of manganese in blood after an intratracheal instillation of manganese(II) chloride ($MnCl_2$) peaked within 30 min; following the less soluble manganese dioxide (MnO_2) instillation, the peak was observed at 168 h. The peak after MnO_2 instillation was 25% higher than that after $MnCl_2$ instillation. Brain levels were comparable

except for the striatum, which had much more manganese after $MnCl_2$ instillation than after MnO_2 instillation (Roels et al., 1997).

The olfactory tract provides an alternative route of passage of Mn^{II} into the brain, which can bypass the blood–brain barrier system (Tjalve & Henriksson, 1999; Dorman et al., 2002a). The total manganese concentration in the brain was significantly higher in rats exposed to manganese phosphate (hureaulite) $[Mn_5H_2(PO_4)_4 \cdot 4H_2O]$ and to a mixture of this and $MnSO_4$ than in rats exposed to manganese metal (Normandin et al., 2004).

Gastrointestinal absorption

Homeostatic mechanisms (notably dose-dependent biliary excretion) regulate the gastrointestinal absorption of dietary manganese compounds, compensating for differences between different manganese compounds. However, at high dietary manganese concentrations, the capacity of the homeostatic regulation may be exceeded, thus revealing differences in absorptive potential among dietary species (Windisch, 2002). Manganese concentrations in the liver and kidney were significantly higher following oral administration of manganese(II) acetate $[Mn(CH_3\text{-}COO)_2]$ or manganese(II) carbonate ($MnCO_3$) than following oral administration of $MnCl_2$ or MnO_2. Chemical species can influence manganese absorption through complex interactions with dietary chelators that can increase or reduce the formation of complexes with varying degrees of solubility: for instance, the absorption was greater for $MnCl_2$ in water than in food. Manganese ions (Mn^{2+}) may form poorly soluble complexes with dietary phytate, the absorption of which is very limited. In animals, $MnCl_2$ orally administered in water produced a peak in blood within 30 min, whereas the peak after ingestion of MnO_2 in water occurred 144 h later. In contrast, 35% of MnO_2 was absorbed after intraduodenal instillation compared with only 15% of an equivalent dose of $MnCl_2$ (Roels et al., 1997; Windisch, 2002).

Manganese absorption is mediated by proteins in the intestinal brush-border membrane that transport divalent cations. It has been suggested that the divalent metal transporter DMT-1 mediates gastrointestinal manganese absorption, even if the carrier was not exactly identified (Leblondel & Allain, 1999; Trinder et al., 2000; Windisch, 2002).

Dermal absorption

The gasoline additive 2-methylcyclopentadienyl manganese tricarbonyl (MMT) is well absorbed through intact skin when applied in concentrated solutions (ACGIH, 1991).

6.2.3 Iron

Gastrointestinal absorption

Fe^{2+} is generally absorbed from the gastrointestinal tract more readily than Fe^{3+}, probably because of its greater solubility. In addition, dietary chelators may increase or reduce the formation of insoluble complexes with Fe^{2+} ions and thus affect Fe^{2+} absorption. For example, EDTA significantly increased the bioavailability of Fe^{2+} in bread; in contrast, phytates can form insoluble complexes at gut lumen pH that are not absorbed. In the presence of phytase, inorganic Fe^{2+} is released and is then available for absorption as a divalent cation (Beliles, 1994; Whittaker et al., 2002; Windisch, 2002; Hurrell et al., 2003).

6.2.4 Cobalt

Respiratory absorption

Although limited data are available in humans, animal studies suggest that approximately 30% of the cobalt in an inhaled dose of cobalt(II/III) oxide is absorbed by the lung (ATSDR, 2004).

Gastrointestinal absorption

Studies in the rat show that complexation of Co^{II} with compounds such as histidine, lysine, glycine, caseine, and EDTA reduce the uptake. There was no difference in absorption between cobalt(II) chloride ($CoCl_2$) and cobalt(III) chloride ($CoCl_3$), but Co^{II} complexed with glycine was absorbed in greater amounts than Co^{III} similarly complexed (Taylor, 1962).

Dermal absorption

Sweat is capable of oxidizing metallic cobalt to Co^{2+} cations, and it has been demonstrated that when metallic cobalt powder was applied on the skin as dispersions in synthetic sweat, cobalt could penetrate the skin as a result of such oxidation (Larese et al., 2004). Similarly, in in vitro studies, Co^{2+} ions were observed on both the receptor and donor side of the apparatus upon sweat-induced oxidation of metallic cobalt powder.

6.2.5 Nickel

Respiratory absorption

Soluble nickel salts rapidly dissociate in aqueous medium, releasing Ni^{2+} ions that can penetrate cellular membranes. The water solubility of nickel compounds appears to be a good indicator of the rate of absorption into the blood of Ni^{II} from nickel-containing particles deposited at the alveolar level. Nickel(II) carbonyl $[Ni(CO)_4]$ is absorbed to a high degree; by evaluating the amount of nickel excreted via the urine in 4 days, at least 50% of the inhaled dose is estimated to have been absorbed. Seventy-five per cent of nickel deposited in the lung of rats by an intratracheal instillation of $NiCl_2$ was absorbed within 3–4 days, whereas 80% of deposited NiO aerosol remained in hamster lung 10 days later. The half-lives of nickel in rat lung following inhalation of nickel(II) sulfate ($NiSO_4$), nickel(II) subsulfide (Ni_3S_2), and nickel(II) oxide (NiO) were about 30 h, 4–6 days, and 120 days, respectively (Clary, 1975; Czerczak & Gromiec, 2001).

Gastrointestinal absorption

Oral nickel absorption is greater from more soluble compounds: 34% for nickel(II) nitrate ($NiNO_3$), 11% for $NiSO_4$, 10% for $NiCl_2$, 0.5% for Ni_3S_2, 0.09% for metallic nickel, 0.04% for black nickel oxide, and 0.01% for green nickel oxide. Absorption was reduced by some ligands, such as cysteine and histidine, and, to lesser extent, proteins (Ishimatsu et al., 1995; Templeton et al., 2000). A study measured an oral absorption of 27 ± 17% (mean ± standard deviation) for $NiSO_4$ given in drinking-water to fasted human subjects; absorption was only 0.7 ± 0.4% when the $NiSO_4$ was given in food (Sunderman et al., 1989).

Dermal absorption

Measurement of the depth–concentration profiles of a number of different nickel salts in the stratum corneum of human volunteers showed a difference in penetration as a function of the counterion (acetate > nitrate > sulfate > chloride) (Hostynek et al., 2001).

In studies using excised human skin under occlusion, penetration of the Ni^{2+} ion from $NiCl_2$ through the skin was about 0.23% of the applied dose after 144 h and 40–50 times quicker than from $NiSO_4$. Without occlusion, the permeation of $NiCl_2$ was reduced by more than 90%, and no absorption was detectable using $NiSO_4$. These observations are in agreement with test results wherein occlusion and the use of $NiCl_2$ rather than $NiSO_4$ were likely to produce a positive reaction in nickel-sensitive patients (Fullerton et al., 1986).

6.2.6 Copper

Gastrointestinal absorption

Approximately 30% of copper(II) sulfate ($CuSO_4$) is absorbed from the gastrointestinal tract in humans. Increasing luminal pH reduces the metal absorption. This is probably due to decreased Cu^{2+} and to a predominance of copper(II) hydroxide [$Cu(OH)_2$] and basic copper salts, which tend to precipitate out of aqueous solution (Wapnir, 1998; Windisch et al., 2001).

A fraction of the copper in cereal grains is thought to be chelated to lectins and glycoproteins, which dissociate at low pH and form insoluble complexes. Copper in complexes, such as copper methionine, is more readily absorbed than copper in inorganic salts, such as $CuSO_4$. Amino acid copper chelates are thought to be absorbed by specific absorption systems. Cysteine and ascorbic acid, in contrast, reduce copper bioavailability, probably by reducing Cu^{II} to Cu^{I} (Wapnir & Stiel, 1986; Baker & Czarnecki-Maulden, 1987; Aoyagi & Baker, 1994; Windisch, 2002).

In cattle, the relative rates of absorption of copper compounds were copper(II) carbonate ($CuCO_3$) > copper(II) nitrate [$Cu(NO_3)_2$] > $CuSO_4$ > copper(II) chloride ($CuCl_2$) > copper(I) and copper(II) oxides (Cu_2O and CuO) (Pott et al., 1994).

6.2.7 Arsenic

Respiratory absorption

Marafante & Vahter (1987) reported that the extent of absorption of inorganic arsenicals from the lungs of hamsters after intratracheal instillation was directly correlated with their water solubility. The lung retentions of elemental arsenic (2 mg/kg of body weight) 3 days after an intratracheal instillation of sodium arsenite ($NaAsO_2$), sodium arsenate (Na_2HAsO_4), arsenic(III) trisulfide (As_2S_3), and lead arsenate ($PbHAsO_4$) were, respectively, 0.06%, 0.02%, 1.3%, and 45.5% of the dose. Similar observations have been reported by Buchet et al. (1995). Sodium arsenate and sodium arsenite (doses of 5 mg/kg of body weight) had a relative bioavailability 10-fold greater than that of the largely water-insoluble gallium arsenide (GaAs) after intratracheal instillation in hamsters (Rosner & Carter, 1987). Also, in humans, sodium arsenate is better absorbed than the highly insoluble arsenic(III) trisulfide. Pershagen et al. (1982) found that there was much more rapid clearance from the lungs of arsenic(III) trioxide (As$_2$O$_3$) than of arsenic(III) trisulfide or calcium arsenate [Ca$_3$(AsO$_4$)$_2$]. This reflects the fact that arsenic(III) trioxide is much more soluble than the other two arsenicals. The authors further suggested that the clearance of calcium arsenate was much slower than that of arsenic(III) trisulfide, because the former was being transported to the alveolar regions of the lung, where clearance is slower.

The relationship of urinary arsenic excretion to air concentrations in several studies indicated that the urinary arsenic output for workers exposed to arsenic at 10 μg/m^3 was more than one third lower for boiler maintenance workers in a coal-fired power plant than it was for copper smelter workers. This finding was attributed to the fact that the arsenic in coal fly ash in their study was predominantly in the form of calcium arsenate, whereas in the copper smelter work environment, the arsenic was in the form of arsenic(III) trioxide (Yager et al., 1997).

Mann and his colleagues (Mann et al., 1996a,b) developed a physiologically based pharmacokinetic model describing the absorption, distribution, metabolism, and excretion of arsenate, arsenite, MMA, and DMA in the hamster, rabbit, and human. The model allows for simulation of human exposure to arsenic aerosols of different particle size distribution in situations with differing physical workload (Mann et al., 1996a,b). In addition, the model can be used to incorporate arsenic dosimetry from all potential exposure routes (oral, dermal, and inhalation).

Gastrointestinal absorption

Water-soluble forms of inorganic arsenic are almost completely absorbed from the gastrointestinal tract of humans and many laboratory animals. It is estimated that humans absorb at least 95% of an oral dose of soluble arsenite, based on the amount of arsenic recovered in faeces (Bettley & O'Shea, 1975; ATSDR, 2005a). At lower doses (e.g. 0.4 mg of arsenic per kilogram of body weight), arsenite may be more extensively absorbed from the gastrointestinal tract than arsenate, whereas the reverse appears to occur at higher doses (e.g. 4.0 mg of arsenic per kilogram of body weight) (Vahter & Norin, 1980). Approximately 55–80% of daily oral doses of soluble arsenate or arsenite have been recovered in the urine of human volunteers (Crecelius, 1977; Mappes, 1977; Tam et al., 1979; Buchet et al., 1981a,b; ATSDR, 2005a). MMA, DMA, and trimethylated arsenic species are also well absorbed (at least 75–85%) across the gastrointestinal tract (Buchet et al., 1981b; Marafante et al., 1987; Yamauchi et al., 1989, 1990). In studies on animals, at least 75% absorption has been observed for DMA (Stevens et al., 1977; Yamauchi & Yamamura, 1984; Marafante et al., 1987) and MMA (Yamauchi et al., 1988). Arsenobetaine undergoes rapid and almost complete absorption from the gastrointestinal tract (WHO, 2001).

Dermal absorption

Dermal exposure to environmental arsenicals has been considered to be a relatively minor route of exposure compared with oral or inhalation exposure (Hrudey et al., 1996), but this may be wrong. It is possible that significant absorption can occur from water during prolonged exposure (Bernstam et al., 2002). In vitro dermal absorption of DMA (10 µg) into mouse skin and receptor fluid was observed and ranged from <1% to 40% of the dose in experiments with three exposure scenarios (solid compound, aqueous solution, or soil). The absorption varied according to the exposure conditions in the following order: 20 µl water > 100 µl water > solid > 250 µl water > soil. No dose or pH effects on absorption of DMA were observed (M.F. Hughes et al., 1995).

6.2.8   Selenium

Gastrointestinal absorption

Selenomethionine is absorbed by an active transport system shared with methionine, while absorption of inorganic selenium as selenate or selenite is a passive process. The percentage of oral absorption of selenium varies from 90–98% for organic L-selenomethionine and selenate to 60% for selenite. The absorption is higher for sodium selenate (Na_2SeO_3) than for methyl selenocysteine, whereas elemental selenium and selenium(II) sulfide (SeS_2) are poorly absorbed (ATSDR, 2003a).

6.2 9   Cadmium

Respiratory absorption
The initial clearance due to mucociliary activity of an insoluble cadmium compound (like cadmium(II) oxide, CdO) from the lungs was greater than that of water-soluble cadmium(II) chloride ($CdCl_2$). For exposure to 760–930 $\mu g/m^3$, however, the long-term clearance of CdO and $CdCl_2$ was similar, with a lung half-life of 70 days (Hirano et al., 1990).

Gastrointestinal absorption
Intestinal absorption rates of Cd^{2+} between 0.5% and 12% (on average 2%) have been reported, depending on the species and age of the animals. $CdCl_2$ appears to be much better absorbed than cadmium(II) sulfide (CdS) and cadmium(II) sulfoselenide (ATSDR, 1999a). In humans with depleted iron stores, up to 8.9% absorption of $CdCl_2$ has been observed; the absorption was up to 4 times higher than in humans with normal iron stores (Flanagan et al., 1978).

6.2.10 Mercury

Mercury is found in living organisms in several chemical species, the most studied of which are the metallic form (Hg^0), Hg^+ and Hg^{2+} ions, methylmercury (CH_3Hg^+) compounds, and dimethylmercury (CH_3HgCH_3).

Respiratory absorption
At moderate ventilation rates and mercury air concentrations, metallic mercury vapour readily crosses biomembranes and is rapidly absorbed in blood and distributed to tissues. Approximately 70–80% of mercury vapour is absorbed in humans (Hursh, 1985; Sandborgh-Englund et al., 1998).

For inorganic mercuric compounds, absorption via the lungs is low, probably due to deposition of particles in the upper respiratory system and subsequent clearance by the mucociliary escalator (Friberg & Nordberg, 1973).

Human and experimental data obtained with methyl- and ethylmercury compounds demonstrated a pulmonary absorption of around 80% of the deposited dose. The absorption is probably lower for other organic mercury species, such as phenyl- or methoxyethyl-mercury (Toll & Hurlbut, 2002).

Gastrointestinal absorption

Only about 0.01% of elemental mercury is absorbed from the gastrointestinal tract, probably due to its physical state, low solubility, formation of a sulfide layer covering the droplet, or binding to sulfhydryl groups (Friberg & Nordberg, 1973; WHO, 2003). The absorption estimates for Hg^I and Hg^{II} salts range from 2–38% to <10% to ~10–15%. Hg^{II} salts (e.g. $HgCl_2$, mercury(II) cyanide [$Hg(CN)_2$], mercury(II) oxide [HgO], and mercury(II) nitrate [$Hg(NO_3)_2$]) may have higher absorption than Hg^I salts (e.g. mercury(I) acetate (CH_3-COOHg), mercury(I) chloride [Hg_2Cl_2], mercury(I) nitrate [$HgNO_3$], and mercury(I) oxide [Hg_2O]) (Sin et al., 1983; Klaassen, 2001).

Using whole-body retention data, estimated $HgCl_2$ absorptions of 3–4%, 8.5%, and 6.5% were calculated for single oral doses of 0.2–12.5 mg/kg of body weight, 17.5 mg/kg of body weight, and 20 mg/kg of body weight, respectively, in rats (Piotrowski et al., 1992). However, also using whole-body retention data to indicate absorption, an estimated absorption of 20–25% was calculated from single oral doses of 0.2–20.0 mg of mercury per kilogram of body weight as $HgCl_2$ in mice by comparing retention data after oral and intraperitoneal dosing and taking excretion and intestinal reabsorption into account (Nielsen & Andersen, 1990). Humans absorbed approximately 15% of the mercury in a trace dose of $Hg(NO_3)_2$ that was given orally either in an aqueous solution or in calf liver protein (Rahola et al., 1973). Several studies suggest that mercury in the form of mercury(II) sulfide (HgS), a relatively water insoluble divalent inorganic mercury compound, has a much lower bioavailability than mercury in the water-soluble $HgCl_2$ (ATSDR, 1999b).

Methylmercury compounds administered as the salt or bound to fish protein are 90–100% absorbed in the gastrointestinal tract. In contrast, aryl- and alkoxyalkylmercury compounds are about 50% absorbed. However, 100% absorption has been reported for phenylmercury in mice. Methylmercury and phenylmercury are absorbed more rapidly than inorganic mercury salts (Yannai & Sachs, 1993; Sue, 1994).

Methylmercury cysteine, a complex structurally similar to methionine, is transported across the gut wall into the circulation by a neutral amino acid carrier (Kerper et al., 1992; Clarkson, 1994). Methylmercury is probably reabsorbed as a sulfhydryl complex by a transport system, while inorganic mercury is not reabsorbed (Langford & Ferner, 1999).

Dermal absorption
The absorption of metallic mercury is thought to be very low (ATSDR, 1999b; WHO, 2003). The rate of skin uptake was estimated to be 2.6% of lung uptake (Hursh et al., 1989; Hostynek, 2003).

Up to 8% of mercury applied as $HgCl_2$ to the skin was absorbed in 5 h. Methylmercury compounds and phenylmercuric salts penetrate intact skin readily. Dimethylmercury rapidly penetrates gloves and is nearly completely absorbed (Nierenberg et al., 1998). A case of fatal dimethylmercury poisoning has been reported after dermal exposure (Smith, 1997; Toribara et al., 1997). A single exposure through latex gloves to 0.1–0.5 ml pure dimethylmercury raised the mercury concentration in whole blood to 4000 µg/l, far above both the normal range (<10 µg/l) and the usual toxic threshold (50 µg/l). On this basis, 40 µl of dimethylmercury applied to skin would be a severely toxic dose. The skin application of mercury-containing drugs, such as thiomersal (sodium ethylmercurithiosalicylate), has been demonstrated to produce an increase in serum mercury levels (USFDA, 1983; Gosselin & Smith, 1984), although there is no evidence of toxicity in adults or children exposed to thiomersal in vaccines (WHO, 2000b).

6.2.11 Lead

Respiratory absorption
The bioaccessibility/bioavailability of lead from inhalation exposure to inorganic lead compounds is highly dependent on particle size (Hrudey et al., 1996). For example, lung deposition fractions of inhaled lead range from 34% to 60% for particle sizes less than 0.05 µm and from 10% to 30% for particle sizes ranging from 0.05 to 0.5 µm (Booker et al., 1969; Hursh & Mercer, 1970; Chamberlain et al., 1975; Koplan et al., 1977; James, 1978; Morrow et al., 1980; Gross, 1981; Chamberlain, 1985). For the smaller

particles, lead bioavailability ranged from 48% to 77% (Booker et al., 1969; Hursh & Mercer, 1970; Koplan et al., 1977). Once deposited in the lower respiratory tract, particulate lead is almost completely absorbed, and all chemical forms of lead also seem to be absorbed (Morrow et al., 1980; USEPA, 1986).

Alkyl lead compounds, such as tetraethyl- and tetramethyl lead, are readily absorbed from the lungs and have caused severe, even fatal, intoxications (see chapter 8) (Chamberlain et al., 1975).

Gastrointestinal absorption
The water solubility of different chemical species of lead is one of the main determinants of gastrointestinal absorption. In rats that received diets containing 17–127 mg of lead per kilogram in the diet for 44 days in the form of lead(II) acetate [$Pb(CH_3COO)_2$], lead(II) sulfide (PbS), or lead-contaminated soil, bone and tissue lead levels increased in a dose-dependent manner (Freeman et al., 1996). Estimated bioavailability of lead sulfide was approximately 10% of that of lead acetate.

Particle size influences the degree of gastrointestinal absorption of lead (USEPA, 1986; Grobler et al., 1988). An inverse relationship between absorption in rats and particle size was found in diets containing metallic lead of particle sizes <250 μm. There was a 2.3-fold increase in tissue lead concentration when animals ingested an acute dose of 37.5 mg/kg of body weight with a particle size of <38 μm (diameter) compared with a particle diameter of 150–250 μm (Barltrop & Meek, 1979). Dissolution kinetics experiments with lead-bearing mine waste soil suggest that surface area effects control dissolution rates for particle diameters of <90 μm; however, dissolution of 90–250 μm particle size fractions appeared to be controlled more by surface morphology (Davis et al., 1994).

Dermal absorption
It is generally assumed that absorption of inorganic lead compounds through the skin is negligible in comparison with that via the oral or inhalation route (ATSDR, 2005b). However, skin penetration, which was low for lead(II) oxide (PbO) and lead(II) acetate, was much more pronounced for organolead compounds (reflecting their relative lipid solubility) (Table 7; Bress & Bidanset, 1991). Exposure via the skin to alkyl lead compounds has also caused severe intoxications (see chapter 8).

Table 7. Diffusion of lead compounds through 2 cm^2 of human skin in vitro over 24 h[a]

Compound (10 mg lead)	Amount of lead absorbed (µg)
Tetrabutyl lead	632 ± 56
Lead nuolate[b]	130 ± 15
Lead naphthenate[c]	30 ± 3
Lead acetate	5.0 ± 0.9
Lead oxide	<1.0

[a] From Bress & Bidanset (1991).
[b] A lead linoleic and oleic acid complex.
[c] Lead salt of cyclohexane carboxylic acid.

6.3 Disposition, excretion, and protein binding

Metallic elements may be stored in tissues/organs both as inorganic species or salts and as species chelated to proteins and other organic compounds.

Excretion depends on the speciation, on the route of absorption, and on other toxicokinetic pathways. The excreted species are either inorganic or organic and frequently at the lowest oxidation state. The elements ingested with food or water are excreted through the bile and faeces; minor routes of excretion include breath, milk, sweat, hair, and nails. The excretion of essential elements is regulated by homeostatic mechanisms (Apostoli, 1999).

Metallic elements form complexes with proteins, including enzymes, such as the essential elements associated with ferritin (iron, copper, and zinc), α-amylase (copper), alcohol dehydrogenase (zinc), and carbonic anhydrase (copper, zinc). Homeostatic control, metabolism, and detoxification of elements such as cadmium and mercury by their interaction with metallothioneins have been the focus of interest of toxicologists and clinical chemists for a long time (Stillman et al., 1992; Spuznar, 2000). Peptide-complexed metal ions are known to perform a wide variety of specific functions (regulatory, catalytic, in transport and storage) associated with life processes.

Peptides contain several groups in their side-chains that are particularly well suited for metal coordination. They include, in particular, cysteine ($-CH_2SH$) and methionine ($-CH_2CH_2SCH_3$), which bind metals with sulfur affinity (cadmium, copper, and zinc); and histidine, whose nitrogen atoms become available for coordination after metal-induced deprotonation (e.g. copper and zinc in superoxide dismutase). In contrast, the carboxamide function of peptide bonds [$-C(=O)-N(-H)-$] is only a poor metal coordination site.

6.3.1 Chromium

The distribution of chromium reflects the difficulty of Cr^{3+} ions in permeating biological membranes as compared with chromate anions and the rapid intracellular reduction of Cr^{VI} to Cr^{III}, with its subsequent binding to macromolecules. The diffusion of Cr^{3+} ions through biological membranes is not, however, negligible and can take place through the red blood cell membranes (Finley et al., 1997).

In blood, Cr^{III} is bound to plasma proteins (transferrin, albumin, others) and to an oligopeptide (molecular mass about 1500 daltons) called low molecular mass chromium-binding substance (Vincent, 1999). Approximately 10% of the cellular chromate content is nuclear. Chromate is taken up by the red blood cells through the anion membrane channels and further reduced to react with haemoglobin and cannot be exchanged in other body compartments (Langård & Norseth, 1986).

The offspring of pregnant rats given $^{51}Cr^{III}$ chloride by gavage 5 days per week through pregnancy exhibited about 1% of the level of radioactivity found in the mother. In another experiment, $^{51}Cr^{III}$ synthesized into "glucose tolerance factor" by brewer's yeast was given to pregnant rats by gavage in 3–5 doses. In this case, chromium label passed the placenta to the extent that the newborn rats exhibited 20–50% of the mothers' radioactivity (Mertz et al., 1969). Cr^{VI} (CrO_4^{2-}) crossed the placenta faster than Cr^{III} (Danielsson et al., 1982).

The accumulation of chromium in tissues depends on its form and exposure route. Soluble chelated compounds of chromium are in part cleared rapidly, whereas the chromium taken up by tissues may stay in the body for some months. If chromium forms colloids or is olated[1] to polynuclear complexes, it is trapped by the reticulo-endothelial system in the liver, spleen, and bone marrow (Burrows, 1983; Langård & Norseth, 1986). After gastrointestinal exposure, chromium thus tends to accumulate in tissue like lung, spleen, kidney, and liver. In workers exposed by inhalation to particulate chromium, the metal accumulates mainly in the lung, as seen in welders (Aitio & Jarvisalo, 1986), demonstrating that species and route of absorption, together with dose, are critical aspects in tissue chromium deposition.

Following intravenous administration, 40% of the injected dose of Cr^{3+} ions was excreted in the urine and 5% in the faeces, and 40% of the injected dose of chromate was excreted equally in urine and faeces over a 4-day period (Langård & Norseth, 1986).

Sayato et al. (1980) compared the urinary elimination of chromium from rats injected with ^{51}Cr-labelled sodium chromate and rats injected with ^{51}Cr-labelled chromium(III) chloride ($CrCl_3$). They found that the ^{51}Cr from chromates was excreted more rapidly than the ^{51}Cr from the trivalent chromium cation.

After inhalation exposure, around 50% of respiratory absorbed chromium is excreted via urine as Cr^{3+} ions; faecal excretion accounts for 5%. In both animals and humans, elimination by urine is biphasic, with a rapid phase, representing clearance from the blood, and a slower phase, representing clearance from tissues. Following intravenous administration, half-lives around 22 days for chromate and 92 days for Cr^{3+} ions for whole-body chromium elimination have been estimated. Among leather tanners whose exposure to basic chromium(III) sulfate [$CrOH(SO_4)$] had ceased, the elimination half-time of chromium in urine was about 1 month (Aitio et al., 1984). Chromium measurements from retired tannery workers showed that no long-term body burden had been developed (Simpson & Gibson, 1992). By contrast, a worker involved for 7 years in cutting stainless steel by plasma exhibited long elimination half-times (serum chromium 40 months, urinary chromium 129 months) (Petersen et al., 2000). The rate-limiting factor may

---

[1] Metal ions linked by hydroxyl bridges; with increasing hydroxyl content, there is a tendency to insolubility (olation).

have been a slow mobilization of the insoluble form of chromium from the lungs.

Mertz et al. (1965) reported a triphasic elimination pattern based on the whole-body counting of chromium in rats that received single doses of $CrCl_3$ by intravenous injection. The half-times for the three components of the elimination pattern were 0.5, 5.9, and 83.4 days, respectively.

6.3.2   *Manganese*

Manganese travels into the blood bound to transferrin in the trivalent state and to α_2-macroglobulin in the divalent state (Gibbons et al., 1976). The percentage of manganese bound to transferrin may increase over time as manganese is oxidized to Mn^{III}. A small fraction is bound to unknown proteins (Harris & Chen, 1994).

The chemical speciation of manganese affects its distribution to the brain, but it is not clear whether there is a predominant manganese species crossing the blood–brain barrier (Roels et al., 1997; Dorman et al., 2001a,b, 2002a,b; Normandin et al., 2004). The oxidation state of the manganese ion determines its mode of transport at the brain barrier system. Mn^{III}, a major form of manganese ions in the circulation, enters the brain via a transferrin receptor–mediated mechanism, whereas Mn^{II} is readily taken up into the central nervous system, most likely as a free ion or as a nonspecific protein-bound species (Zheng et al., 2003). It is suggested that manganese citrate may be a major species entering the brain (Crossgrove et al., 2003). The zinc transporting protein ZIP (ZRT and IRT-like protein) can also transport manganese (Qin et al., 2003; Kambe et al., 2004).

The major route of manganese excretion is the gastrointestinal tract via the bile. However, under overloading conditions, other gastrointestinal routes may be involved in the excretion. The urinary excretion ranges from 0.01% to 1% of the absorbed dose; in contrast, following exposure to MMT, the manganese excretion was mainly by urine. This has been attributed to MMT biotransformation in the kidney.

In cows, it has been demonstrated that clearance of manganese(II)- $_2$-macroglobulin was much more rapid than that of manganese(III) transferrin (Gibbons et al., 1976).

6.3.3 Copper

A carrier-mediated facilitated diffusion system for uptake of copper complexes, amino acids, and small peptides into rat hypothalamus has been identified. The system has a broad ligand specificity with respect to amino acids (histidine, cysteine, threonine, glycine) and polypeptides (glycine–histidine–lysine, glutathione), but will not transport albumin-bound copper (WHO, 2000a).

After oral administration, copper is initially bound to albumin, partially to amino acids. About 5% of plasma Cu^{II} is bound in low molecular mass complexes. After entering hepatocytes, copper is then bound to caeruloplasmin and re-enters the circulation (Figure 6). About 65% of circulating copper is irreversibly bound to caeruloplasmin, and approximately 15% is bound to the N-terminus of albumin, containing an aspartic acid–alanine–histidine sequence with a specific Cu^{II} binding site. Another protein fraction called "transcuprein" appears to be involved in the copper chelating system.

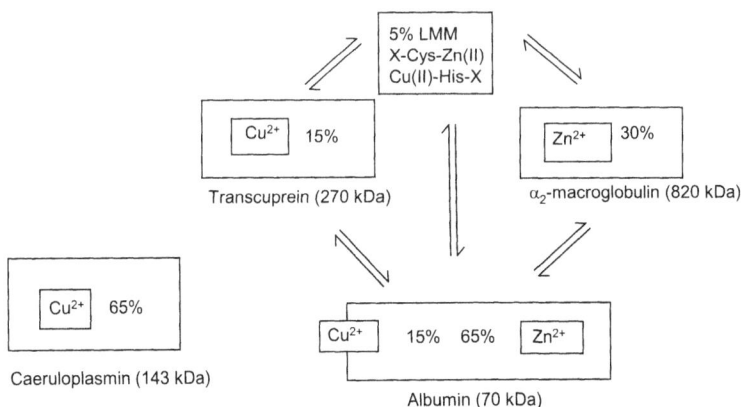

5% LMM
X-Cys-Zn(II)
Cu(II)-His-X

Cu^{2+} 15%

Zn^{2+} 30%

Transcuprein (270 kDa)

α_2-macroglobulin (820 kDa)

Cu^{2+} 65%

Cu^{2+} 15% 65% Zn^{2+}

Caeruloplasmin (143 kDa)

Albumin (70 kDa)

Fig. 6. Distribution of Cu^{2+} and Zn^{2+} among low molecular mass amino acid complexes and binding proteins in normal human blood plasma. LMM = low molecular mass (adapted from Templeton, 2003).

In hepatocytes, histidine binds copper in the presence of albumin. The resulting copper–histidine complex $[Cu(His)_2]$ interacts with a transport protein and then releases Cu^{II} into the cell (McArdle et al., 1990). A metallothionein has been identified as a possible cellular protein storage for copper. The erythrocyte chloride–bicarbonate anion exchanger can mediate Cu^{II} uptake, as $[Cu(OH)_2Cl]^-$ and $[Cu(OH)_2HCO_3]^-$ (Alda & Garay, 1990; Cherian & Chan, 1993; Lee et al., 2002).

6.3.4 Zinc

Zinc is an essential trace element in all biological systems studied and plays a fundamental role in the structure and function of numerous proteins, including metalloenzymes, transcription factors, and hormone receptors. After ingestion, zinc in humans is initially transported to the liver and distributed throughout the body, where it is found in all tissues, organs, and fluids (WHO, 2001).

The main zinc species in plasma is the albumin-bound Zn^{II}.

6.3.5 Arsenic

Inorganic arsenic is rapidly cleared from the blood in humans and most common laboratory animals, including mice, rabbits, and hamsters. The notable exception to this is the rat, in which the presence of arsenic is prolonged owing to accumulation in erythrocytes. Inorganic arsenic, administered orally or parenterally in either the trivalent or pentavalent form, is rapidly distributed throughout the body. Many of these studies have used radiolabelled arsenic, and it is noteworthy that arsenic-derived radioactivity is generally present in all tissues examined (WHO, 2001).

Intravenous administration of arsenate to mice resulted in much lower arsenic concentrations in liver and gall-bladder but higher concentrations in kidney compared with intravenous administration of arsenite to mice. In general, concentrations of arsenic in organs tended to be higher after administration of arsenite than of arsenate, with the notable exception of the skeleton. This latter finding was ascribed to arsenate being a structural analogue of phosphate and substituting for it in the apatite crystal of bone. The greater retention of arsenite in tissues is a consequence of its reactivity and binding with tissue constituents, most notably sulfhydryl groups (WHO, 2001).

The main route of excretion of arsenic after exposure to inorganic or organic arsenic species is urine, both in humans and in experimental animals. Excretion is more rapid after exposure to arsenate than after exposure to arsenite, owing to the greater arsenite binding to protein thiol groups (WHO, 2001). For the speciation of the urinary excretion, see section 6.4.

6.3.6   Selenium

Selenium after absorption appears to be rapidly distributed as water-soluble selenium compounds or selenium-containing plasma proteins. Selenocysteine is the predominant selenium-containing amino acid in animals given inorganic selenium; selenomethionine is not synthesized in higher animals and is thus an essential amino acid (Whanger, 2002; Schrauzer, 2003). Selenocysteine-containing proteins translocate selenium from liver to other organs (Motsenbocker & Tappel, 1982; Thomson et al., 1982).

The inorganic selenium species are rapidly excreted in urine, in contrast to selenomethionine, which is retained. The total recovery in the urine and faeces of selenate and selenite was 82–95% of the total dose, whereas only 26% of the selenomethionine was recovered. Methylated species, such as trimethylselenonium, contribute to only a minor fraction of selenium in urine, in variable amounts (Sun et al., 1987; Neve, 1991; Thomson, 1998). Selenium is excreted into the urine in the form of monomethylated selenium (selenosugar) when rats are fed a diet with selenium sources at an adequate concentration (Suzuki & Ogra, 2002). A small portion of selenium is excreted into the hair.

6.3.7   Silver

The well known silver deposition is the result of precipitation of insoluble silver salts. Silver appears firstly to be biotransformed into soluble silver sulfide albuminates, which bind to complexes with amino or carboxyl groups of proteins or other organic compounds or are reduced to metallic silver. Metallic silver is the species preferentially deposited, together with silver(I) sulfide (Ag_2S), silver(I) selenide (Ag$_2$Se), and other compounds, such as silver(I) chloride (AgCl) and silver(I) phosphate (Ag$_3$PO$_4$). Some species may undergo a photoreduction in the skin to elemental silver, producing the blue/grey discoloration of skin when exposed to UV light (Danscher, 1981; Juberg & Hearne, 2001).

6.3.8 Cadmium

Cadmium absorption via the lung or gastrointestinal tract results in transport of cadmium in blood, in the initial phase, mainly by high molecular mass proteins (albumin). In blood, cadmium is distributed to red blood cells (90%) and bound to albumin in plasma. Albumin–cadmium is taken up mainly in the liver, but also in other organs. It induces the expression of metallothionein (Nordberg et al., 1978; WHO, 1992; Nordberg, 1998), which sequesters Cd^{2+} ions up to a saturation level (Nordberg et al., 1982). The cadmium–metallothionein complex released from the liver is filtered through the glomeruli, because of its low molecular mass, and then reabsorbed by the proximal tubules, where the cadmium–metallothionein complex is dissociated in lysosomes (Figure 7). Current models assume that Cd^{II}–metallothionein is taken up at the apical membrane of proximal tubule cells by receptor-mediated endocytosis and sorted to the lysosomal compartment. A crucial step in the cascade of events leading to cellular toxicity is induced by Cd^{II}–metallothionein, which releases free Cd^{II} from the lysosomes into the cytosol; in the cytosol, Cd^{II} generates reactive oxygen species, which deplete endogenous radical scavenger (Thévenod, 2003). Cadmium interferes with basolateral calcium pumps, leading to cellular toxicity with dearrangement of calcium homeostasis (Leffler et al., 2000) (Figure 7).

Cadmium accumulation in alveolar macrophages also induces metallothionein synthesis. The capability of the lung to detoxify cadmium by synthesizing metallothionein may be an important mechanism in limiting potential lung toxicity (Nordberg et al., 1975; Nordberg, 1984; Grasseschi et al., 2003).

Cadmium tends to concentrate in the liver and kidneys, and concentrations are generally higher in older organisms.

Cadmium is eliminated from the organism mainly via urine and faeces. The amount of cadmium excreted daily in urine is, however, very small; it represents only about 0.005–0.01% of the total body burden, which corresponds to a biological half-life for cadmium of about 20–40 years. In subjects non-occupationally exposed to cadmium, the urinary excretion of cadmium is usually less than 2 µg/g of creatinine (Sartor et al., 1992). In urine, cadmium is partly bound to metallothionein (Bernard & Lauwerys, 1986).

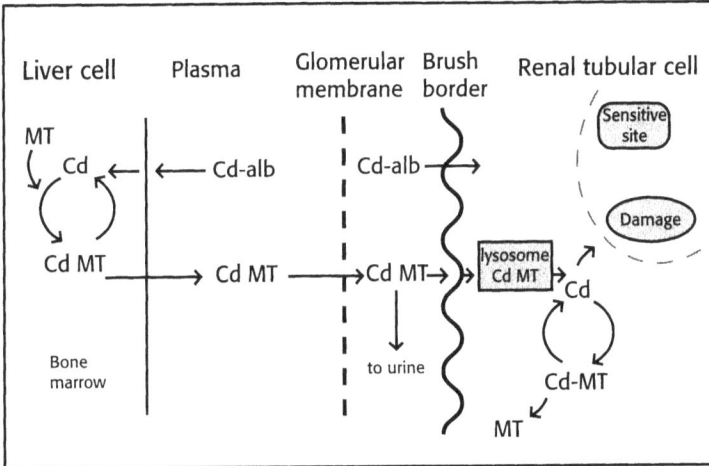

Fig. 7. Schematic diagram of cadmium binding and flow between plasma, liver, blood cells, and kidney. MT = metallothionein; alb = albumin (adapted from Nordberg, 1984; Nordberg & Nordberg, 1987).

A physiologically based multicompartment model of cadmium kinetics in humans was developed by Kjellstrom & Nordberg (1978) and has recently been amended by Choudhury et al. (2001). The latter authors showed that there is a good agreement between levels of cadmium in urine measured in the population of the United States and levels predicted by the model.

6.3.9 *Mercury*

Distribution of mercury in different tissues depends on its species, and many species may undergo conversion to each other. Only non-oxidized forms can pass the blood–brain barrier (see Figure 8).

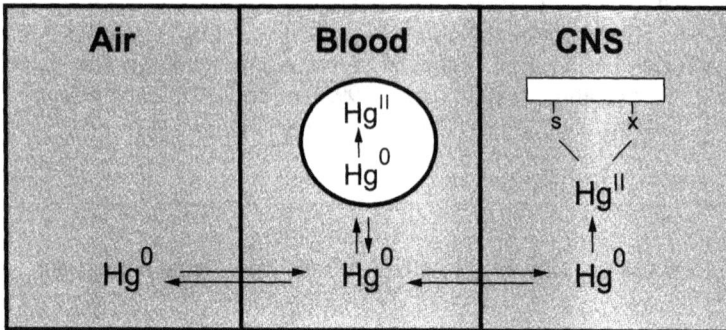

Fig. 8. Absorption and transport of inhaled mercury species (adapted from Clarkson, 1979). CNS = central nervous system.

Hg^0 readily passes biological membranes, including the blood–brain barrier and the placenta. Although its oxidation to Hg^{II} is rapid (see section 6.4), some elemental mercury remains dissolved in the blood long enough (a few minutes) for it to be carried to the blood–brain barrier and the placenta. Mercury ionic species tend to bind to plasmatic protein and are therefore not available for transport across the blood–brain barrier (Berlin et al., 1986; WHO, 1991b; Baselt & Cravey, 1995).

Following exposure to inorganic mercury, mercury tends to distribute to all tissues and organs, although higher amounts are deposited in kidney and muscles. Accumulation of mercury also occurs in the epithelial cells, such as those of the mucous membranes of the gastrointestinal tract, although a significant part of this accumulation is later eliminated by cell shedding.

Distribution of methylmercury to all tissues takes place via the bloodstream. The pattern of this distribution is much more uniform than following inorganic mercury exposure, except in red cells, where the concentration is 10–20 times greater than the plasma concentration. The half-life of methylmercury is 1.5 months; consequently, methylmercury tends to accumulate in the body (WHO, 1990a). Methylmercury readily crosses the blood–brain and placental barriers; the passage across the blood–brain barrier is helped by an active transport mechanism, which is dependent on the formation of an L-cysteine complex. Low molecular mass complexes, formed in the liver from methylmercury secreted in bile and reabsorbed into the bloodstream, may represent an important mobile form (Rowland et al., 1978; Ballatori & Clarkson, 1982).

The pharmacokinetic profile of ethylmercury is substantially different from that of methylmercury. The half-life of ethylmercury is short, less than 1 week, making exposure to ethylmercury in blood comparatively brief. Unlike methylmercury, ethylmercury is actively excreted via the gut (WHO, 1990a).

The passage of ethylmercury through the blood–brain barrier is hindered by its larger size and fast decomposition. Ethylmercury does not form an L-cysteine complex necessary for active transport across the blood–brain barrier, and the slower diffusion results in a different blood–brain concentration ratio for ethylmercury than for methylmercury (Magos, 2001). In ethylmercury-treated rats, higher total or organic mercury concentrations in blood and lower concentrations in kidneys and brain were observed than in methylmercury-treated rats. The higher tissue levels of inorganic mercury seen with ethylmercury indicate that ethylmercury breaks down to inorganic mercury more rapidly than methylmercury.

Methylmercury accumulates in hair during its process of formation. The hair/blood concentration ratio is approximately 250:1 in humans at the time of incorporation into hair. Methylmercury is accumulated and concentrated in the fetus, especially in the brain (Langford & Ferner, 1999).

After short-term exposure to Hg^0, mercury is mainly excreted in the faeces and exhaled air; after long-term exposure, excretion is mainly via faeces and urine. After exposure to inorganic Hg^{II}, the principal pathways of excretion are the urine and faeces (Clarkson et al., 1988; WHO, 1991b).

Organic mercury is predominantly excreted in faeces after conversion to inorganic species. For example, mercury excreted by humans who ate methylmercury in tuna fish was essentially all in the faeces as inorganic mercury. The kinetics of mercury excretion are influenced by the compound administered and animal species studied. Inorganic mercury and arylmercury are more rapidly excreted than methylmercury (Turner et al., 1975; Foulkes, 2001).

Urinary mercury excretion was similar after phenylmercury and $HgCl_2$ administration, consistent with rapid biotransformation of arylmercury compounds to inorganic mercury. For example, 90% of a single intravenous dose of phenylmercury or inorganic mercury was eliminated in 20 days in the rat, whereas this required more than 150 days for methylmercury. In all animal species studied, short-chain alkyl mercurials were excreted at a slower rate than other compounds. The elimination half-life of methylmercury ranged from 8 days in the mouse to ~1000 days in some fish and shellfish species. Methylmercury is excreted in the bile as a complex with glutathione; such complexes undergo reabsorption in the gastro-intestinal tract. Such low molecular mass complexes, formed within the liver, secreted in bile, and reabsorbed into the bloodstream, may represent an important mobile form of the metal in the body, allowing the metal to reach its site of action (Ozaki et al., 1993).

Faecal excretion reflects the active transport of mercury across hepatocyte membranes into bile canaliculi as glutathione complexes. Inorganic mercury is more readily eliminated in breast milk than methylmercury, and it was hypothesized that inorganic mercury enters the mammary gland by carrier-mediated transport that is saturated at high plasma inorganic mercury concentrations (Foulkes, 2001).

Glutathione and cysteine are small enough to be filtered freely at the glomerulus. They are avidly reabsorbed along the proximal tubule. Therefore, Hg^{II}–cysteine and Hg^{II}–glutathione complexes are also small enough to be easily filtered by the glomerulus (Silbernagl, 1992; Sundberg et al., 1998).

6.3.10 Lead

More than 99% of lead in blood is within the red blood cells, while the diffusible fraction of the metal present in the plasma lead is the relevant species from a toxicological point of view. Plasma lead is in equilibrium with the extracellular pool and is directly involved in all the exchange between the different biological compartments.

The three major compartments for the distribution of lead are blood, soft tissue, and bone. Almost all blood lead is associated with erythrocytes, and 50% of erythrocyte lead is bound to haemoglobin.

The biological half-life of blood lead is 25–28 days when blood lead is in equilibrium with the other compartments. Blood lead levels change rapidly with exposure and are used as an index of recent exposure. The small fraction of lead in the plasma and serum is in equilibrium with soft tissue lead. Soft tissues that take up lead are liver and kidney, with smaller amounts taken up by the brain and muscle. The lead content in the kidney increases with age and may be related to dense inclusion bodies seen in the renal cell nuclei. The greatest amount of lead found in the brain is localized in the hippocampus, followed by the cerebellum, cerebral cortex, and medulla. The largest fraction of lead retained in the body is found in the bone. About 95% of total body lead in adults is in the bone, compared with only 73% in children. Although bone lead is a large, relatively inert fraction, with a half-life for lead greater than 20 years, there is a "labile" fraction that is in equilibrium with soft tissue lead (ATSDR, 2005b).

Free Pb^{2+} ions may diffuse across the intestinal membrane. Lead phosphate complexes are larger (compared with Pb^{II}) and more hydrophilic and therefore unable to cross the membrane by passive diffusion. The lead complexes present in the bile may diffuse across the luminal membrane based on this mechanism; an increasing lead accumulation in the cells is expected for increasing bile levels, since these complexes can dissociate and the free lead ions thus produced can be absorbed as well. Under these conditions, not only the free metal ions but also those rapidly dissociating (i.e. labile) metal species contribute to the metal flux across the biological membrane, although only lead in the form of Pb^{II} is transported across the luminal membrane (Oomen et al., 2003).

6.4 Biotransformation

In general, the removal of electrons from or addition of electrons to the atom influences the chemical activity and therefore the ability of metallic elements to interact with tissue targets (ligands). Examples of charge relevance in crossing lipid barriers are represented by Fe^{2+}/Fe^{3+} and Hg^{+}/Hg^{0} passages (Misra, 1992).

Among the other metabolic transformations, the most important is bioalkylation, which mercury, tin, and lead undergo in microorganisms, whereas arsenic and selenium are additionally bioalkylated as part of their metabolic pathways in higher organisms (Templeton, 2003).

Alkylation reactions produce more hydrophobic species, leading to an increased bioavailability, penetration to cells and through the blood–brain barrier, as well as accumulation in fatty tissues.

6.4.1 Chromium

Cr^{VI} is rapidly reduced in vivo to Cr^V, which in turn is rapidly converted to Cr^{IV} and then to Cr^{III}. Whereas Cr^{III} compounds in general represent the most stable form of chromium in the environment, the aromatic bidentate picolinate ligand in chromium(III) picolinate (a widely used nutritional supplement) may result in a shift of the redox potential of the complex, such that the Cr^{III} can be reduced to Cr^{II} by biological reductants (Speetjens et al., 1999).

Hepatic and, to a lesser extent, pulmonary cells and gastrointestinal juice have some capacity to reduce in vitro Cr^{VI} to Cr^{III} (Petrilli & Deflora, 1978; USEPA, 1984).

6.4.2 Manganese

Manganese may undergo oxidation or reduction: in several enzymes, the form of manganese has been demonstrated to be Mn^{III}, whereas the intake of manganese was in the form Mn^{II} or Mn^{IV}. Following $MnCl_2$ administration, manganese was detected as Mn^{III} and/or Mn^{II} complexed with proteins (Sakurai et al., 1985).

Oxidation of Mn^{II} to Mn^{III} was reported to be catalysed in vivo by caeruloplasmin and during dismutation reactions with superoxide (Archibald & Tyree, 1987). The methyl side-chain of MMT is rapidly metabolized in rat liver and lung microsomes to an alcohol, hydroxymethylcyclopentadienyl manganese tricarbonyl, and an acid, carboxycyclopentadienyl manganese tricarbonyl, by a cytochrome P-450 monooxygenase (Lynam et al., 1990).

6.4.3 Arsenic

Biotransformation of arsenic involves methylation, leading to the formation and excretion of monomethylated and dimethylated compounds. In most mammals, only trivalent arsenic species are methylated — i.e. in the metabolism, reduction and methylation alternate (Figure 9). Possibly, As^{III} is bound to a dithiol, a carrier protein, before the methyl groups are attached. *S*-Adenosyl methionine is the main methyl donor in arsenic methylation (Vahter, 2002).

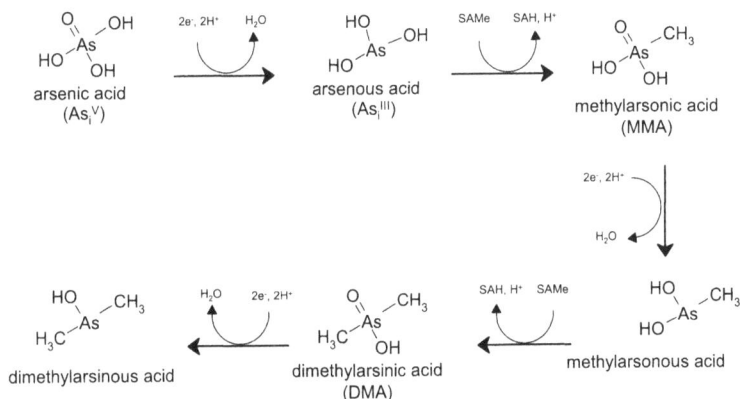

SAMe: *S*-adenosyl-L-methionine   **SAH**: *S*-adenosyl-L-homocysteine

Fig. 9. Arsenic metabolism (adapted from Buchet, 2005)

Experimental studies have indicated that the liver is an important site of arsenic methylation, especially following ingestion, when the absorbed arsenic initially passes the liver. This is supported by studies showing a marked improvement in the methylation of arsenic in patients with end-stage liver disease following liver transplantation (Geubel et al., 1988). However, arsenic may also be methylated in other tissues, as methylating activity has been detected in several different tissues of male mice. The highest activity was detected in the testes, followed by kidney, liver, and lung (Vahter, 2002).

Experimental findings with rat liver preparations suggest that two different enzymatic activities are involved in the methylation of inorganic arsenic in mammals (Buchet & Lauwerys, 1985). Moreover, observations in humans repeatedly ingesting low inorganic arsenic doses or acutely intoxicated by As_2O_3 also suggest a different rate for two methylation steps and an inhibitory effect of the trivalent inorganic form for the second methylation step leading to DMA.

According to the suggested mechanism of arsenic methylation, the methyl groups react with arsenic in its trivalent form. Experimental studies have shown that a major part of absorbed As^V as arsenate is rapidly reduced to As^{III} as arsenite, probably mainly in the blood. Because arsenite is more toxic than arsenate, this initial step in the biotransformation of arsenate may be regarded as a bioactivation. However, much of the formed arsenite is distributed to the tissues, where it is methylated to MMA and DMA. It has been shown that arsenite is taken up in hepatocytes much more readily than arsenate. At physiological pH, arsenites are present mainly in undissociated form, which facilitates passage through the cellular membrane, whereas arsenate is in an ionized form (Lerman et al., 1983).

Glutathione and probably other thiols serve as reducing agents for arsenate and MMA (Buchet & Lauwerys, 1985). Depletion of hepatic glutathione in rats and hamster by buthionine sulfoximine was shown to decrease the methylation of inorganic arsenic. Arsenate reductase activity has been detected in human liver (Radabaugh & Aposhian, 2000).

The population variation in arsenic metabolite production indicates a genetic polymorphism in the regulation of enzymes responsible for arsenic methylation. Genetic polymorphism has been demonstrated for other human methyltransferases (Weinshilboum et al., 1999).

The role of speciation in arsenic metabolism in a case of arsine intoxication was assessed by examining the urinary arsenic species of the patient for 1 month (Apostoli, 1997; Apostoli et al., 1997). As shown in Figure 10, MMA, DMA, and arsenite were the most excreted species, with quite different excretion patterns among species: arsenite excretion followed an exponential curve; an important elimination of MMA was observed early on day 1 or 2, while DMA elimination increased progressively and culminated on day 5, when MMA excretion tended to decrease. Less than 5% of the total amount was excreted as arsenate, and it disappeared after day 10. The conversion of arsenate to arsenite seemed to be influenced by the amount of arsenite and by synthesis of other metabolites. The fact that DMA excretion culminated after only a few days, while MMA excretion was still elevated, seems to confirm the existence of two different methylating enzymatic systems. Arsenobetaine seemed to be excreted independently of other species, being probably linked to uptake of arsenic from meals. The amount of arsenobetaine measured in food does not seem, however, sufficient to justify the amount of arsenic metabolite measured.

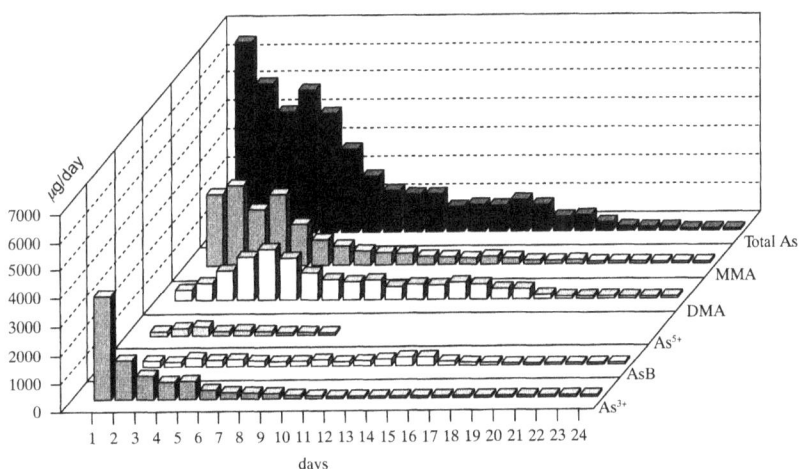

Fig. 10. Excretion of arsenic species in a case of acute arsine intoxication. As^{3+} in arsenite, As^{5+} in arsenate, MMA (methylarsonic acid), DMA (dimethylarsinic acid), AsB (arsenobetaine) (adapted from Apostoli et al., 1997).

Irrespective of the type and extent of exposure, the average relative distribution of arsenic metabolites in the urine of various population groups seems to be fairly constant (e.g. 10–30% inorganic arsenic, 10–20% MMA, and 60–70% DMA). However, there are certain exceptions. Indigenous people living in the Andes, mainly Atacameños, excrete less MMA in urine, often only a few per cent. In contrast, people living in certain areas of Taiwan, China, seem to have an unusually high percentage of MMA in urine, 20–30% on average. Interestingly, the Atacameños people have lived in the north of Chile and Argentina, areas with high arsenic levels in the groundwater, for thousands of years (Vahter et al., 1995; Vahter, 1999).

6.4.4 Selenium

The key reactions in selenium metabolism can be divided into three types: namely, reduction, selenoprotein synthesis, and methylation (Figure 11) (Itoh & Suzuki, 1997). Inorganic selenium is reduced stepwise by cellular glutathione to hydrogen selenide (H_2Se), and it, or a closely related species, is either incorporated into selenoproteins after being transformed to selenophosphate and selenocysteinyl transfer RNA or excreted into urine after being transformed into methylated metabolites of selenide. As a result, selenium is present mostly in the forms of covalent C–Se bonds in mammals. It is known that humans exposed to high concentrations of the element develop a garlicky breath odour characteristic of dimethyl selenide.

6.4.5 Mercury

Hydrogen peroxide catalase oxidizes elemental mercury to Hg^{II} in erythrocytes and tissues. Hg^{II} is highly reactive, readily binding to thiols. Hg^0 oxidation converts it to a more toxic species. The oxidation of Hg^0 takes a few minutes in blood, providing time for Hg^0 to cross membranes (e.g. the blood–brain and placental barriers) (Halbach et al., 1988).

Intracellular Hg^{II} binds to metallothionein in the cytosol (Ogata et al., 1987; Liu et al., 1991); the toxicity of the metallothionein complex is less than that of Hg^{II}. Exposure to inorganic mercury or elemental mercury Hg^0 induces metallothionein in the kidney, the major site of inorganic mercury deposition in the body. Hg^I is rather unstable; in the presence of sulfhydryl groups, it undergoes disproportionation to one atom of Hg^0 and to one ion of Hg^{II}. The actions of Hg^+ ions have been attributed to their oxidation to Hg^{II} species (Foulkes, 2001).

The ubiquitously distributed enzyme superoxide dismutase can catalyse Hg^{II} reduction to Hg^0.

Methylmercury, in experimental animals and humans, is slowly converted to inorganic mercury in all organs, except skeletal muscle, and it passes through the renal tubule as inorganic Hg^{II} (Clarkson et al., 1988; WHO, 1990a).

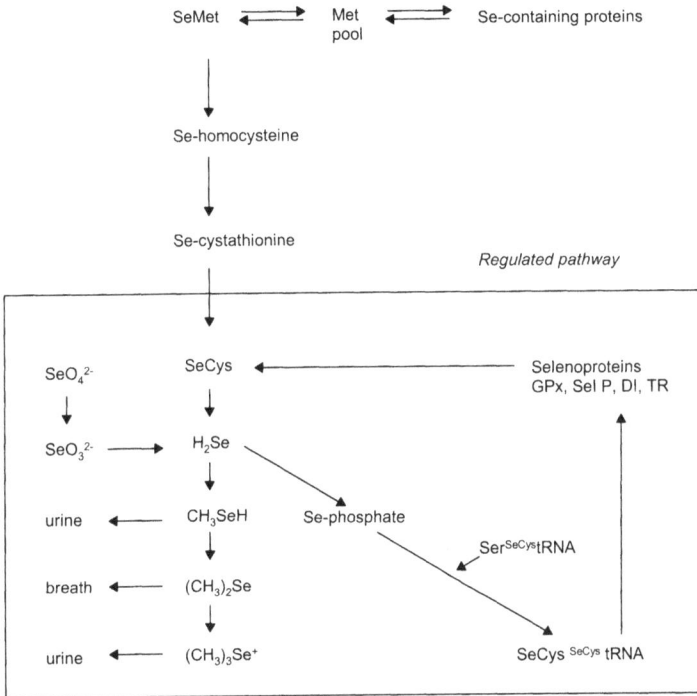

Fig. 11. The metabolic fate of selenium in the human body. Cys = cysteine; Met = methionine; tRNA = transfer RNA; GPx = glutathione peroxidase; Sel P = selenoprotein P; DI = type 1-iodothyronine de-iodinase; TR = thioredoxin reductase (adapted from Lobinski et al., 2000). © IUPAC

Ethylmercury compounds are more readily dealkylated than methylmercury compounds. In monkey brain, the concentration of Hg^{II} increased and the concentration of methylmercury decreased over time after methylmercury exposure (Charleston et al., 1996; Foulkes, 2001; Magos, 2003). Thiomersal is metabolized to ethyl-mercury and then to inorganic mercury.

A small amount of methylmercury is converted to Hg^0 in the gastrointestinal tract. The conversion of methylmercury to inorganic mercury may result in biliary mercury excretion. This conversion may be the rate-limiting step in methylmercury elimination. Methylmercury is excreted in bile as a sulfhydryl (-SH) complex, the conjugation being catalysed by glutathione transferase. These complexes may be reabsorbed from the gastrointestinal tract (Clarkson, 1979; WHO, 1979).

Dimethylmercury is demethylated to methylmercury within the first few days after exposure. Phenylmercury and methoxyethylmercury are rapidly converted to inorganic Hg^{2+} ions, since their Hg–C bonds are more readily cleaved than those in other alkylmercury compounds (Clarkson, 1979). For more details, see chapter 8.

6.5 Exposure assessment and biological monitoring

6.5.1 Exposure assessment

For human health risk assessment, it is important to determine to which species humans are exposed. Speciation deeply affects the bioavailability of elements (see chapter 6); thus, ideally, exposure assessment should be based on speciation analysis or at least fractionation. To some extent, this has been done in experimental studies, such as those on inorganic cadmium compounds (CdO, $CdCl_2$, cadmium(II) sulfate [$CdSO_4$], and CdS), and in epidemiological studies, such as those on inorganic arsenic, chromium, and nickel. However, epidemiological studies have usually been limited just to the element, due to the lack of reliable information on the specific species involved (K. Hughes et al., 1995).

Most data on concentrations of arsenic in relevant environmental media refer to total arsenic. However, for the purposes of estimating population exposure, it was assumed that most of the arsenic in ambient air, drinking-water, and soil is present in the inorganic form (Mukai et al., 1986). While limited available data indicate that the proportion of inorganic arsenic in various food groups ranges from 0% in saltwater fish to 75% in dairy products, beef, and pork (Weiler, 1987), both trivalent and pentavalent arsenic may be present in air, drinking-water, and soil.

Data on exposure to inorganic arsenic in relevant environmental media (air, drinking-water) in available surveys are usually of total inorganic arsenic rather than of individual inorganic arsenic compounds. In the occupationally exposed cohorts, exposure was probably mostly to As_2O_3, since arsenic is principally emitted to the air from anthropogenic sources in this form.

While only total chromium was measured in most surveys on the effects of chromium, a fractionation in Cr^{III} and chromate (Cr^{VI}) was done based on information on the process in many occupational epidemiological studies (IARC, 1990; Gibb et al., 2000). As to the environmental exposure, it is likely that nearly all of the chromium present in soils, except in areas contaminated with chromate, and in foodstuffs is trivalent (Barlett & James, 1991).

Similarly, in the epidemiological studies on nickel-induced cancer at work, most of the studies depend on information on the process chemistry (IARC, 1990). An international collaborative analysis of mortality in cohorts of workers in nickel production and use was able to assess separately the effects of four groups of inorganic nickel compounds (oxidic, sulfidic, soluble, and metallic) and consequently to assess a more specific risk due to exposure to nickel species (International Committee on Nickel Carcinogenesis in Man, 1990).

6.5.2 *Speciation in biological monitoring*

The main goal of biological monitoring is to unequivocally establish an exposure, to reduce or prevent misclassification in epidemiological studies, and to determine the internal dose. In addition, biomarkers allow a focus on the body burden (or the total absorbed dose); on integrated sources, routes, and patterns of exposure; and on genetic and behavioural differences between individuals (WHO, 1996b). Major goals of many of the research programmes are to develop and validate biomarkers that reflect specific exposures and permit the prediction of the risk of disease in individuals and population groups (Mutti, 1995, 1999; Groopman & Kensler, 1999; Bartsch, 2000; Trull et al., 2002).

In this context, the speciation may be approached on three different levels: analysis of specific element species (practically limited to arsenic), fractionation by chemical analytical means to organic and inorganic species (mainly mercury, lead in blood), or application to the analysis of information on the differences in the distribution of different species of an element (mercury in plasma, blood cells, urine; chromium in erythrocytes/plasma).

In biological monitoring, the matrix choice may contribute to better understanding of the toxicokinetics of some elements. Inorganic and alkyl lead compounds show different kinetics; the latter are extensively and rapidly excreted in the urine. Thus, exposure to alkyl lead is best reflected in the urinary lead concentration, whereas for inorganic lead, most useful information is gained from the analysis of lead in blood (Skerfving, 1992).

Mercury can be measured in different biological matrices and in particular in blood, urine, and hair (Clarkson et al., 1988). The determination of mercury in blood and urine is very important in order to assess occupational and non-occupational exposure, while mercury in hair is used for evaluating exposure in the general environment due to mercury stably binding to -SH groups of keratine. The two biomarkers most frequently used to determine individual exposure to methylmercury are the mercury concentrations in scalp hair and in whole blood. The known toxicokinetics fate of methylmercury suggests that the air mercury concentration reflects a longer-term average than the blood. Because absorbed methylmercury is detectable in hair beyond the scalp after a lag time of 1–2 months, the two biomarkers are not affected by the same biological fluctuations on a temporal scale (Budz-Jørgensen et al., 2004).

In the last decade, attempts were made to introduce plasma lead determination in order to improve the biological monitoring of lead exposure, facilitated by the introduction of new analytical techniques such as ICP-MS (Smith et al., 1998).

There are some studies in humans that did not show a weak association between blood lead and plasma lead, while other authors have indicated a curvilinear relationship between blood lead and plasma lead (Desilva, 1981). The correlation between blood lead and plasma lead is probably conditioned by saturation of lead binding sites in the erythrocytes (Lolin & O'Gorman, 1988).

Bergdahl & Skerfving (1997) investigated the relationship of plasma lead, blood lead, and lead in bone and reported significant correlation only between the ratio of plasma lead to blood lead and blood lead. The determination of plasma lead is a potentially useful biomarker, to complement the toxicological information that usually is obtained from the lead determination in blood.

The chromium speciation carried out by determining chromium in plasma and in red blood cells provides useful information, since chromium measured in red blood cells reflects the amount of chromate absorbed, whereas the plasma fraction better reflects the distribution of absorbed Cr^{III}. The concentration of chromium in erythrocytes was elevated among workers exposed to hexavalent chromium (Lukanova et al., 1996).

Aitio et al. (1984) found high chromium concentrations in the blood (where the chromium was completely confined to the plasma) and urine of two tannery workers who fed soaking wet hides into a roller press. The chromium species used in tanning was trivalent basic chromium sulfate [CrOH(SO$_4$)]. In chromium lignosulfonate production, five packaging workers exhibited increased concentrations of chromium in urine, and there was a correlation between the levels of urinary chromium and airborne chromium for the individuals (Kiilunen et al., 1983). Chromium was rapidly absorbed, since the peak of urinary excretion occurred immediately after exposure, and the rate of excretion dropped to a low level by the next morning (elimination half-time varied between 4 and 10 h). There was no indication of accumulation of chromium in the body.

The different kinetics (most importantly, absorption and deposition in the lungs after inhalation exposure) of elements have important implications in the interpretation of biological monitoring. The concentration of cobalt in urine at the end of the work week is considered to be a good indicator of very recent exposure to this element in case of exposure to cobalt metal, soluble cobalt salts, and hard metals, but not in the case of exposure to cobalt oxide, which is much less soluble in biological media and probably persists longer in the lung compartment (Lison et al., 1994).

For the biological monitoring of exposure to inorganic arsenic, speciation has provided the best information.

An investigation carried out in workers employed in a glass manufacturing plant (urinary inorganic arsenic ranging from 10 to

360 µg/l) demonstrated that the most excreted species were As^{III}, As^V, DMA, MMA, and arsenobetaine (Apostoli, 1999).

The urinary excretion of arsenite, arsenate, MMA, and especially DMA for biological monitoring of exposure to arsenite, arsenate, or arsenic(III) trioxide was measured, avoiding the confounding effect of arsenic species from other sources. In those subjects who drank water contaminated with arsenic, the excretion of MMA and DMA increased (from a median of 0.5 µg/day to 5 µg/day for MMA and from 4 µg/day to 13 µg/day for DMA). From the data in this study, it can be estimated that at exposure concentrations of 10 µg/m^3, the following concentrations of urinary arsenic species can be expected: As^{III}, 4.3 µg/l; As^{III} + As^V, 5.3 µg/l; MMA, 7.5 µg/l; DMA, 26.9 µg/l; inorganic arsenic + MMA + DMA, 43.7 µg/l. The concentrations of the sum of urinary inorganic arsenic, MMA, plus DMA varied among the groups of exposed subjects (mean 106 µg/l, SD 84, median 65 µg/l). Arsenobetaine was the most excreted species (34% of total arsenic), followed by DMA (28%), MMA (26%), and As^{III} + As^V (12%) (Apostoli et al., 1999).

The significance of measurement of the inorganic arsenic species in urine must also be emphasized. From a toxicological point of view, As^{III} is the most critical species, owing both to its reactivity with thiol groups and to the easy diffusion of arsenite through biological membranes. As a consequence of the progressive saturation of methylation capability, an increase in arsenic exposure would lead to an increase of inorganic arsenic in tissues and urine. It has been postulated that decreased As^{III} methylation might be related to the appearance of effects, such as cancer, since methylation is considered to be a detoxifying mechanism (Carlson-Lynch et al., 1994).

Knowledge of chemical composition, particle size distribution, and the bioavailability of manganese aerosol in industry is still limited. The speciation of manganese may be of interest not only for oxidation state (among 11 theoretical oxidation states, only the 2+ and the 3+ are currently of biological interest), but also for the range of metal–protein complexes. Metal–protein complexes are important in transport and distribution mechanisms. For manganese, several protein complexes have been suggested: metallothionein, albumin, transferrin, and monoglobulin. The measurement of different fractions and species of manganese will become an important tool for understanding the element's toxicity (Apostoli et al., 2000).

Baker et al. (1990) carried out an investigation to determine the sensitization to platinum and its salts in a group of workers employed in a precious metals refinery. Maynard et al. (1997) examined some cases of respiratory sensitization to soluble platinum arising from a platinum group elements industry. Many studies on animals have confirmed the association of acute toxic effects with the metallic platinum, while soluble compounds are much more toxic. For instance, ammonium tetrachloroplatinate [(NH$_4$)PtCl$_4$] has been reported to induce acute poisoning in rats, with hypokinesia, diarrhoea, convulsions, and respiratory impairment, whereas hexa-chloroplatinic acid (H$_2$PtCl$_6$) was found to be highly nephrotoxic (Ward et al., 1976). Nephrotoxicity is also well documented in anticancer chemotherapy using complex halide platinum salts, such as cisplatin and its analogues (Ludwig & Oberleithner, 2004; Uehara et al., 2005).

The use of antineoplastic drugs is increasing, and nursing staff are evidently concerned about the risk of hazardous exposure. Air sampling in the workroom as well as analysis of blood and urine samples from the exposed subjects were carried out during the process of handling of drugs. No increased airborne platinum levels were found. However, increased platinum blood levels were found. Staff nurses had a higher mean level than graduate nurses, which indicates that possible exposure occurs while attending treated patients rather than during the preparation and administration of drugs. There was a noticeable variation in the mean blood level for the investigated groups as a whole (Nygren & Lundgren, 1997). Biomonitoring of this metal in human fluids is also recommended to evaluate individual platinum exposure and to prevent allergenic effects of platinum salts in catalyst production plants (Merget et al., 2000; Petrucci et al., 2005).

In the last few years, several elements have been speciated in biological matrices, and progress in this field of investigation is regularly reported (e.g. Taylor at al., 2005).

From this evaluation, it can be observed that arsenic and mercury are the most speciated elements, followed by chromium, selenium, lead, and cadmium, in blood, serum, and urine, while tissues were relevant media for copper, cadmium, and zinc; about 20 oxidation states and organic compounds, such as ethyl, methyl, and aryl compounds, have been analysed for arsenic, mercury, lead, selenium, vanadium, and antimony; other organic compounds (complexes with amino acids, proteins, macromolecules) have been demonstrated for silver, cadmium, copper, chromium, lead, selenium, zinc, vanadium, platinum, and aluminium.

An important target for future studies on biological monitoring is a better understanding of the elemental species to be measured, on a group or individual basis, in order to accurately follow the stages of absorption, deposition, distribution, metabolism, toxicity, and, finally, excretion. This will facilitate the identification of better biomarkers of exposure and effect. This will require the development of standardized methods for analysis of elemental species in biological matrices. Such methods will have to cope with low or very low species concentrations, changes in species induced by sample treatment, and interference from the biological matrix.

7. MOLECULAR AND CELLULAR MECHANISMS OF METAL TOXICITY

7.1 Introduction

To understand the biological activity of a toxic element requires examination of events at the molecular level, and this of course involves chemical processes that are dependent on the element's speciation. In this chapter, we will consider mechanisms by which metals cause human toxicity, to provide a framework for understanding how different metal species may produce different effects. Important mechanisms include DNA damage, protein binding, generation of reactive oxygen species, immunosensitization, and immunosuppression.

7.2 Mechanisms of DNA damage and repair

DNA provides phosphate anions and nitrogen and oxygen ligands suited to binding cationic metals. Oxidation of DNA by metal-catalysed HO$^\bullet$ production (see below) produces a characteristic pattern of oxidation products (Dizdaroglu, 1991), including 5-hydroxy-6-hydrothymine, 5,6-dihydrothymine, thymine glycol, cytosine glycol, 5-hydroxy-6-hydrouracil, 5-hydroxyuracil, 5,6-dihydroxyuracil, 5-hydroxyhydantoin, and the purine derivatives 8-hydroxyadenine and 8-hydroxyguanine. Isolated chromatin in the presence of hydrogen peroxide shows this pattern after addition of Ni^{II} or Co^{II} salts (Nackerdien et al., 1991) or Cu^{II} and Fe^{III} compounds (Dizdaroglu et al., 1991). In the latter study, ascorbate increased damage due to an iron(III) chloride (FeCl$_3$)/hydrogen peroxide mixture, probably by reducing Fe^{3+} to Fe^{2+}. Damage increased in the order iron–nitrilotriacetate (NTA) > iron–EDTA > FeCl$_3$ (all in the presence of hydrogen peroxide), and the chelates showed different patterns of oxidized products. CuSO$_4$ alone caused damage that was suppressed by NTA, and CuSO$_4$ plus hydrogen peroxide caused comparatively extensive damage. In contrast to Fe^{3+}, chelation of Cu^{2+} with EDTA and NTA suppressed oxidation in the presence of hydrogen peroxide, compared with CuSO$_4$ plus hydrogen peroxide alone. Nickel had a similar oxidative effect with or without the addition of peroxide (Nackerdien et al., 1991), suggesting reaction of DNA-bound Ni^{2+} directly with oxygen. 8-Oxo-2'-deoxyguanine was isolated from kidneys of rats treated with Fe^{III}–NTA, but not $FeCl_3$ (Umemura et al., 1990a,b); 8-oxo-2'-deoxyguanine is itself a mutagenic substance.

Metals can cause protein–DNA cross-links by forming metal bridges, but they can also form covalent cross-links — for example, when chromatin is incubated with Fe^{II}–EDTA and hydrogen peroxide (Lesko et al., 1982). Thymine–tyrosine cross-links were identified in chromatin treated with hydrogen peroxide in the presence of Fe^{3+} or Cu^{2+}. As noted for oxidative damage, chelation with EDTA or NTA increased thymine–tyrosine cross-links produced by Fe^{3+} and suppressed those forming in the presence of Cu^{2+} (Dizdaroglu, 1992). DNA cleavage also occurs. Strand breaks were produced in cultured cells by $NiCl_2$, Ni_3S_2, and crystalline NiS, but not by amorphous NiS (Sunderman, 1989). Chromosome breaks and sister chromatid exchange have been observed in peripheral lymphocytes of workers exposed to chromium and nickel compounds (Sunderman, 1989). Ni^{II}-mediated DNA cleavage with oxidants shows selectivity based on the ligand (Mack & Dervan, 1992; Muller et al., 1992). Important factors are the availability of free coordination sites, Ni^{2+}/Ni^{3+} redox potential, and charge of the complex (Muller et al., 1992). Depurination following metal exposure has been described. In a model system, chromate released guanine, whereas Cu^{2+} and Ni^{2+} released adenine (Schaaper et al., 1987). There was also species dependence; whereas chromic acid or chromium(VI) trioxide (CrO_3) caused a significant release of guanine, none was detected with $CrCl_3$. The mechanism appears to involve coordination of the metal to the N-7 position of the purine, with subsequent scission of the glycosidic bond linking the purine to the sugar-phosphate backbone.

DNA repair mechanisms are necessary to maintain genome integrity. DNA is under continual insult from endogenously generated reactive oxygen species as well as exogenous toxicants, chemicals, and mechanical stresses. Therefore, mechanisms have evolved to repair DNA continuously or, alternatively, to eliminate cells, by apoptosis, in which DNA is irreversibly damaged. Both DNA repair and apoptosis are targets of toxicity. One of the main mechanisms for repairing damaged DNA is to excise the altered, oxidized, or cross-linked bases — so-called excision repair. The reparative machinery responds both to the altered nucleotide and to the resulting conformational change in the DNA. Mismatch repair of replication errors and recombinational repair of cross-links and double strand breaks are also potential targets of toxic metals (Hartwig et al., 2002), but most information has been derived concerning excision repair.

Two types of excision repair can be distinguished, based on excision of the base or the nucleotide. Both types of excision repair are inhibited by low concentrations of Ni^{2+}, Co^{2+}, Cd^{2+}, and As^{3+} (Hartwig et al., 2002). The involvement of the metal ions is complex. Base excision repair following damage from nitrosourea analogues is inhibited by arsenite (Li & Rossman, 1989). Cadmium and nickel inhibit base excision repair following photolytic damage (Dally & Hartwig, 1997). Ni^{2+} and Cd^{2+} can interfere with nucleotide excision repair by affecting the initial step of recognition of DNA damage (Hartmann & Hartwig, 1998), whereas Co^{2+} affects both incision and reparative polymerization (Kasten et al., 1997). Arsenite impairs incision at lower concentrations and ligation at higher concentrations (Hartwig et al., 1997). Hartwig et al. (2002) have used a model of benzo[a]pyrene-induced DNA damage to study the effects of nickel species. Both $NiCl_2$ and NiO inhibited removal of adducts in cultured cells, with NiO being slightly more effective. The metal species differences were rather subtle, however, and, as Hartwig et al. (2002) note, "do not provide an explanation for the marked differences in carcinogenic potencies between water-soluble and particulate nickel compounds". Inhibition of DNA repair by Pb^{2+} and Cd^{2+} following injury to bacteria or cultured mammalian cells by various carcinogens, alkylating agents, and UV radiation has been reviewed (Hartwig, 1994). Some species differences are suggested — for example, between an inhibitory effect of lead(II) chloride ($PbCl_2$) and a lack thereof with lead acetate on DNA repair in X-ray-irradiated HeLa cells.

Metals may also cause cancer through non-mutagenic, or epigenetic, mechanisms (Klein & Costa, 1997) that alter the structure of DNA without changing the base sequence itself. Two major mechanisms are DNA methylation and heterochromatin formation. Methylation primarily affects the C5 position of cytosine in 5'-CpG-3' (and, to a lesser extent, in CpNpG) sequences that cluster in so-called CpG islands in regulatory regions of many genes.

Hypermethylation leads to gene silencing and regulates processes of differentiation and development and cell-specific gene expression (Cedar & Razin, 1990). Loss of normal methylation can reactivate the gene. Heterochromatin is composed of protein-rich regions of the chromosome that normally remain condensed and transcriptionally silent through the cell cycle and contain late-replicating DNA. Spreading of heterochromatin to adjacent chromosomal regions silences the gene in those regions. Histone deacetylation and chromatin-associated non-histone protein, HP-1, are involved in heterochromatin spreading, and the methylation status of the DNA may also be important (Klein & Costa, 1997).

Even in its carcinogenic species, nickel is a weak mutagen. Costa and co-workers (reviewed in Klein & Costa, 1997) have produced several lines of evidence showing an epigenetic mechanism. Carcinogenic nickel compounds were hypothesized to induce methylation silencing of an X-linked senescence gene, contributing to cell immortalization (Klein et al., 1991). In another model, DNA condensation and coordinate hypermethylation by carcinogenic nickel compounds silenced a mutagenic target sequence transgene (Lee et al., 1995).

7.3 Metal–protein interactions

Proteins are a major target for interaction with toxic metals and metalloids. Again, the availability of the element to exchange with the ligands provided by amino acid side-chains, to transfer or accept electrons, or to form covalent adducts with thiols will all be determined by the element's speciation. A full consideration of metal–protein interactions would include the rich chemistry of metalloenzymes, central to the field of bioinorganic chemistry. Many enzymes exploit metal ions for structural stability, thermodynamic effects (e.g. the entatic state [Williams, 1985]; allostery), acid–base catalysis, or redox properties (Williams, 1981, 1985; Nieboer & Fletcher, 1996). All such properties are influenced by speciation. In some instances, the same element can serve multiple roles in the same enzyme. An example is the occurrence of two Zn^{2+} ions in alcohol dehydrogenase, one of which stabilizes protein structure while the other serves as a Lewis acid polarizing the substrate oxygen atom (Walsh, 1979). This is a good example of speciation at the macromolecular level (see chapter 2), but raises the question of whether the complex represents a single species in the aggregate or two species of the zinc atom.

Another important aspect of metal–protein interactions is the selective passage of ions such as Ca^{2+}, Na^+, and K^+ through protein-based ion channels. Several excellent reviews cover these points (Catterall, 1995, 2000; Roden & George, 1996). In addition to passive conductance down a concentration gradient, energy-dependent protein transporters pump ions against gradients. Of numerous examples, the copper transporters ATP7A and ATP7B have been particularly well characterized (Iida et al., 1998; La Fontaine et al., 1998; Payne & Gitlin, 1998; Forbes et al., 1999). These are the protein products of the genes mutated in Menkes and Wilson diseases, respectively. Interaction of copper with thiol groups in the "tail" of the protein delivers the ion to an ATP-dependent transport domain for export from the cell or delivery to intracellular organelles. A channel that conducts down a concentration gradient can nevertheless be energy dependent, an example being the cystic fibrosis transmembrane conductance regulator, which uses ATP hydrolysis to regulate chloride ion channel opening (Riordan, 1993). Despite their impressive specificity, competition at ion channels with unphysiological metals is well known. For example, the lanthanum ion, La^{3+}, is a calcium channel blocker (Spedding & Cavero, 1984; Raeburn, 1987). The species dependence of poisoning or blocking of channels and transporters by competing metals seems to be an area that is quite underinvestigated, however.

Several examples of macromolecular metal–protein speciation will be considered here. Three major macromolecular species in human tissues and fluids are diferric transferrin, cadmium/zinc/copper–metallothioneins, and the copper protein caeruloplasmin. Transferrin and metallothioneins have sufficiently high stability constants with the indicated metals that they dominate the speciation of iron in the blood and copper and cadmium in tissues such as liver, respectively. They, along with caeruloplasmin, are used frequently as standards in developing speciation methods based on hyphenated chromatographic techniques. Zn^{2+} plays an important role in biology and serves as a particularly challenging example for speciation; present in microgram per millilitre concentrations in plasma (and higher in many tissues) and mainly protein bound, its protein complexes are nevertheless of sufficiently low stability that its speciation profile is seldom well defined. Selenium is an essential element that is covalently incorporated into proteins as the amino acids selenocysteine and selenomethionine, a permanent part of the protein's structure. Selenium serves as an interesting example of speciation of the element in the diet affecting the ultimate distribution of selenoproteins (see below).

In the plasma of a healthy individual, essentially all detectable iron will be associated with transferrin (stability constants $\log K_1 = 22.7$ and $\log K_2 = 22.1$; Martin et al., 1987). Only about one third of the available transferrin is bound to iron, presenting a safety margin for scavenging potentially harmful redox-active species that invariably have lower stability constants. However, in patients with iron overload disorders (e.g. primary haemochromatoses or secondary to chronic transfusion therapy in thalassaemia), iron levels can exceed the saturation capacity of the transferrin pool, and the excess is referred to as non-transferrin-bound iron. The nature of non-transferrin-bound iron is itself an interesting problem in speciation, but most is probably non-protein bound, with iron(III) citrate as a major species (Grootveld et al., 1989; Hider, 2002). This raises the point that it is a Fenton-active complex, and the precise species present will determine the potential for generating harmful reactive oxygen species (Graf et al., 1984). Estimates of <1 µmol/l up to >10 µmol/l have been reported for non-transferrin-bound iron in plasma of iron-overloaded patients (Parkes & Templeton, 2002). There may be a specific transport mechanism for clearing these harmful species into the soft tissues (Randell et al., 1994), and such a mechanism itself would be species dependent, including a dependence on redox state (Parkes & Templeton, 2002).

In tissues, iron is found in three major species. Most is deposited in the mineral core of ferritin, the major storage form of tissue iron (Harrison & Arosio, 1996). A variable pool is transferrin bound and depends on the extent to which transferrin-bound iron is being taken up (by receptor-mediated endocytosis) in the tissue at that time. Depending on the degree of iron loading, a pool of insoluble iron(III) oxide and hydroxide species, collectively termed haemosiderin, will deposit. Normally a small amount of the iron in liver, haemosiderin can reach 90% of total tissue iron in severe iron overload (Stuhne-Sekalec et al., 1992). A small but important cellular iron pool is termed the labile iron pool (Kruszewski, 2003). Present at comparatively low concentrations that are difficult to characterize or measure reliably, the labile iron pool is generally thought to represent the pool of low molecular mass, kinetically exchangeable species that may determine cellular responses to iron overload through signalling to iron regulatory proteins (Cairo & Pietrangelo, 2000) and availability for Fenton activity.

A number of issues in the design of effective therapeutic iron chelators, and their safe implementation, require attention to details of speciation of the resultant iron chelates (Templeton, 1995). Denticity of chelators determines the stoichiometry of the complex, with, for example, bidentate hydroxypyridones having possible equilibria in which less than full 3:1 coordination is possible. These bidentate chelators may show increased Fenton activity compared with a hexadentate like deferoxamine, which forms complete octahedral coordination in the 1:1 complex. The nature of the chelator also determines redox potential and hence the propensity to redox cycle. Complexes with a molecular weight less than approximately 400–500 daltons pass more readily through cell membranes. The hydrophobicity and charge of the chelator and the chelate are also important. If the species is too hydrophilic, it will not enter or exit cells, but if it is too lipophilic, it will partition into the membrane. Octanol–water partition coefficients (K_{ow}) between 0.5 and 1.5 for both chelator and complex are optimal. Permeability of the blood–brain barrier is proportional to $K_{ow}/(M_r)^{1/2}$ (where M_r is molecular mass) up to about 400 daltons (Templeton, 1995).

Metallothioneins are a group of low molecular mass, cysteine-rich proteins that bind a number of divalent and monovalent metal ions, notably Cu^+, Zn^{2+}, Cd^{2+}, Hg^{2+}, and Ag^+. Comprehensive reviews on metallothionein appear in a number of monographs and reports of international symposia, such as Elinder & Nordberg (1985) and Nordberg & Nordberg (2002), and reports of international symposia, such as Klaassen (1999) and Kägi & Nordberg (1979). Although we often think of binding of metals to proteins, other than the directed formation of metalloenzymes, for instance, as at least potentially toxic, formation of the metallothionein species generally seems to detoxify a toxic metal, at least temporarily (Templeton & Cherian, 1991); it shares with transferrin the property of sequestering a toxic metal in an inert species in tissue. However, it is also recognized that extracellular cadmium–metallothionein in the blood is more toxic to the kidney than cadmium salts (Nordberg et al., 1975; Templeton & Cherian, 1991; Nordberg & Nordberg, 2000).

While about 80% of copper in normal human plasma is bound to albumin (exchangeable fraction) and caeruloplasmin (non-exchangeable), another protein fraction termed "transcuprein" has been described (Wirth & Linder, 1985). About 5% of plasma copper exists in low molecular mass complexes. Modelling based on stability constants predicts that this fraction will be dominated by histidine and histidine-containing bis-peptide species (May, 1995). In Wilson disease, caeruloplasmin is frequently decreased and plasma copper can be increased because of increased tissue stores. The fraction of copper bound to non-caeruloplasmin species is therefore increased (Barrow & Tanner, 1988); as non-ceruloplasmin species potentially cause oxidative stress, as they increase, so potentially does oxidative stress to the erythrocyte, leading to haemolysis.

Selenium substitutes for sulfur in cysteine and methionine, which become covalently incorporated into proteins. In blood, most selenium is in haemoglobin in the erythrocyte, albumin and selenoprotein P in plasma, and glutathione peroxidase in both sites. Selenoproteins have been divided into those where the incorporation is specific during transcription, the TGA codon coding for selenocysteine, and those where the incorporation of selenomethionine instead of methionine is incidental (Behne & Kyriakopoulos, 2001). Glutathione peroxidase is an example of the former, haemoglobin and albumin of the latter. Additional selenium-binding proteins occur that bind the element specifically, but little is known of their structure or function (Behne & Kyriakopoulos, 2001).

Humans take in various species of organic and inorganic selenium in the diet and biotransform them to selenocysteine and selenomethionine. The final distribution of selenium among proteins depends on these dietary species in ways that are poorly understood; it also depends on the animal species concerned. In humans, intake of selenomethionine results in most erythrocyte selenium incorporating into haemoglobin, whereas selenite deposits more erythrocyte selenium in glutathione peroxidase. Selenate produces a roughly equal distribution. Comparing selenium content in erythrocytes of two populations, Oregon, USA, residents had about 3 times the level of those from New Zealand, but functional glutathione peroxidase was similar in both populations (Whanger et al., 1994).

Inconsequential incorporation into haemoglobin was higher in the Oregon population. In rats, both dietary selenite and seleno-methionine distribute plasma selenium into 50–60% selenoprotein P, 20–30% glutathione peroxidase, and 20–25% albumin (Whanger et al., 1994).

7.4 Generation of reactive oxygen species

Damage to DNA, proteins, and lipid membranes by reactive oxygen species is of central importance in metal toxicology, with generation of the reactive hydroxyl radical (HO$^{\bullet}$) being the greatest concern (Halliwell & Gutteridge, 1990; Kasprzak, 1996). HO$^{\bullet}$ is produced from peroxide in the Fenton reaction:

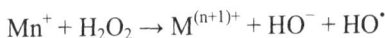

$$M^{n+} + H_2O_2 \rightarrow M^{(n+1)+} + HO^- + HO^{\bullet}$$

If superoxide is available to reduce the metal back to M^{n+} according to

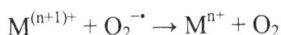

$$M^{(n+1)+} + O_2^{-\bullet} \rightarrow M^{n+} + O_2$$

then the reaction is a metal-catalysed cycle generating HO$^{\bullet}$ in the overall reaction

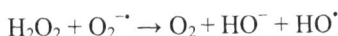

$$H_2O_2 + O_2^{-\bullet} \rightarrow O_2 + HO^- + HO^{\bullet}$$

known as the Haber-Weiss process.

The ability of the metal to act as a Fenton catalyst is sensitive to its species. In the absence of chelators, Cu^+, Fe^{2+}, and Co^{2+}, for instance, can drive the process, whereas some other metals catalyse the process after appropriate chelation. Several good examples are cited by Kasprzak (1996). Thus, autoxidation of Fe^{2+} is enhanced by EDTA and NTA but suppressed by *o*-phenanthroline and deferoxamine. Deferoxamine also inhibits HO$^{\bullet}$ generation by Cr^V species. Stable inorganic Co^{2+} becomes reactive with atmospheric oxygen in the presence of organic ligands. Kasprzak (1996) also compiled a list of amino acids and peptides that confer reactivity of the resulting Ni^{2+} species towards oxygen and oxygen intermediates.

7.5 Effects on the immune system

7.5.1 *Mechanisms of sensitization*

A number of metallic elements can act as sensitizers. This is frequently dependent on the chemical form and is true of certain species of nickel, cobalt, chromium, copper, mercury, beryllium, platinum, palladium, iridium, indium, and gold (Templeton, 2004). In general, allergy occurs when T cells recognize a metal ion species. In contrast to antibodies that bind tightly to epitopes on the surfaces of protein antigens, T cell receptors bind to small peptides present on the surfaces of antigen-presenting cells bound to major histocompatibility complex class I or class II molecules (Hennecke & Wiley, 2001). The antigenic peptide is bound to the antigen-presenting groove in the major histocompatibility complex molecule. The immune response is initiated by recognition of the antigen by $CD4^+$ T cells, which then become activated. There is no evidence for metal ion binding to antigen-presenting groove. Rather, metal species act by bringing about conformational changes in endogenous proteins that in turn result in recognition by specific subsets of T cells (Sinigaglia, 1994).

There is good evidence that recognition of metals by the immune system is restricted to T cells. The major histocompatibility complex consists of an antigenic peptide bound to a human leukocyte antigen (HLA) class I (HLA-A, HLA-B, HLA-C) or class II (HLA-DR, HLA-DP, HLA-DQ) molecule and complexed to the T cell receptor. $CD4^+$ T cell clones were isolated from patients sensitized to nickel or gold and tested against a series of antigen-presenting cells expressing different HLA isotypes (Sinigaglia et al., 1985; Emtestam et al., 1989; Sinigaglia, 1994). T cells were activated by Ni^{2+} when it was presented by cells expressing HLA-DRw11 and by gold presented by HLA-DR4. These associations argue that recognition depends on HLA isotype, and therefore likely on the major histocompatibility complex. The idea that the antigenic metal acts as a hapten has led to discussion of four possibilities (Templeton, 2004): 1) The metal might bind to the antigenic peptide before it associates with the HLA component, changing the presentation or conformation of the peptide; 2) it might bind to the antigenic peptide after it associates with the HLA component, with similar consequences; 3) it might interact with the major histocompatibility complex class II molecule before peptide binding; and 4) it might interact with the intact complex, perhaps requiring ligands from both the peptide and the major histocompatibility complex protein. Two HLA-DRw11-restricted T cell clones were selected that proliferate in response to different antigenic peptides. Ni^{2+} inhibited proliferation in one clone when treating the intact complex, but not when the antigen-presenting cell was treated with Ni^{2+} before exposure to the peptide (Romagnoli et al., 1991; Sinigaglia, 1994). Binding was shown to involve a specific histidine residue in the peptide. While in this case binding was inhibitory of T cell activation, it establishes the principle of peptide–metal hapten binding to influence T cell recognition.

7.5.2 *Immunosuppression*

Proper functioning of the immune system involves complex interactions among a variety of cells and signalling molecules. Identifying specific sites of toxicity is difficult, and few data are available on this topic. In general, most metals will cause some degree of immunosuppression at high concentrations (Zelikoff & Thomas, 1998). One means of assessing host defences is to examine the effect on resistance to experimental infection in test animals. A number of studies with cadmium, reviewed by Koller (1998), illustrate the complexity of this approach. Various animal species have been infected with bacteria or viruses, and host resistance has been examined after treatments by various routes of exposure with $CdCl_2$, cadmium(II) acetate, CdO, and $CdSO_4$. $CdCl_2$ was generally the most toxic, but effects were variable. Thus, intraperitoneal $CdCl_2$ in mice showed an increase in virulence with *Listeria mono-cytogenes* but not with *Klebsiella pneumoniae* or *Pseudomonas aeruginosa*. In another study, mice showed increased mortality with Japanese encephalitis virus given together with a single injection of $CdCl_2$, but not if the same dose of cadmium was given 10 days earlier. In contrast, $CdSO_4$ tends to increase host resistance. Cadmium acetate decreased infectivity of encephalomyocarditis virus in mice but increased lethality of *Escherichia coli* in rats. Mice infected with either bacteria or virus were exposed to CdO by inhalation; death rates increased in the bacterially infected mice and decreased in the virally infected rodents. Clearly, complex factors of interaction of the metal with both host and infectious agent come into play, which are dependent on dose, route of exposure, and metal species.

8. HEALTH EFFECTS

8.1 Introduction

The evaluation of the toxicity of an inorganic element is often reported as if it would apply similarly to all compounds of the element as a whole (e.g. in early generic evaluations by the International Agency for Research on Cancer) or assumes that all the biological effects of a compound are mediated by the soluble ionic species (i.e. the "ion theory"). In the scientific literature, there exist, however, a number of very well documented examples indicating that toxicity may vary significantly according to the oxidation state, the formation of complexes, and the biotransformation of the element. Moreover, in recent years, the introduction of modern analytical techniques that better allow investigators to perform a speciation of toxic elements has focused new interest on this topic. We discuss here a selection of the most significant examples where the relevance of speciation to health effects in humans has been demonstrated. An evaluation of these data indicates that, where appropriate, the consideration of speciation allows a better understanding of the mechanism of toxicity of an element and a refinement in the risk assessment by directing exposure evaluation at the most relevant species.

8.2 Acute toxicity

8.2.1 Chromium

The chemical and toxicological properties of chromium differ markedly, depending on the valence state of the metal. Hexavalent chromium (chromate) is much more toxic than trivalent chromium, which is an essential species. In contrast to trivalent chromium compounds, hexavalent chromium compounds are oxidizing agents capable of directly inducing tissue damage. Hexavalent compounds appear to be 10–100 times more toxic than the trivalent chromium compounds by the oral route (Katz & Salem, 1993). Among hexavalent compounds, water-soluble compounds such as CrO_3, sodium dichromate ($Na_2Cr_2O_7$), and potassium dichromate ($K_2Cr_2O_7$), which are substantially absorbed systemically, are much more toxic than less water-soluble salts; they are strong irritants of mucosal tissue. Systemic toxicity may occur following the ingestion of a chromate salt, from chromate-induced skin burns, or from acute inhalation of chromate occurring occupationally. Chromates may cause severe eye, skin, digestive tract, and respiratory tract irritation with possible burns. Caustic burns in the gastrointestinal tract can result in thirst, vomiting, abdominal pain, severe haemorrhage, cardiovascular collapse due to severe hypovolaemia, acute tubular necrosis with oliguria/anuria, severe liver damage, coagulopathy, convulsions, coma, and death (WHO, 1988; ATSDR, 2000). Typically, the kidney and liver effects develop 1–4 days after ingestion of a sublethal dose (Varma et al., 1994; Kurosaki et al., 1995; Loubieres et al., 1999; Stift et al., 2000). An adult respiratory distress syndrome is also possible following ingestion of potassium dichromate (Iserson et al., 1983). Acute poisoning due to insertion of a potassium dichromate crystal in the nose has also been reported (Andre et al., 1998). Intact or damaged skin contact with chromate compounds can result in severe systemic toxicity (Harry et al., 1984; Laitung & Earley, 1984; Terrill & Gowar, 1990). Chromium intoxication can occur from the cutaneous absorption of chromium following chromic acid burns to as little as 1% of the total body surface area (Matey et al., 2000). Fatalities have been reported in cases with chromium-induced corrosions covering less than 10% of the body surface area (Schiffl et al., 1982).

8.2.2   *Nickel*

Although exposure to zinc oxide fumes is the most common and best characterized cause of metal fume fever, other metal oxides, including those of nickel, have been suggested to cause the disease. The condition is very common among welders, with onset of symptoms typically 4–12 h after the inhalation of high levels of respirable oxide particles. Symptoms begin with a sweet or metallic taste in the mouth, throat irritation, cough, dyspnoea, malaise, fatigue, myalgias, and arthralgias. Later, fever develops, associated with profuse sweating and shaking chills. The syndrome may last 24–48 h (Kelleher et al., 2000). A case of death from adult respiratory distress syndrome has been reported following acute inhalation of a large amount of metallic nickel of very small particle size. It was estimated that almost 65% was in the form of particles less than

1.4 μm in diameter, the majority being 50 nm in diameter (Rendall et al., 1994).

The ingestion of soluble nickel salts such as $NiSO_4$ and $NiCl_2$ may cause an irritation of the gastrointestinal tract, with symptoms such as nausea, vomiting, abdominal discomfort, and diarrhoea. Giddiness, lassitude, headache, cough, and shortness of breath can also develop (Sunderman et al., 1988; WHO, 1991a; ATSDR, 2003b).

In terms of human health, the most acutely toxic nickel compound is nickel carbonyl [$Ni(CO)_4$]. This colourless, highly volatile liquid is extremely toxic and induces systemic poisoning, with the lungs and brain being especially susceptible targets (Sunderman & Kincaid, 1954; Vuopala et al., 1970; Shi, 1986, 1994; Kurta et al., 1993). The acute toxic effects occur in two stages: immediate and delayed. An immediate acute stage lasting 4–5 h is often observed, followed by a remission period, which generally lasts 12 h but may extend for 2–3 days, before the onset of the delayed stage. The immediate symptomatology includes frontal headache, vertigo, nausea, vomiting, insomnia, irritability, dizziness, sleeplessness, dysphoria, and irritation of the upper respiratory tract. The delayed stage is characterized by the appearance of symptoms such as constrictive chest pains, dry coughing, occasional gastrointestinal symptoms, sweating, visual disturbances, and weakness. In more severe cases, dyspnoea, cyanosis, tachycardia, chemical pneumonitis, and pulmonary oedema may develop. Cerebral oedema and punctuate cerebral haemorrhages were noted in men dying after inhalation of nickel carbonyl. Other affected organs included the liver, kidneys, adrenal glands, and spleen, where parenchymal degeneration was observed.

8.2.3   Arsenic

The degree of toxicity of arsenic is basically dependent on the form (e.g. inorganic or organic) and the oxidation state of the arsenical compounds. It is generally considered that inorganic arsenicals are more toxic than organic arsenicals; within these two classes, the trivalent forms are more toxic than the pentavalent forms, at least at high doses (WHO, 2001). Arsine (AsH_3) containing arsenic in the oxidation state 3− is by far the most acutely toxic species.

The toxicity of inorganic arsenic compounds is generally linked to the soluble inorganic trivalent forms. The greater toxicity of arsenic(III) trioxide (As_2O_3) may be attributed to its greater solubility, enabling it to distribute throughout the organism and reach target organs at a sufficient concentration to elicit a toxic response. Trivalent inorganic arsenicals, such as arsenite, readily react with sulfhydryl groups, such as glutathione and cysteine. The complex between arsenic and vicinal sulfhydryl reagent is particularly strong. The activity of enzymes or receptors is due in part to the functional groups on amino acids, such as the sulfhydryl group on cysteine or coenzymes such as lipoic acid, which has vicinal thiol groups. Thus, if arsenite binds to a critical thiol or dithiol, the enzyme may be inhibited. Arsenite inhibits pyruvate dehydrogenase, a lipoic acid–dependent enzyme involved in gluco-neogenesis. The acute toxicity of inorganic arsenic may result in part from inhibition of gluconeogenesis and ultimately depletion of carbohydrates from the organism. However, binding of arsenite to protein at non-essential sites may be a detoxification mechanism (WHO, 2001).

Acute gastrointestinal syndrome is the most common presentation after acute arsenic ingestion. This syndrome starts with a metallic or garlic-like taste associated with dry mouth, burning lips, and dysphagia. Violent vomiting may ensue and may eventually lead to haematemesis. Gastrointestinal effects, which are caused by paralysis of the capillary control in the intestinal tract, may lead to a reduction of blood volume, lowered blood pressure, and electrolyte imbalance. Thus, after the initial gastrointestinal disorders, multi-organ failure may occur, including renal and respiratory failure, depression of vital cardiovascular and brain functions, and death. Survivors of the acute toxicity often develop bone marrow suppression (anaemia and leukopenia), haemolysis, hepatomegaly, melanosis, and polyneuropathy resulting from damage to the peripheral nervous system. Polyneuropathy is usually more severe in the sensory nerves, but may also affect the motor neurones (WHO, 2001).

Seafood frequently contains high concentrations of arsenic, occurring predominantly as arsenosugars and arsenobetaine, generally considered to be non-toxic. In fish and most shellfish, the predominant arsenical is arsenobetaine; in edible seaweed (algae), the arsenic is primarily bound to carbohydrate compounds, termed arsenosugars. While arsenobetaine is excreted rapidly and unchanged in urine, arsenosugars appear to be metabolized to several arsenic compounds, such as DMA, which is more toxic than arsenosugars.

The enzymatic conversion of inorganic arsenic to mono- and dimethylated species (see chapter 6) has long been considered a major mechanism to detoxify inorganic arsenic species. The picture appears much more complex now, since experimental data obtained from several laboratories indicate that biomethylation is a process that produces reactive intermediates, particularly methylated metabolites that contain As^{III}, which may contribute to the biological reactivity of arsenic. One of these intermediates, monomethylated As^{III} or methylarsonous acid, has been shown to be several orders of magnitude more toxic than inorganic As^{III} (Mass et al., 2001; Nesnow et al., 2002; Styblo et al., 2002; Aposhian et al., 2003).

The most acutely toxic form of the arsenic compounds is AsH_3, a potent haemolytic gas. Following exposure to AsH_3, there is generally a delay (2–24 h) before the occurrence of the acute clinical manifestations, including fever, chills, shivering, thirst, malaise, nausea, vomiting, jaundice, dizziness, headache, confusion, weakness, shortness of breath, and red or dark-coloured urine. In most severe cases, these symptoms are accompanied by a haemolytic reaction, with intravascular haemolysis and acute renal tubular necrosis leading to oliguric/anuric kidney failure (Teitelbaum & Kier, 1969; Phoon et al., 1984; Hesdorffer et al., 1986; Romeo et al., 1997).

8.2.4   Tin

Inorganic tin is of low toxicity; acute ingestion of inorganic tin salts may produce nausea, vomiting, diarrhoea, stomach cramps, fatigue, and headache (WHO, 2005).

Symptoms of organotin toxicity are determined by the nature and complexity of the alkyl and aryl groups, as well as by the activity of products formed by biotransformation. Alkyltin compounds are classified into four large groups, which are represented by the general formulae $RSnX_3$, R_2SnX_2, R_3SnX, and R_4Sn, where R is an alkyl group and X an anion. The toxicity of these compounds depends more on the number and species of the alkyl group than on the nature of X. Monoalkyltins have low toxicity and are not activated by biotransformation. Some trisubstituted compounds (trimethyltin, triethyltin) have a specific effect on the central nervous system, whereas disubstituted compounds do not produce this effect but are potent irritants that can induce an inflammatory reaction in the bile duct. Toxicologically, the tetraalkyltin compounds resemble trisubstituted compounds; they are, as such, relatively inactive, but are biotransformed to the trialkyltins (WHO, 1980; Feldman, 1999).

Dermal and conjunctival exposures to tributyltin cause irritation and inflammation; inhalation of its vapours causes pharyngeal irritation, coughing, nausea, and vomiting. Exposure to trimethyltin and triethyltin results in acute symptoms of general malaise, nausea, epigastric discomfort, visual disturbances, and shortness of breath. However, much more serious manifestations of central nervous system impairment are seen after several days of exposure to trimethyltin and triethyltin, including headache, apathy, somnolence, memory loss, convulsions, coma, and death (Feldman, 1999) (see section 8.5).

Acute systemic effects reported to have followed both dermal and inhalation exposure to triphenyltin acetate also include general malaise, nausea, gastric pain, dryness of the mouth, vision disturbance, and shortness of breath. Hepatomegaly and elevated levels of liver transaminase activity have been found in some cases (WHO, 1980, 1997).

8.2.5 *Barium*

Ingestion of high levels of soluble barium salts — e.g. barium(II) carbonate ($BaCO_3$), chloride ($BaCl_2$), sulfide (BaS) — may cause gastroenteritis (vomiting, diarrhoea, abdominal pain), hypokalaemia, hypertension, cardiac arrhythmias, myoclonus, and skeletal muscle paralysis. The muscular paralysis appears to be related to severe hypokalaemia (WHO, 1990b; Johnson & VanTassell, 1991; Schorn et al., 1991; Downs et al., 1995; Thomas et al., 1998; Centers for Disease Control and Prevention, 2003). Acute systemic poisoning caused by a barium chloride burn is also possible (Stewart & Hummel, 1984). Explosion of the propellant, barium styphnate, leading to transcutaneous and pulmonary absorption, resulted in a similar clinical picture (Jacobs et al., 2002).

Insoluble barium compounds, such as sulfate used as radio-opaque agent in radiodiagnostic testing, being poorly absorbed, are inefficient sources of the toxic Ba^{2+} ion and have minimal toxicity. However, accidental barium(II) sulfate ($BaSO_4$) intravasation during radiological examinations can result in acute barium intoxication (Gray et al., 1989; Pelissier-Alicot et al., 1999; Takahashi et al., 2004).

8.2.6   *Mercury*

Acute inhalation exposure to high levels of elemental mercury may lead to respiratory and central nervous system effects, but ingestion does not present a hazard, because elemental mercury is poorly absorbed (WHO, 1991b, 2003; Bluhm et al., 1992; USEPA, 1997; ATSDR, 1999b). Acute inhalation of elemental mercury vapours is irritating to the upper respiratory tract and causes the onset of symptoms such as cough, shortness of breath, chest tightness, or burning and fever. In more severe cases, respiratory distress, pulmonary oedema, lobar pneumonia, fibrosis, and desquamation of the bronchiolar epithelium may occur. Central nervous system effects such as delirium, tremor, hallucinations, and suicidal tendency can also occur. Less dramatic acute symptoms are irritability, lethargy, confusion, emotional lability, mood changes, and slowed sensory and motor nerve function. Neuromuscular symptoms include myoclonus and fasciculations. Inflammation of the oral mucosa (stomatitis), a metallic taste in the mouth occasionally accompanied by excessive salivation or difficulty swallowing, abdominal pain, nausea, vomiting, and diarrhoea may also follow acute exposure to high concentrations of elemental mercury vapours. Finally, kidney effects ranging from mild transient proteinuria to acute renal failure can result from acute inhalation exposure to metallic mercury.

Acute exposure to inorganic mercury compounds is usually through ingestion. Inorganic divalent mercury compounds are corrosive poisons and affect initially the gastrointestinal tract and later the kidney. Acute single oral doses of Hg^{II} compounds, in particular mercuric chloride ($HgCl_2$), can induce gastrointestinal lesions ranging from stomatitis and mild gastritis causing nausea, vomiting, and abdominal pain to severe necrotizing ulceration of the mucosa. Acute tubular necrosis leading to renal failure, cardio-vascular collapse, and systemic shock may ensue. Ingestion of mercury(I) chloride (Hg$_2$Cl$_2$) has generally not been reported to cause the magnitude of gastrointestinal effects attributed to mercury(II) chloride.

The toxicity of organic mercury depends on the type of mercury compound involved. The toxicity of long-chain alkyl- and arylmercury compounds such as phenylmercury mimics the toxicity of inorganic mercury salts. The short-chain alkyl compounds, particularly mono- and dimethylmercury, are considered the most toxic of the organomercurials. Acute exposure to these compounds results in severe central nervous system effects (see section 8.5). Devastating neurological damage and death due to spilling of only a few drops of dimethylmercury have been reported (Nierenberg et al., 1998). The primary route of exposure was probably dermal, but dimethylmercury is also highly volatile, and inhalation might also have occurred. In fact, methylmercury is not a compound in itself but a cation, which forms one part of methylmercury compounds, usually methylmercury salts. Dimethylmercury is not a salt. Ethylmercury is a cation that forms organic mercury compounds, such as ethylmercury chloride. Thiomersal is also an ethylmercury salt: sodium ethylmercuric thiosalicylate. In the case of ethylmercury poisoning, gastrointestinal and renal effects are more prominent than neurological symptoms (Feldman, 1999).

Dimethylmercury has been absorbed transdermally with fatal consequences for a university scientist (Smith, 1997; Toribara et al., 1997). A single exposure through latex gloves to 0.1–0.5 ml pure dimethylmercury raised the mercury concentration in whole blood to 4000 µg/l, far above both the normal range (<10 µg/l) and the usual toxic threshold (50 µg/l). On this basis, 40 µl of dimethylmercury applied to skin would be a severely toxic dose.

8.2.7   Lead

Acute poisoning from a single exposure to metallic/inorganic lead is extremely rare but may result from the ingestion of solutions of soluble lead salts (lead acetate, lead(II) carbonate [PbCO$_3$]). (Sub)acute inhalation exposure to inorganic lead dust or fumes such as lead oxide or lead sulfide may also occur. Lead is a cumulative poison, and the acute symptoms are more commonly a manifestation of (sub)chronic poisoning. Symptoms are nonspecific and include malaise, abdominal colicky pains, constipation, anorexia, nausea, vomiting, headaches, light-headedness, dizziness, forgetfulness, anxiety, depression, irritability, and sleep disturbance. Numbness of the extremities, muscle and joint pain, lower back pain, and limb weakness are common complaints. In extreme cases, convulsions, severe encephalopathy, and/or coma may occur (Pollock & Ibels, 1986, 1988; Marino et al., 1989; Rae et al., 1991; Grimsley & Adams-Mount, 1994; WHO, 1994).

While metallic lead and inorganic lead salts are not significantly absorbed via the skin, acute poisoning may occur from dermal exposure to organic lead compounds, such as tetraethyl and tetramethyl lead. Acute inhalation of tetraethyl and tetramethyl lead vapours, resulting in a high absorption rate of both compounds, can also cause severe toxicity. There is often a latent period between exposure and onset of symptoms, which varies from a few hours in the most severe cases to as much as 10 days. The initial effects are anorexia, nausea, vomiting, insomnia, fatigue, weakness, headache, tremulousness, aggression, depression, irritability, restlessness, hyperactivity, disorientation, confusion, and disturbing dreams. Severe effects include acute mania, convulsions, hallucinations, delirium, coma, and death. Severe tremulousness with choreiform movements and associated gait disturbances is frequently seen in the most severe cases of acute organic lead poisoning. Constipation, abdominal colic, pallor, peripheral neuropathy, and myalgia typical of inorganic lead poisoning are not as common following exposure to organic lead (WHO, 1994; Feldman, 1999).

8.3 Sensitization and irritation

Several elements, generally metals, are known to be allergenic, including beryllium, cobalt, chromium, nickel, platinum, and palladium. The clinical manifestations associated with allergic reactions to these metals include bronchial asthma (essentially occupational asthma, generally type I reaction) and allergic contact dermatitis (occupational or environmental, typically type VI reaction).

It is well demonstrated that, for a given element, not all chemical species are equivalent in terms of allergenic potential. We review here some examples that have been very well characterized experimentally and/or clinically.

8.3.1   Chromium

Chromium is another illustration of the importance of chemical speciation for toxicity in general, and for allergenicity in particular. Besides its capacity to induce primary skin irritation and corrosion, direct contact with small amounts of chromium may be the cause of an allergic contact dermatitis. It is clear that hexavalent chromium compounds are responsible for the majority of the cases of allergy to chromium in cement workers, housewives, leather workers, etc. This is most likely explained by the fact that Cr^{VI} penetrates the skin tissue better and is therefore more able than trivalent chromium to induce an allergic reaction. The role of the oxidation state of chromium in allergy is, however, complex. Experimental studies have shown that an allergic response can be elicited in animals sensitized with Cr^{III} or Cr^{VI} compounds, when challenged with any species (Gross et al., 1968; Jansen & Berrens, 1968). In humans, the minimum elicitation thresholds (MET) were recently determined for trivalent chromium chloride and hexavalent potassium dichromate in Cr^{VI}-sensitive patients with mainly a leather-related history of previous chromium dermatitis but no active eczema (Hansen et al., 2003). The concentration of either Cr^{III} or Cr^{VI} that resulted in 10% or 50% of the patients with a positive skin reaction was calculated from the dose–response curves. For Cr^{III}, the $MET_{10\%}$ and $MET_{50\%}$ concentrations were 6 times and 18 times, respectively, higher than the corresponding concentrations for Cr^{VI}. The general view to interpret these data is that Cr^{VI} is reduced in the skin to Cr^{III}, which, in turn, acts as a hapten. Clinically, Cr^{VI} compounds are considered as strong sensitizers and Cr^{III} compounds as moderate (Kligman, 1966) or poor sensitizers (Samitz et al., 1969). Metallic chromium, such as present in stainless steel, is not an allergen.

In 1981, Denmark was the first country to take action to prevent occupational chromium sensitization from cement by adding iron(II) sulfate ($FeSO_4$) to the product. $FeSO_4$ is used to reduce Cr^{VI} to Cr^{III} (the remaining concentration of Cr^{VI} is below 2 mg/kg). Subsequent epidemiological studies from Denmark show that chromium dermatitis due to occupational cement contact has become much less frequent (Skoet et al., 2004).

Clinical reports on 19 patients have in each case documented chromate-induced asthma by controlled bronchial challenge testing in the laboratory (Bernstein et al., 1999). In another study, a bronchial provocation test with nebulized chromium(III) sulfate [$Cr_2(SO_4)_3$; hydrate] solution elicited clear asthmatic responses in four persons with clinical asthma from occupational exposure to chromates (Park et al., 1994).

Occupational exposure to Cr^{VI} compounds (electroplating and chromate production) has also been associated with the occurrence of ulcerative lesions of the skin and nasal septum (Katz & Salem, 1993). The irritative/corrosive action of chromium is specific to Cr^{VI} compounds, as demonstrated experimentally by Samitz & Epstein (1962) in guinea-pigs: ulcers were produced by the application of potassium chromate (K_2CrO_4) on the depilated and abraded dorsal skin, but not by chromium(III) sulfate [$Cr_2(SO_4)_3$].

8.3.2 *Nickel*

Nickel is one of the most common contact allergens on the skin, not only in industrial settings, but also in the general population exposed via direct contact of the skin with nickel-containing items (watches, jewellery, coins, etc.). Sensitized individuals can be detected by eliciting an allergic reaction through the dermal application of Ni^{II} compounds, such as $NiCl_2$ or $NiSO_4$. The mechanisms, and the exact species, involved in nickel sensitization remain, however, incompletely understood, in part because it appears extremely difficult to sensitize experimental animals with Ni^{II} compounds, except when strong adjuvants are injected concomitantly. An experimental study has shown that, in the absence of adjuvants, Ni^{II} and Ni^{IV} compounds were more effective to induce sensitization in mice than Ni^{2+} ions (Artik et al., 1999). Since these higher oxidation species of nickel can be generated from the reaction of Ni^{II} with reactive oxygen species released during an inflammatory reaction, the authors speculated that these results may explain why nickel sensitization develops much more readily in irritated than in normal skin.

8.3.3 *Palladium*

Palladium, together with iridium, is chemically very close to platinum, and allergic reactions have been reported in individuals with dental prostheses or jewellery made of palladium-based alloys. Palladium allergy seems to occur mainly in patients who are very sensitive to nickel. Dentistry patients mainly reported stomatitis or oral lichenoid reactions.

The allergenic potential seems to be associated with the ionic palladium species, which form complexes able to react with endogenous proteins, and not with metallic palladium (Santucci et al., 1995). A case of occupational asthma has been reported in a worker exposed to palladium in a galvanoplasty plant (Daenen et al., 1999). In remarkable contrast with platinum (see next section), in this case, sensitization to tetraamine palladium(II) chloride $[(NH_3)_4PdCl_2]$ was documented, but not to ammonium tetrachloro-palladate $[(NH_4)_2PdCl_4]$. The chemical and biological bases for this contrast between platinum and palladium compounds remain elusive.

8.3.4   Platinum

Platinum compounds provide an excellent illustration of the need to differentiate the chemical species of an element when evaluating its allergenic potential. Allergic symptoms including rhinitis, asthma, and urticaria have been reported after World War II in workers employed in platinum refineries and in secondary users, mainly for the manufacture or recycling of catalysts (Cristaudo et al., 2005). The allergic reaction seems to be mediated by immuno-globulin E (immediate or type I), and a skin prick test is available to detect sensitized subjects (Calverley et al., 1995). Quite remarkably, this allergenic potential is restricted to soluble halogenated platinum salts such as ammonium chloroplatinate $[(NH_4)_2PtCl_6]$, in which the leaving halides determine the biological reactivity and the capacity to bind to methionine groups of proteins like human serum albumin. Neutral platinum compounds or salts without a halide ligand do not induce allergic reactions (Cleare et al., 1976). The comprehension of the mechanistic basis of the allergenic potential of chloroplatinates has allowed the industry to develop less toxic platinum compounds for substitution. It has, for instance, been shown that tetraamine platinum dichloride $([(NH_3)_4Pt]Cl_2)$, in which the halide is present as an ion and not as a ligand coordinated to platinum, does not induce sensitization in exposed workers, although it is even more soluble than chloroplatinates (Linnett & Hughes, 1999).

Other platinum compounds used as chemotherapeutic agents in the treatment of certain forms of cancer (*cis*-platinum, carboplatinum, oxaliplatin) may also induce hypersensitivity reactions ranging from facial flushing or itching to seizures, dyspnoea, and even anaphylaxis. Immediate type I reactions mediated by immunoglobulin E have been incriminated, but non-allergic reactions (idiosyncratic reactions) also seem to exist. Skin prick or patch testing demonstrates the sensitization of a patient and allows the therapy to be adapted. There does not seem to exist a cross-reactivity among the three platinum drugs, and substitution has been recommended in sensitized patients (Khan et al., 1975; Brandi et al., 2003; Ottaiano et al., 2003). The exact biochemical mechanisms of the allergenicity of the platinum-containing drugs have not been elucidated; in view of their high chemical reactivity, however, it seems plausible that they also act as haptens.

8.4 Lung toxicity

8.4.1 Cobalt

The various respiratory disorders caused in occupational settings by the inhalation of metallic cobalt–containing particles have been extensively reviewed (Balmes, 1987; Cugell, 1992; Lison, 1996; Barceloux, 1999). These particles may cause nonspecific mucosal irritation of the upper and lower airways, leading to rhinitis, sinusitis, pharyngitis, tracheitis, or bronchitis, but the main diseases of concern are bronchial asthma and fibrosing alveolitis. Asthma seems to be caused by Co^{2+} ions acting as hapten to elicit a type I reaction (immunoglobulin E–mediated immediate hypersensitivity), and cases of occupational asthma have been reported in almost all settings where workers are exposed to cobalt-containing particles, irrespective of the species involved (Roto, 1980; Gheysens et al., 1985; Kusaka et al., 1996).

The occurrence of a fibrosing alveolitis seems to be almost exclusively limited to the hard metal industry (hard metal disease), where exposure is to cobalt metal mixed with tungsten carbide particles (Lison, 1996). A similar condition has not been reported in other occupational settings, where exposure is to cobalt metal alone (Swennen et al., 1993; Linna et al., 2003). The enhanced inflammatory and fibrosing activity of cobalt metal when mixed with tungsten carbide particles has been reproduced experimentally in the rat (Lasfargues et al., 1992, 1995), and a physicochemical mechanism accounting for this interaction has been proposed (Lison et al., 1995). Through the mutual contact between cobalt metal and tungsten carbide particles, the reduction of ambient oxygen by cobalt metal particles is catalysed at the surface of tungsten carbide particles. Cobalt metal has also been shown to interact in a similar manner with other carbides, such as those of niobium, titanium, and chromium. Through this reaction, cobalt metal is rapidly oxidized to Co^{2+} ions, but this species is not the main source of free radicals and, hence, is not responsible for the toxic reaction causing the fibrosing alveolitis. Further investigations on the surface interaction between cobalt metal and tungsten carbide particles (Zanetti & Fubini, 1997) indicated that the association of the two solids behaves like a new chemical entity, with physicochemical properties different from those of the two individual components; this new entity provides a long-lasting source of reactive oxygen species as long as metallic cobalt is present. Radical generation originates from superoxide ions formed at the carbide surface. When compared with other metals (iron, nickel), cobalt metal was the most active in the above reaction (Fenoglio et al., 2000).

Collectively, together with the genotoxic and carcinogenic effects discussed below, there is strong evidence that hard metals, by their association of cobalt metal and tungsten carbide particles, constitute a unique chemical and toxicological entity (see Table 8).

Table 8. Summary of effects caused by cobalt metal compared with hard metal

	Geno-toxicity	Carcino-genicity	Asthma	Fibrosing alveolitis	Reactive oxygen species production
Cobalt metal	+	?	+	−	+
Hard metal	+++	+	+	+	+++

8.5 Neurotoxicity

8.5.1 Manganese

Manganese is an essential nutrient that, in case of excessive absorption via inhalation or ingestion, can act as a potent neurotoxicant in humans. "Manganism" is a progressive, disabling neurological syndrome characterized by extrapyramidal dysfunction and neuropsychiatric symptomatology (WHO, 1981, 1999a). The clinical syndrome of manganese-related neurotoxicity may be broadly divided into three stages, depending on the predominant manifestations: 1) behavioural changes, 2) parkinsonian features, and 3) dystonia with severe gait disturbances (Pal et al., 1999). There are similarities between Parkinson disease and manganism, notably the presence of generalized bradykinesia and widespread rigidity. There are also dissimilarities, notably the following in manganism: 1) less frequent resting tremor, 2) more frequent dystonia, 3) a particular propensity to fall backward, and 4) failure to achieve a sustained therapeutic response to levodopa. Pathological findings in manganism and Parkinson disease also differ. In humans with chronic manganese poisoning, lesions are more diffuse, found mainly in the pallidum, the caudate nucleus, the putamen, and even the cortex. In people with Parkinson disease, lesions are found in the substantia nigra and other pigmented areas of the brain. Magnetic resonance imaging of the brain reveals accumulation of manganese in cases of manganism, but little or no changes in people with Parkinson disease. Fluorodopa positron emission tomography scans are normal in cases of manganism, but abnormal in people with Parkinson disease (WHO, 1981, 1999a; Calne et al., 1994).

The extent of the neurotoxicity appears to be determined by its oxidation state. Mn^{III} appears to be more cytotoxic than Mn^{II}, and its greater relative toxicity has been related to its greater oxidative reactivity (Chen et al., 2001; Reaney et al., 2002). It is also suggested that manganese neurotoxicity is dependent on the ease with which simple Mn^{III} complexes are formed under physiological conditions and the efficiency with which they destroy catecholamines (Archibald & Tyree, 1987). However, the extent to which Mn^{III} would act as an oxidant in vivo remains unknown, as one would expect Mn^{III} to be largely, if not completely, coordinated with biological ligands (Reaney et al., 2002).

Little is known about the relative neurotoxicity of different manganese compounds. Available evidence indicates that various manganese compounds can induce neurological effects (WHO, 1981, 1999a). First described by Couper in 1837 in workers exposed to dust while grinding manganese oxide, manganism has been documented in welders and in workers exposed to high levels of inorganic manganese dust or fumes in mines or foundries (e.g. Archibald & Tyree, 1987; Roels et al., 1987, 1992; Iregren, 1990; Chia et al., 1993; Mergler et al., 1994; Lucchini et al., 1995; Huang et al., 1997; Pal et al., 1999; Myers et al., 2003). Sustained ingestion of potassium permanganate ($KMnO_4$) has also been implicated in the development of a similar syndrome (Holzgraefe et al., 1986).

Several studies have reported an association between chronic exposure to an organic manganese compound, manganese ethylene-bisdithiocarbamate (maneb, a dithiocarbamate fungicide), and neurological symptoms (Ferraz et al., 1988; Meco et al., 1994; Ruijten et al., 1994), but the effects could not be conclusively attributed to maneb alone (WHO, 1999a). MMT, another organic manganese compound, is a fuel additive that raises the octane of gasoline. Although the ability of MMT to induce seizure activity, brain neurotransmitters, and enzyme imbalances has been shown in rats and mice, data in humans are lacking (Gianutsos & Murray, 1982; Fishman et al., 1987; McGinley et al., 1987; Komura & Sakamoto, 1991, 1994). The experimental data suggest that MMT or a closely related metabolite and not elemental manganese itself is responsible for the seizure activity observed (Fishman et al., 1987).

8.5.2 Tin

Whereas inorganic tin compounds do not appear to elicit a neurotoxic effect, some organic tin compounds are potent neurotoxicants. Trialkyltin compounds with short carbon chains, such as trimethyltin and triethyltin, are the most toxic. Trimethyltin and triethyltin each have their own cellular targets, mechanism of neurotoxicity, and presentation of predominant clinical features (Feldman, 1999). Trimethyltin affects neurons and causes neurobehavioural changes; it is a neurotoxin that damages areas of the limbic system, cerebral cortex, and brainstem. Depending on the dose, signs and symptoms may appear from a few hours up to 3 days following administration. Neurological and psychiatric symptoms, such as headache, insomnia, fatigue, tinnitus, defective hearing, blurred vision, memory impairment, confusion, disorientation, aggressiveness, attacks of rage, bouts of depression, and psychotic behaviour, are symptoms of trimethyltin intoxication. Some patients also develop epileptic equivalents. Coma, respiratory depression requiring artificial central ventilation, and death follow severe intoxications (Fortemps et al., 1978; WHO, 1980, 1999b; Rey et al., 1984; Besser et al., 1987; Kreyberg et al., 1992).

Triethyltin attacks myelin, produces brain oedema, and impairs motor function (Arakawa et al., 1981; Feldman, 1999). The hazard associated with the use of organotin compounds was actually discovered by an episode of intoxication in 1954 involving over 200 cases, 100 of which were fatal. The cause was the ingestion of an oral preparation containing diethyltin diiodide intended as a treatment for boils and other staphylococcal skin infections. The oral preparation contained impurities, including triethyltin iodide, believed to be the primary agent of intoxication (Alajouanine et al., 1958; WHO, 1980, 1997). Symptoms and signs mainly ascribed to cerebral oedema of the white matter included diffuse headache, sometimes intolerably severe and appearing a few days after ingestion of the compound, nausea and vomiting, visual disturbances (mainly photophobia, but also double vision, abnormal colour vision, and blindness), stupor, meningeal irritation, somnolence, insomnia, convulsions, constipation, and bradycardia. Other frequent symptoms and signs were urinary incontinence, vertigo, loss of weight, and abdominal pains. Absence of fever and a tendency towards hypothermia were also noted. Transitory paralysis lasting 5–6 h and even persisting paresis were common in patients poisoned. Death occurred during coma or from respiratory or cardiac failure and in some cases during convulsions (Alajouanine et al., 1958; Cossa et al., 1958, 1959).

8.5.3 Mercury

The central nervous system is the critical target organ for exposure to mercury vapour and some organic mercury compounds.

Although the oxidation of metallic mercury vapour to Hg^{2+} ion takes place very soon after absorption, some elemental mercury remains dissolved in the blood long enough (a few minutes) for it to be carried to the blood–brain barrier (WHO, 1991b) (see Figure 8 in chapter 7). In vitro studies on the oxidation of elemental mercury in blood indicate that because of the short transit time from the lungs to the brain, almost all the mercury vapour arrives at the brain unoxidized (Hursh et al., 1988). Because of its lipid solubility and high diffusibility, mercury vapour easily crosses the blood–brain barrier to be oxidized to divalent mercury in the brain tissue. As the passage of the Hg^{2+} ion through this barrier is impeded, mercury is steadily accumulated in the brain tissue. Both acute exposure to high levels (see section 8.2.6) and long-term exposure to lower levels of mercury vapour cause effects on the central nervous system. Symptoms of chronic poisoning vary, but they prominently include tremor (initially affecting the fingers and hands, then the eyelids and the face, and sometimes spreading to other parts of the body), psychological changes (emotional lability characterized by irritability, excitability, timidity, mood changes, confidence loss, withdrawal from social interactions), performance deficits in tests of cognitive function (poor concentration, memory loss), and insomnia, fatigue, and headache. The peripheral nervous system may also be involved, as evidenced by paraesthesia (a sensation of pricking on the skin), stocking-glove sensory loss, weakness, muscle atrophy, hyperactive tendon reflexes, decreased sensory and motor nerve conduction velocities, and electromyographic abnormalities. Changes in vision, such as blurred vision, narrowing of the visual field, and loss of colour discrimination, are also possible.

The central nervous system is not considered to be a target organ of inorganic mercury compounds. Hg^{2+} ions have a limited capacity for penetrating the blood–brain barrier. The concentration of mercury in the brain was found to be about 10 times higher after mercury vapour exposure than after administration of a corresponding dose of divalent mercury (Berlin & Johansson, 1964; Magos, 1968; Berlin et al., 1969). However, animal investigations on some inorganic compounds such as mercury(II) chloride ($HgCl_2$) have shown that the compounds can act as direct blood–brain barrier toxicants (Peterson & Cardoso, 1983). Cases of central nervous system disorders and polyneuropathy have been ascribed to the ingestion of herb drugs that contained mercury(II) sulfate ($HgSO_4$) (Chu et al., 1998), the topical application of ammoniated mercury ointment (Kern et al., 1991; Deleu et al., 1998), or the use of skin-lightening cream or soap containing inorganic mercury salts (mercury iodide, mercury(II) ammonium chloride [$HgNH_2Cl$], mercury(I) chloride [Hg_2Cl_2]) (Dyall-Smith & Scurry, 1990; Harada et al., 2001).

The primary effect from acute or chronic exposure to methylmercury is damage to the central nervous system. Ingestion of fish or grain contaminated with methylmercury resulted in epidemics of severe neurotoxicity and death in Japan in the 1950s and 1960s and in Iraq in 1972. The central nervous system is particularly vulnerable to the toxic effects of methylmercury; this is attributed to its high lipid solubility, resulting in rapid transfer across the blood–brain barrier. However, methylmercury appears to be present in the body as water-soluble complexes mainly attached to the sulfur atom of thiol ligands (Clarkson, 2002). Its uptake from blood plasma into these cells is mediated in part by an amino acid carrier that transports the methylmercury–L-cysteine complex; complexation with glutathione and subsequent transport of the complex by an ATP-independent mechanism may be involved in the transport of methylmercury out of brain capillary endothelial cells into brain interstitial space (Kerper et al., 1992, 1996). $HgCl_2$ and methylmercury can inhibit the binding of radioligands to the muscarinic acetylcholine receptor, $HgCl_2$ being the more potent inhibitor of the two (Basu et al., 2005). It is thought that Hg^{II} is the toxic species of mercury to astrocytes and microglia in the nervous system after exposure to methylmercury (Charleston et al., 1996).

In methylmercury toxicity, the sensory, visual, and auditory functions, together with those of the brain areas, especially the cerebellum, concerned with coordination, are the most common functions to be affected. The earliest effects are nonspecific symptoms, such as complaints of paraesthesia, malaise, and blurred vision. Subsequently, signs such as concentric constriction of the visual field, deafness, dysarthria (speech difficulties), and ataxia appear. In the worst cases, the patient may go into a coma and ultimately die. Methylmercury poisoning has several important features: there is a long latent period, usually lasting several months; damage is almost exclusively limited to the nervous system, especially the central nervous system; areas of damage to the brain are highly localized (focal) — for example, in the visual cortex and the granular layer of the cerebellum, especially in the infolded regions (sulci); effects in severe cases are irreversible due to destruction of neuronal cells; and the earliest effects are nonspecific subjective complaints, such as paraesthesia, blurred vision, and malaise. The peripheral nervous system may also be affected, especially at high doses, but usually after effects have already appeared in the central nervous system (WHO, 1990a).

Dimethylmercury appears to be even more dangerous than monomethylmercury compounds. The physical properties of dimethylmercury permit transcutaneous absorption, and the volatility of this liquid permits toxic exposure through inhalation. Very small amounts of this highly toxic chemical can result in devastating neurological damage and death. A fatal case was described in a scientist after a few drops of dimethylmercury solution were spilled on her disposable gloves. The compound permeated the latex gloves and was absorbed through the skin, causing severe and fatal central nervous system toxicity (Byard & Couper, 1998; Nierenberg et al., 1998; Siegler et al., 1999).

Brain damage was less severe and kidney damage greater after ethylmercury administration to rats compared with methylmercury administration. However, when the dose of ethylmercury was increased by only 20%, the brain damage was similar to or slightly more severe than that seen from the lower dose of methylmercury (Magos et al., 1985). Actually, severe cases of ethylmercury poisoning can result in the same neurological signs and symptoms associated with methylmercury poisoning (e.g. constriction of the visual fields). Occupational exposure to ethylmercury, ingestion of rice or grains treated with the chemical, or ingestion of meat of a hog inadvertently fed seed treated with fungicides containing ethylmercury chloride resulted in severe neurotoxic effects (Hay et al., 1963; Hilmy et al., 1976; Zhang, 1984). Effects on spinal motor neurons, peripheral nerves, skeletal muscles, and myocardium were also described (Cinca et al., 1980). In contrast to methylmercury, signs of renal damage in humans are found in severe cases of ethylmercury intoxication (Magos, 2001). Ethylmercury poisoning is also characterized by a latent period of several weeks between first exposure and onset of the first symptoms of poisoning, as observed for monomethyl- and dimethylmercury.

8.5.4   Thallium

Thallium is one of the most toxic metals. It affects several tissues and systems, such as the epidermal, gastrointestinal, cardiovascular, and renal systems. The major manifestations of toxicity consist of a rapidly progressive, ascending, extremely painful sensory neuropathy and alopecia. Many other findings, such as an autonomic neuropathy, cranial nerve abnormalities, altered mental status, motor weakness, and cardiac, hepatic, and renal effects, are described, but are less specific (Saddique & Peterson, 1983; WHO, 1996a; Hoffman, 2003). Thallium has two oxidation states, 1+ and 3+. Tl^I, which is more stable, resembles potassium and is available in a number of soluble salts (e.g. sulfate, acetate, and carbonate), which are extremely toxic; the toxic element is rapidly absorbed, distributed, and accumulated in all organs and tissues and crosses the blood–brain barrier (Rios et al., 1989; Galvan-Arzate & Rios, 1994; Galvan-Arzate et al., 2000). Tl^{III} is a strong oxidant and behaves like aluminium. Both Tl^I and Tl^{III} are protoplasmic toxicants that mainly affect the central and peripheral nervous systems, the skin, the gastrointestinal tract, the cardio-vascular system, and the kidney (Diaz & Monreal, 1994; Villaverde & Verstraeten, 2003). The more water-soluble salts are considered to have higher toxicity than the salts of lower solubility, such as thallium(III) hydroxide [$Tl(OH)_3$], which is one of the least soluble among metal hydroxides (Lin & Nriagu, 1998). However, it has recently been suggested that the noxious effects of $Tl(OH)_3$ could have been overlooked, since it has been demonstrated that the effects of $Tl(OH)_3$ on the physical properties of liposome membranes were only slightly lower than those observed for Tl^{3+}. Even when the amount of Tl^{3+} available in water solutions is low, it produces significant effects on membrane physical properties and could contribute to the neurotoxicity associated with thallium poisoning (Villaverde & Verstraeten, 2003).

8.5.5   Lead

The central nervous system is probably the most sensitive target of lead. Both inorganic and organic lead are neurotoxic, but the clinical patterns of injury are different (Feldman, 1999).

From subtle effects on intellectual functioning and deficits in memory, attention, concentration, psychomotor performance, and intelligence to severe encephalopathy, a broad range of central nervous system effects is associated with inorganic lead exposure, depending on the degree of intoxication. Early clinical features of lead toxicity are nonspecific and subjective: headache, dizziness, poor attention, insomnia, asthenia, lethargy, irritability, dullness, loss of memory, anxiety, depression, and general malaise. Overt/acute severe lead encephalopathy associated with hallucinations and, in most serious cases, delirium, convulsions, coma, and death is a condition seen in children, but rarely in adults. Acute lead toxicity to the nervous system is characterized by oedema or swelling of the brain due to altered permeability of capillary endothelial cells. Cerebral oedema, associated with arterial hypertension and purpuric haemorrhagic extravations, is the principal gross neuropathological finding in individuals dying from inorganic lead encephalopathy.

Of particular concern are the possible neurotoxic effects on the developing child. The higher vulnerability of the fetus/child to the neurotoxic effects of lead is well documented. Long-term exposure to low lead levels has been shown to cause subtle effects on the central nervous system, which manifest as deficits in intelligence, poorer school performance, impaired neurobehavioural functioning, and even delinquent behaviour (Needleman et al., 1996, 2002; Mendelsohn et al., 1998; Lanphear et al., 2000; Counter et al., 2005).

Trimethyl and triethyl lead, trialkyl metabolites of tetramethyl and tetraethyl lead, are potent neurotoxicants (Tilson et al., 1982; Hong et al., 1983; Walsh et al., 1986; Verity et al., 1990; Yagminas et al., 1992). The clinical picture typically includes marked irritability, insomnia, disturbing dreams, hallucinations, anorexia, nausea, vomiting, tremulousness, and ataxia (WHO, 1997; Feldman, 1999).

The acute inhalation of leaded gasoline, containing tetraethyl lead, induces euphoria, dizziness, slurred speech, ataxia, and hallucinations. In some individuals, the abuse of leaded gasoline can also induce a severe encephalopathy that is characterized by decreased conscious state, tremor, myoclonus or chorea, limb and gait ataxia, hyperreflexia, motor impairment, nystagmus, and convulsive seizures. Chronic gasoline abuse is associated with cognitive impairment and mild movement disorders. In subjects with leaded gasoline encephalopathy, additional severe neurological abnormalities are present. These are characterized by the cerebellar features of ataxia, nystagmus, and poor hand and foot coordination. In addition, hyperreflexia and the presence of primitive reflexes suggest cortical damage (Cairney et al., 2002, 2004, 2005). It is suggested that many of the symptoms and signs are due to the hydrocarbons of gasoline, while the tetraethyl lead contributes to the altered mental status and is responsible for the persistent psychosis (Tenenbein, 1997).

Peripheral neuropathy develops insidiously during (sub)chronic exposure to inorganic lead and reflects the accumulation of lead in the body. It is typically a motor neuropathy, although sensory changes may be present. Inorganic lead can cause primary segmental demyelination and secondary axonal degeneration. The amount of lead intake generally correlates with the gradual progression in severity of the neuropathy from the subclinical stages to overt clinical signs and symptoms. Weakness in the upper or lower limbs is a common sign of chronic, high-level lead exposure (WHO, 1995). In adults, median and ulnar nerves appear to be affected preferentially (Feldman, 1999). The clinical distal motor neuropathy manifested as wrist drop is currently rare (Barats et al., 2000).

Peripheral neuropathy and myalgia are not as common following exposure to inorganic lead (Feldman, 1999). Symmetric sensorimotor neuropathy is described among gasoline sniffers; however, this neuropathy can occur despite the absence of tetraethyl lead in modern gasoline mixtures (Burns et al., 2001).

8.6 Nephrotoxicity

8.6.1 Cadmium

Long-term exposure to cadmium has caused severe chronic effects in the kidneys among the exposed workers and also in the general population. The accumulation of cadmium in the renal cortex leads to renal tubular dysfunction with impaired reabsorption of, for instance, proteins, glucose, and amino acids. A characteristic sign of tubular dysfunction is an increased excretion of low molecular mass proteins in urine. In some cases, the glomerular filtration rate decreases. An increase in urinary cadmium correlates with low molecular weight proteinuria and, in the absence of acute exposure to cadmium, may serve as an indicator of renal effect. In more severe cases, there is a combination of tubular and glomerular effects, with an increase in blood creatinine in some cases. For most workers and people in the general environment, cadmium-induced proteinuria is irreversible (WHO, 1992).

Among other effects are disturbances in calcium metabolism, hypercalciuria, and formation of renal stones. High exposure to cadmium, most probably in combination with other factors, such as nutritional deficiencies, may lead to the development of osteoporosis or osteomalacia (WHO, 1992).

Cadmium toxicity appears in critical organs only when the chelation capability of metallothionein in critical organs or tissues is completely used up; intracellular metallothionein production is an important biochemical mechanism for reducing the intracellular bioavailability/toxicity of cadmium by sequestering the Cd^{2+} ion in both liver and kidney (Squibb & Fowler, 1984).

Kidney proximal tubule cells take up cadmium–metallothionein highly efficiently; depending on the concentration of cadmium–metallothionein in the glomerular ultrafiltrate, there is a development of proximal tubule cell damage and low molecular mass tubular proteinuria following lysosomal degradation of the cadmium–metallothionein complex, to yield non-thionein-bound Cd^{2+} prior to induction of renal metallothionein (Nordberg et al., 1975, 1982; Garvey & Chang, 1981; Nordberg, 1984). Most evidence available at present indicates that toxicity to the kidney is related to the balance between toxic "free" non-metallothionein-bound cadmium and cadmium–metallothionein in renal cells. When metallothionein synthesis was induced by pretreatment of animals with repeated small doses of $CdCl_2$, the kidney was protected against a nephrotoxic dose of cadmium–metallothionein (Jin et al., 1998).

8.7 Reproductive toxicity

8.7.1 Nickel

Although data on nickel-induced reproductive/developmental effects in humans are lacking, a variety of developmental, reproductive, and teratogenic effects have been reported in animals exposed to soluble nickel compounds via oral and parenteral administration. Experimental data on rats and mice indicate that the male reproductive system is a sensitive target of soluble nickel compounds, such as $NiCl_2$ and $NiSO_4$, by ingestion, but also via dermal exposure (Mathur et al., 1977; Das & Dasgupta, 1997, 2000, 2002; Kakela et al., 1999; Pandey et al., 1999; Pandey & Srivastava, 2000; Pandey & Singh, 2001). In vitro studies with $NiSO_4$ and $NiNO_3$ have confirmed this effect (Jacquet & Mayence, 1982; Forgacs et al., 1998).

Serious developmental effects have also been reported in animals exposed to soluble nickel compounds (WHO, 1991a). Stillbirth and postimplantation/perinatal lethality have been consistently observed in several studies that involved $NiCl_2$ and $NiSO_4$ exposure prior to mating and during gestation and lactation (Sunderman et al., 1978; Lu et al., 1979; Smith et al., 1993; Kakela et al., 1999). Decreased pup survival has also been observed in a study in which nickel-exposed males were mated with unexposed females (Kakela et al., 1999). Nickel chloride caused an increased incidence of malformations in mice (Lu et al., 1979), and a teratogenic effect of this compound was confirmed in chicken embryo (Gilani & Marano, 1980). Moreover, an oxytoxic action of $NiCl_2$ has also been shown in vitro (Rubanyi & Balogh, 1982).

Nickel carbonyl $[Ni(CO)_4]$ is teratogenic and embryotoxic in rats and hamsters (Sunderman et al., 1978, 1979, 1980).

8.7.2 Mercury

Studies on the reproductive and developmental effects of elemental mercury in humans have yielded mixed results (WHO, 1991b, 2003; ATSDR, 1999b).

Experimental exposures of pregnant animals to mercury vapour have shown that although elemental mercury (Hg^0) is rapidly oxidized to ionic mercury (Hg^{2+}), some Hg^0 readily crosses the placental barrier and is taken up by fetal tissues (Clarkson et al., 1972; Khayat & Dencker, 1982; Yoshida et al., 1986; Warfvinge et al., 1994). Mercury vapour metabolism in fetuses appears to be quite different from that in their mothers. This might prevent the fetal brain, which is rapidly developing, and thus vulnerable, from being exposed to excessive elemental mercury (Yoshida et al., 1986). Mercury exposure during gestation may result to some extent in the appearance of the element in the central nervous system (Khayat & Dencker, 1982), but the uptake in the fetal central nervous system differs with gestational age and is markedly less than in adults (Yoshida et al., 1986; Takahashi et al., 2001). A significantly increased level was found in kidney, lung, and brain in neonate guinea-pigs, compared with fetuses, and there was a progressive decrease in liver concentration, with diminishing hepatic metallo-thionein levels, in the neonates. These results suggest a redistribu-tion of mercury to other tissues in the neonate (Yoshida et al., 1987). Metallic mercury is rapidly oxidized to Hg^{2+} in the fetal liver, where it accumulates and binds to a metallothionein-like protein (Yoshida et al., 2002). The oxidization of mercury prevents it from affecting the vulnerable fetal brain, as the blood–brain barrier prevents ionic mercury from entering the brain tissues (Takahashi et al., 2003). It is suggested that the binding to the fetal metallothionein-like protein might also play a role in preventing further distribution of mercury from the liver to the brain (Yoshida et al., 1987, 2002, 2005).

Only limited information is available regarding the developmental toxicity of inorganic mercury salts. Animal experiments have shown that the placental membrane constitutes an efficacious barrier against the penetration of Hg^{II} into the fetus (Berlin & Ullberg, 1963; Yang et al., 1996). Hg^{II} appears to accumulate in the placenta, thereby limiting the amount reaching the fetus (Clarkson et al., 1972; Khayat & Dencker, 1982). Mercury levels in the fetuses of rats exposed to mercury vapour were 10–40 times higher than in animals exposed to equivalent doses of $HgCl_2$ (Clarkson et al., 1972).

Methylmercury easily passes both the placental and the blood–brain barriers, and exposure of the fetus constitutes a main concern. Its toxic action on the developing brain differs in both mechanism and outcome from its action on the adult brain. The prenatal period is the stage of human life most susceptible to methylmercury expo-sure. Why the fetus displays different neuropathological effects and a higher sensitivity to methylmercury relative to the adult is still unknown. The clinical picture is dose dependent: methylmercury may result in effects ranging from fetal death to subtle neuro-developmental delays. In infants exposed to high maternal blood levels of methylmercury, the picture is that of cerebral palsy. Microcephaly, hyperreflexia, and gross motor and mental impair-ment, sometimes associated with blindness or deafness, compose the main pattern. Milder degrees of the affliction are not easy to diagnose during the first few months of life, but they later become clear (WHO, 1990a).

8.8 Genotoxicity

Genotoxicity is defined as the capacity of an agent to cause damage to the genetic material (DNA, chromosomes, mitotic spindle, etc.) either directly (e.g. by binding covalently to DNA) or indirectly (e.g. by inducing the production of reactive oxygen species that will attack DNA or by interfering with DNA repair systems). Genetic damage, when insufficiently repaired, will be converted into a mutation that can be expressed at the DNA sequence (gene mutation), chromosome (chromosomal mutation), or genome level (genomic mutation).

The evaluation of the genotoxic activity of a chemical is important, because it may help to explain or predict its capacity to cause genetic diseases or cancers (genotoxic carcinogens).

8.8.1 Chromium

An increased risk of occupational cancers has been reported in several industrial settings, mainly involving exposure to Cr^{VI} compounds (see below). It is widely accepted that the carcinogenicity of chromium compounds is closely related to their capacity to cause genotoxic damage. When considering the genotoxicity of chromium compounds, it is necessary to take several properties of the tested compounds into account, including solubility, oxidation state, intracellular stability, and reactivity with cellular components.

There is a wealth of experimental data indicating that, in cellular systems, soluble Cr^{VI} compounds produce genotoxic effects for a variety of end-points, whereas soluble Cr^{III} compounds are generally inactive (De Flora et al., 1990). While in acellular systems (e.g. purified nucleic acids) soluble Cr^{III} compounds produce genotoxic effects, Cr^{VI} itself is unreactive towards DNA at physiological pH and requires reductive activation (e.g. by cysteine) to produce DNA-damaging species (Zhitkovich et al., 2002).

The current understanding of the genotoxicity of chromium compounds is that Cr^{VI} is bioactive because of its capacity to cross biomembranes and enter the cells. When Cr^{VI} is reduced outside the cell (e.g. by ascorbate), its genotoxic activity is suppressed, because Cr^{III} species poorly penetrate cell membranes. The genotoxic activity of Cr^{VI} also depends on its capacity to undergo an intracellular reduction by a variety of systems (ascorbate, glutathione, hydrogen peroxide, cysteine, cytochrome P450 reductases, mitochondrial enzymes). Following intracellular reduction, several reactive intermediates are produced, including Cr^{V}, Cr^{IV}, and Cr^{III}, as well as oxygen radicals. These secondary forms have the capacity to react with macromolecules and cause DNA damage (breaks, cross-links, adducts, etc.) (Shi et al., 1999a) and affect the fidelity of DNA replication (Singh & Snow, 1998).

In an in vitro study comparing the capacity of several transitional metals to produce oxygen radicals in a Fenton reaction (Lloyd et al., 1998), Cr^{III} was the most potent species, followed by Cr^{VI}, V^{III}, Fe^{II}, and Cu^{II}. Cr^{VI} has also been shown to induce in Jurkat cells (a human T cell leukaemia cell line) the expression of the nuclear transcription factor NF kappa-B, which is particularly sensitive to cellular perturbations caused by reactive radicals (Shi et al., 1999b).

In cultured lung cells, the genotoxic activity of the poorly soluble carcinogen lead chromate has been shown to be mediated by the extracellular dissolution of the particles and not their internalization (Xie et al., 2004).

In vivo, it has been shown that intratracheally administered Cr^{VI}, but not Cr^{III}, induced the formation of DNA strand breaks, measured by the alkaline DNA unwinding assay, in peripheral lymphocytes of rats (Gao et al., 1992).

In humans, the importance of chromium speciation for inducing genotoxic effects is not very well documented. Studies in populations occupationally exposed to chromium compounds have shown that electroplating workers exposed to hexavalent chromium had an increased rate of micronucleus formation (Vaglenov et al., 1999) and sister chromatid exchanges (Wu et al., 2001), both assessed in circulating lymphocytes. No change in the rate of chromosomal aberrations could be detected in lymphocytes of workers exposed to Cr^{III} in a ferrochromium factory in Italy (Sbrana et al., 1990). No study comparing, for the same genotoxic end-point, populations exposed to equivalent levels of Cr^{III} and Cr^{VI} is available.

Since Cr^{III} compounds are essential nutrients required for proper insulin function and normal protein, fat, and carbohydrate metabolism, the potential toxicity of several bioavailable ligand species has been investigated. Chromium picolinate has been shown to be mutagenic, and the picolinic acid moiety appears to be in part responsible, as studies show that picolinic acid alone is clastogenic. Niacin-bound Cr^{III} has been demonstrated to be more bioavailable and efficacious as a nutrient, and no toxicity has been reported (Bagchi et al., 2002).

8.8.2 Cobalt

Data accumulated in recent years indicate that, depending on the cobalt species considered (Co^{2+} ions or cobalt metal), different toxicity outcomes can be observed (see also sections 8.4 and 8.9). Regarding genotoxicity, the production of reactive oxygen species by Co^{2+} ions and cobalt metal together with inhibition of DNA repair by Co^{2+} ions appear to be the predominant modes of action (Lison et al., 2001).

In vitro, soluble and insoluble cobalt compounds have shown evidence of genotoxicity. Karyotype analysis after exposure of peripheral blood cells to cobalt(II) chloride ($CoCl_2$) led to the observation of aneuploidy. Poorly soluble cobalt(II) sulfide (CoS) was found to induce DNA strand breaks in Chinese hamster ovary cells (Robison et al., 1982). It was also shown that, in the presence of hydrogen peroxide, micromolar concentrations of Co^{2+} ions are able to mimic Fe^{2+} cations in a Fenton-like reaction and cause damage to DNA bases of human lymphocytes or isolated DNA through the production of hydroxyl radicals (Nackerdien et al., 1991; Kawanishi et al., 1994; Lloyd et al., 1997). DNA damage resulting from the generation of reactive oxygen species by $CoCl_2$ and hydrogen peroxide was further investigated by Mao et al. (1996) with electron spin resonance, electrophoretic assays, and HPLC. They showed that the oxidation potential of Co^{2+} can be modulated by chelators to alter its capacity to generate reactive oxygen species and DNA damage: anserine enhanced the reactivity of Co^{2+} ions, whereas 1,10-phenanthroline and deferoxamine reduced and suppressed it, respectively. Co^{2+} ions were also shown to substitute for zinc in protein–zinc finger domains, which control the transcription of several genes. This substitution may contribute to explain how Co^{2+} generates reactive oxygen species sufficiently close to DNA to cause damage (Sarkar, 1995). In vitro, in human lymphocytes and purified DNA, in the absence of hydrogen peroxide, $CoCl_2$ up to a concentration of 0.1 mmol/l did not induce DNA single strand breaks (Anard et al., 1997), supporting the idea that Co^{2+} ions damage DNA through a Fenton-like reaction. In contrast to Anard et al. (1997), however, DNA breakage was detected by De Boeck et al. (1998) in human lymphocytes incubated with $CoCl_2$.

Until 1997, no report was available on the genotoxicity of cobalt metal particles, and it was assumed to be similar to that of the solubilized species (i.e. the Co^{2+} ion). The current view is that cobalt metal possesses a biological activity independent of its ionic form. Physicochemical studies have shown that cobalt metal, and not its Co^{2+} ionic species, is thermodynamically able to reduce oxygen to form reactive oxygen species. The kinetics of this process are, however, slow as a result of the poor oxygen binding capacity at the surface of cobalt metal particles (Lison et al., 1995). In this system, soluble Co^{2+} ions are produced during, but do not drive, the critical reaction — i.e. reactive oxygen species are not produced by a Fenton-like reaction as for Co^{2+} ions. Meanwhile, the same authors found that the capacity of cobalt particles to produce reactive oxygen species is markedly increased in the presence of tungsten carbide particles, such as in hard metal powders. Anard et al. (1997) demonstrated the capacity of cobalt metal to induce DNA breaks and alkali-labile sites in isolated DNA and human lymphocytes. This damage could be partially blocked by scavenging reactive oxygen species with formate, indicating the possible involvement of the hydroxyl radical. The same authors demonstrated that, when tested in a range of cobalt equivalent concentrations, a hard metal mixture consisting of 94% tungsten carbide and 6% cobalt particles induced significantly more (on average a 3-fold increase) DNA breaks and alkali-labile sites than cobalt particles alone, both in isolated DNA and in cultured human lymphocytes. Scavenging reactive oxygen species with formate completely prevented DNA damage, again consistent with the involvement of hydroxyl radicals in this effect. Similar results were reported by De Boeck et al. (1998). The mechanism of this interaction is most probably associated with an enhanced capacity of the mixture to produce reactive oxygen species (see section 8.4).

A similarly greater genotoxicity of hard metal compared with cobalt particles was found with the cytokinesis-blocked micronucleus test applied on human lymphocytes (Van Goethem et al., 1997). The mechanism by which cobalt and tungsten carbide–cobalt induce micronuclei is not clearly identified; it might be the consequence of the direct clastogenic activity discussed above, but an aneugenic activity should not be overlooked, as centromere-positive micronuclei were detected after in vitro exposure to cobalt (De Boeck et al., 1998). De Boeck et al. (2003) subsequently demonstrated, again in cultured human lymphocytes, that the aneugenic interaction between cobalt and carbide particles previously observed with tungsten carbide also applies to some other metallic carbides (chromium carbide [Cr_3C_2] and niobium(IV) carbide [NbC], but not molybdenum(II) carbide [Mo_2C]).

In addition to the capacity of cobalt metal and Co^{2+} to indirectly cause DNA damage via the production of reactive oxygen species, Co^{2+} ions have been reported to affect DNA repair processes. In vitro, $CoCl_2$ was shown to inhibit nucleotide excision repair after UV irradiation in human fibroblasts (Hartwig et al., 1991). $CoCl_2$ inhibited the incision and polymerization steps of the DNA repair process in human fibroblasts treated with UV-C (Kasten et al., 1997). Since DNA damage repair is an essential mechanism of homeostasis maintenance, its inhibition may also account for a mutagenic or carcinogenic effect of Co^{2+}. Competition with essential Mg^{2+} ions (Kasten et al., 1997) and binding to zinc finger domains in repair proteins were identified as potential modes of indirect genotoxic activity of Co^{2+} ions. It has also been reported that the DNA binding capacity of the p53 protein, which is also a zinc-dependent mechanism, can be modulated by Co^{2+} ions (Palecek et al., 1999; Meplan et al., 2000).

Overall, the available data indicate that an assessment of the genotoxicity of cobalt and its compounds requires a clear distinction between the different species of the element and needs to take into account the different mechanisms involved.

8.9 Carcinogenicity

8.9.1 Chromium

For chromium, the importance of speciation as a determinant of the carcinogenic activity is well documented; there is, indeed, a major difference between chemically stable trivalent species and hexavalent forms, which are strong oxidants.

Most experimental studies with Cr^{III} species have not detected a carcinogenic activity. In contrast, Cr^{VI} species did produce respiratory tumours (strontium chromate [$SrCrO_4$], zinc chromate [$ZnCrO_4$], lead chromate [$PbCrO_4$], and, to a lesser extent, CrO_3) as well as renal tumours ($PbCrO_4$). Cr^{VI} compounds are classified as Group 1 carcinogens by IARC (1990); metallic and Cr^{III} compounds are not classified as to their carcinogenic activity in humans (Group 3) (IARC, 1990).

It is not easy to exactly define industrial activities involving a potential of exposure to each specific species, because both metallic forms are usually mixed. The highest exposures to Cr^{VI} have been recorded in the distal steps of the production of chromates (sodium [Na_2CrO_4], potassium [K_2CrO_4], and calcium chromate [$CaCrO_4$]), plating (CrO_3), and the production and manipulation of paints containing $ZnCrO_4$ or $PbCrO_4$. Exposure to chromate compounds is also possible while welding or cutting chromium-based alloys (e.g. stainless steels). Exposure to Cr^{III} compounds is associated with the proximal steps of chromate production (roasting of iron chromite ores), ferrochromium industries, and tanning operations.

Epidemiological studies have convincingly demonstrated an increased risk of lung cancer associated with inhalation exposure to Cr^{VI} compounds, mainly $ZnCrO_4$ and CrO_3 in chromate production workers (Mancuso & Hueper, 1951; Ohsaki et al., 1978; Davies et al., 1991; Korallus et al., 1993). Chromium platers exposed to soluble CrO_3 also show evidence of an increased risk of lung cancer (Okubo & Tsuchiya, 1977; Franchini et al., 1983; Sorahan et al., 1998; Sorahan & Harrington, 2000). Several studies have also reported an excess mortality from lung cancer associated with mixed exposures (Cr^{VI} and Cr^{III}), but it is impossible to disentangle the respective role of each species (Mancuso, 1997; Gibb et al., 2000).

An excess risk of nasal cancer has also been identified in workers exposed to Cr^{VI} compounds (Rosenman & Stanbury, 1996). Studies in workers from leather tanneries (Cr^{III} species) or from the ferrochromium industry (Cr^{III} and chromium metal) did not detect an increased risk of lung cancer associated with chromium exposure (Pippard et al., 1985; Stern, 2003) or found an increased risk associated with a confounder (e.g. polycyclic aromatic hydrocarbons) (Moulin et al., 1990).

Administration of K_2CrO_4 through drinking-water has been shown to increase the occurrence of UV-induced skin tumours in mice, suggesting that Cr^{VI} compounds may represent a carcinogenic hazard via exposure routes other than inhalation (Davidson et al., 2004). In humans, ingested Cr^{VI} is, however, largely reduced to Cr^{III} species in the gastrointestinal system, and consumption of tap water appears unlikely to pose a health risk when considering the current water standards in the United States (Paustenbach et al., 2003).

8.9.2 *Cobalt*

The importance of considering the varying genotoxic activities of the different cobalt compounds (ions, metal alone or associated with tungsten carbide particles) has already been discussed above (see section 8.8). Concerning carcinogenicity, the picture is more fragmentary, because appropriate (experimental or epidemiological) studies allowing a comparison of the activities of the different cobalt species are lacking.

Long-term inhalation of a cobalt(II) sulfate ($CoSO_4$) aerosol has been shown to induce lung tumours (bronchioalveolar carcinoma) in both rats and mice (Bucher et al., 1999); unfortunately, similar studies with other cobalt species (metal, hard metal mixture) are not available. However, since all soluble cobalt salts, cobalt metal alone, or cobalt metal mixed with tungsten carbide particles will result in the release of Co^{2+} ions in vivo, it has been considered that the carcinogenic activity of the soluble $CoSO_4$ can be extended to all these compounds. Based on this consideration, IARC (2006) has reached a conclusion of "sufficient evidence of carcinogenicity in animals" for $CoSO_4$, all soluble cobalt salts, cobalt metal alone, and cobalt metal mixed with tungsten carbide particles (hard metals) (Table 9). Insufficient experimental data are available to assess the carcinogenic potential of other, less soluble cobalt species, such as cobalt oxides (CoO or cobaltosic oxide [Co_3O_4]) or CoS.

Table 9. International Agency for Research on Cancer (IARC) evaluation of carcinogenic risks to humans of cobalt metal, hard metal, cobalt oxide, and soluble cobalt salts

	Evidence in humans	Evidence in experimental animals	IARC group	Reference
Cobalt metal alone	Inadequate	Sufficient	Possibly carcino-genic to humans (2B)	IARC (2006)
Hard metal	Limited	Sufficient	Probably carcino-genic to humans (2A)	
Soluble cobalt salts	Inadequate	Sufficient	Possibly carcino-genic to humans (2B)	
Cobalt oxide	Inadequate	Sufficient	Possibly carcino-genic to humans (2B)	IARC (1987)

Epidemiological studies have been conducted only in occupational cohorts exposed to cobalt metal alone, and mainly in hard metal workers.

No increased mortality from lung cancer has been found in a cohort of workers employed in an electrochemical plant producing cobalt and sodium (Moulin et al., 1993). In contrast, in hard metal plants, where exposure is to cobalt metal associated with tungsten carbide particles, several studies have reported an increased mortality from lung cancer (Hogstedt & Alexandersson, 1987; Lasfargues et al., 1994; Moulin et al., 1998; Wild et al., 2001); this has led IARC (2006) to conclude that there is "limited evidence" of carcinogenicicity of hard metals in humans (Table 9). These findings are not unexpected, based on the enhanced genotoxic activity of cobalt metal when mixed with tungsten carbide particles, and further support the view that hard metals constitute a distinct entity with a biological activity different from that of cobalt metal or cobalt cations (Lison et al., 2001).

8.9.3   Nickel

Nickel and its compounds have numerous industrial applications, including the production of steels, alloys, and electrical and domestic appliances. Occupational exposure to inorganic nickel compounds occurs during the extraction and purification of ores, during the manufacture of alloys, and in relation to different electrolytic processes where this element is used. Other sources of occupational exposure are the manufacture of batteries, welding, and glass, ceramics, and chemical industries. The chemistry of nickel is complex, and the toxicological properties of the various compounds depend on physicochemical characteristics, surface chemistry, solubility, geological history, etc.

The carcinogenic risk associated with occupational exposure to nickel compounds is difficult to assess exactly, partly because of the involvement of different nickel species with varying and incompletely understood biological activities (Grandjean et al., 1988). Epidemiological studies point to an increased risk of cancer (lung, nasal cavities) associated with a prolonged inhalation exposure to elevated levels of relatively insoluble species (Doll et al., 1970), but also of soluble nickel species (International Committee on Nickel Carcinogenesis in Man, 1990; Anttila et al., 1998; Grimsrud et al., 2005). From the available epidemiological studies, it is, however, difficult to delineate the specific contribution of each species, because exposures were almost always mixed. Nickel compounds are collectively considered by IARC (1990) as human carcinogens (Group 1), and nickel metal is considered as possibly carcinogenic to humans (Group 2B) (IARC, 1990). Respiratory tumours have been induced in early experimental studies with nickel metal, NiO, and Ni_3S_2, but the relevance of the mode of administration used (intratracheal instillation) has been questioned (Oller et al., 1997). More recent experimental studies conducted by inhalation have indicated a clear carcinogenic activity of Ni_3S_2 (insoluble in water), whereas NiO (insoluble in water) and $NiSO_4$ (water soluble) showed, respectively, doubtful and no carcinogenic activity (Dunnick et al., 1995).

The parameters responsible for the carcinogenic activity of nickel compounds have not yet been clearly identified. Three possible modes of action are considered: DNA damage caused by reactive oxygen species produced from Ni^{2+} ions, inhibition of certain steps involved in DNA repair processes, and an aspecific toxic effect that leads to the production of reactive oxygen species by inflammatory cells. It is generally well accepted that the Ni^{2+} ion is the ultimate genotoxic species and that its capacity to produce reactive oxygen species via a Fenton-like reaction (Nackerdien et al., 1991) contributes to causing DNA damage (Kasprzak et al., 1994; Kawanishi et al., 1994; Lloyd & Phillips, 1999). It has also been suggested that Ni^{2+} ions could alter the degree of DNA methylation (Lee et al., 1998). Several nickel compounds also interact with other genotoxic carcinogens to produce lung tumours (Kasprzak et al., 1973), possibly reflecting the capacity of Ni^{2+} ions to inhibit DNA repair processes (Krueger et al., 1999).

DNA damage induced by reactive oxygen species could also be the result of a toxic and aspecific inflammatory reaction induced in the lung by the accumulation of insoluble particles (Driscoll et al., 1994). This mechanism could, in particular, account for the carcinogenic activity of nickel compounds that do not show genotoxic activity in vitro (e.g. NiO).

While the genotoxic activity of the Ni^{2+} ion is almost unanimously accepted, it remains, however, to be explained why the biological activity of nickel compounds (e.g. Ni_3S_2, NiO, and $NiSO_4$) does not vary according to solubility. This paradox is particularly notable in animal carcinogenicity bioassays performed by the United States National Toxicology Program (Dunnick et al., 1995).

The most commonly accepted hypothesis is based on differences in the bioavailability of Ni^{2+} at the nuclear level. In particular, it is known that the capacity of a nickel particle to be phagocytosed/endocytosed is an important determinant of its nuclear bioavailability, because Ni^{2+} ions barely penetrate the cells.

A hypothesis that attempts to integrate all these considerations in an explanation of the varying carcinogenic responses of nickel compounds in experimental and epidemiological studies has been proposed based on three model compounds: Ni_3S_2, NiO, and $NiSO_4$. Ni_3S_2 particles do not seem to accumulate in the lung and are therefore likely to be phagocytosed/endocytosed and solubilized in target cells, allowing the delivery of a sufficient dose of Ni^{2+} ions to exert its genotoxic effects in the nucleus. Epidemiological and experimental studies concur to support a carcinogenic potential of Ni_3S_2. NiO, which is not soluble in biological media, would not provide sufficient Ni^{2+} ion levels at the DNA level. However, owing to its low solubility, its accumulation in the lung would cause an inflammatory reaction capable of producing indirect genotoxic damage. Epidemiological data support a carcinogenic potential of NiO, and recent experimental studies indicate a weak carcinogenic activity. Epidemiological data concerning soluble nickel salts are conflicting, and experimental studies do not indicate a carcinogenic activity of soluble nickel salts (Oller et al., 1997). It should, however, be noted that this view is not consistent with the previous IARC (1990) evaluation that concluded that there was sufficient evidence of carcinogenicity in humans for $NiSO_4$.

Overall, the solubility of nickel compounds is not a predictor of their carcinogenic potential (Haber et al., 2000).

Nickel carbonyl [$Ni(CO)_4$] is a gas formed in the refining process of nickel and used as a catalyst in the production of petroleum, plastic, and rubber. It is extremely toxic and may cause severe acute effects involving the respiratory tract (pneumonitis), the brain, and several other organs. IARC (1990) concluded that there is limited evidence of carcinogenicity for $Ni(CO)_4$ in experimental animals. Inhalation of $Ni(CO)_4$ has been shown to cause a few pulmonary tumours in rats (Sunderman & Donnelly, 1965), and intravenous injections induced an increase in the overall incidence of neoplasms in several organs in rats (Lau et al., 1972). The mechanism possibly responsible for these tumours remains elusive.

8.9.4 Arsenic

The various forms of arsenic to which humans are exposed complicate the issue of hazard evaluation, since these compounds appear to have different effects. Until the end of the previous century, it was believed that only inorganic arsenic species exerted a carcinogenic activity, but this view has been challenged by recent experimental data indicating that some organic species also exert a carcinogenic activity.

Inorganic arsenic is derived from the production of non-ferrous metals, chiefly in primary copper smelters (mainly trivalent but also pentavalent species). Several epidemiological studies have shown a causal relationship between occupational inhalation exposure to inorganic arsenic compounds and the occurrence of respiratory cancers. Other investigations point to an increased risk of cancer (skin, liver, digestive tract, bladder, prostate, kidney) upon environmental exposure, notably via drinking-water. IARC (1987) concluded that inorganic arsenic compounds are carcinogenic to humans (Group 1). More recently, an evaluation specifically focusing on exposure via drinking-water led to similar conclusions (IARC, 2004). Inorganic arsenic is probably the only element classified as a human carcinogen in the absence of strong evidence in experimental animals. Indeed, almost all bioassays did not detect a carcinogenic response to inorganic arsenic compounds alone, except after intra-tracheal instillation of As_2O_3 (Yamamoto et al., 1995). However, other experimental studies point to a co-carcinogenic or promoting activity of some inorganic arsenic compounds (Pershagen et al., 1984; Rossman et al., 2004).

Epidemiological demonstrations of an increased risk of lung cancer originated from a report of copper smelter workers in whom a 3-fold increased mortality by respiratory cancer was found (Pinto & Bennett, 1963; Lee & Fraumeni, 1969). Trivalent (mainly As_2O_3) and pentavalent inorganic compounds were present in these environments, but metallic elements and sulfur dioxide were also present. Several subsequent reports have largely confirmed the increased risk of lung cancer associated with inorganic arsenic exposure, including in other occupational settings involving inhalation exposure to similar arsenic species (pesticide production workers mainly exposed to arsenates such as lead arsenate [$PbHAsO_4$]; tin and gold miners exposed to inorganic arsenic species, but also to radon and crystalline silica). Increased risks of other cancers (skin, digestive) have also been reported in similar settings, but the associations were markedly weaker and less consistent (IARC, 1987; WHO, 2001).

Cases of skin cancers and liver angiosarcomas have been consistently reported in patients treated with trivalent inorganic compounds, particularly Fowler's solution (liquor arsenicalis, which contains 1% potassium arsenite and was used as a tonic and remedy).

Arsenic in drinking-water (primarily inorganic, as arsenate and, to a lesser extent, arsenite) was evaluated by IARC (2004) as carcinogenic to humans (Group 1) on the basis of sufficient evidence for an increased risk of cancer of the urinary bladder, lung, and skin. There is, indeed, extensive evidence of increased risks of urinary bladder, renal, lung, skin, and possibly liver cancers associated with arsenic in drinking-water (IARC, 2004).

The cellular mechanisms by which inorganic arsenic compounds exert a carcinogenic activity remain incompletely understood, and there is a hypothesis that could account for it, although it has not been generally agreed upon. Inorganic arsenic species, mostly As^{III}, generally did not produce gene mutations when tested at non-cytotoxic concentrations. In most in vitro tests, however, they exert a co-mutagenic activity. It has therefore been proposed that mechanisms of arsenic carcinogenesis may involve oxidative stress, damage to DNA and inhibition of repair processes, alteration of DNA methylation, chromosomal aberrations, activation of certain signal transduction pathways leading to aberrant gene expression, and modifications of cell cycle control and/or differentiation.

In contrast to its carcinogenic activity, arsenic(III) trioxide (As_2O_3) was reported in 1930 to be effective for the treatment of certain forms of leukaemia. After a decline in the use of arsenic during the mid-20th century, reports from China described good haematological responses in patients with acute promyelocytic leukaemia treated with As_2O_3. Randomized clinical trials in the United States led to the approval of As_2O_3 for relapsed or refractory acute promyelocytic leukaemia (Antman, 2001).

It has been generally accepted that only inorganic arsenic species have carcinogenic potential. However, recent studies have demonstrated that one of the methylation intermediates, monomethylated As^{III} or methylarsonous acid, not only is several orders of magnitude more toxic than inorganic As^{III}, but also exhibits genotoxic properties (Mass et al., 2001; Nesnow et al., 2002; Styblo et al., 2002; Aposhian et al., 2003).

Furthermore, experimental studies have indicated a carcinogenic potential for the dimethylated metabolite, DMA. After oral administration, DMA produced urinary bladder tumours in rats (Wei et al., 2002). Mechanistic studies have indicated that this damage is due mainly to the peroxyl radical of DMA. Multiorgan initiation–promotion studies have demonstrated that DMA acts as a promotor of urinary bladder, kidney, liver, and thyroid gland cancers in rats and as a promotor of lung tumours in mice (Kenyon & Hughes, 2001). These data suggest that DMA plays a role in the carcinogenesis of inorganic arsenic.

Gallium arsenide (GaAs) is used primarily to make light-emitting diodes, lasers, laser windows, and photodetectors and in the photoelectronic transmission of data through optical fibres. An inhalation study has shown an increased incidence of lung tumours in female, but not male, rats (NTP, 2000). Although human data on its carcinogenic potential are not available, IARC (2006) decided to classify GaAs as a Group 1 carcinogen because, once in the organism, it releases a small amount of its arsenic moiety, which behaves as inorganic arsenic (Webb et al., 1984).

9. CONCLUSIONS AND RECOMMENDATIONS

1.   Consideration of speciation is an important component of both hazard identification and exposure assessment, and hence of risk characterization, of chemicals in the general and work environments. Speciation analysis allows a better understanding of the mechanism of toxicity.

2.   Aspects of speciation to be considered include isotopic composition, electronic and oxidation state, inorganic and organic compounds and complexes, organometallic species, and macromolecular compounds and complexes.

3.   There are important qualitative and quantitative differences in the toxicity of different species of an element (e.g. methylmercury and Hg^{2+} ions, tributyltin and tin ions, chromate and Cr^{III} salts). Thus, when characterizing hazards and risks, the use of generic element names is to be discouraged.

4.   There is no general rule that, across elements, individual species or characteristics of a species (such as water solubility, valence state) are predictive of toxicity.

5.   Grouping together different species of a single element for risk assessment by a common characteristic, such as water solubility, is seldom justified and requires careful consideration of data on the hazards of the members of the proposed group.

6.   Existing practices in risk assessment and management are based on historical availability of analytical methodology that allowed the determination of only the total concentration of elements. Modern methods that can measure elemental species are becoming more affordable. However, their implementation is still an important impediment in the risk assessment and management of most elements.

7.   Great care should be given to sampling, storage, handling, and isolation of the species to ensure that the speciation does not

change. The appropriate sample should be chosen: for example, species can change during processing, cooking, or storing food.

8.   There is a current shortage of reference materials for speciation analysis. However, legal obligation to include speciation in monitoring schemes would promote the development of such reference materials and their use in quality assurance programmes.

9.   Methods for determination of individual species are frequently appropriate and should be applied both in the measurement of external exposure and in biomonitoring.

10.   Where appropriate, risk management guidance (e.g. guidelines for ambient and workplace air) should be related to individual species.

11.   Even when the total concentration of an element is measured for biomonitoring, exposure indices of the individual species to which the population is exposed should be developed and used where appropriate.

12.   Consideration of species of an element may reduce the hazards from exposure, by suggesting substitution of harmful chemicals with less harmful ones: for example, replacement of elemental yellow phosphorus by red (polymeric) phosphorus as a flame retardant; replacement of chromic acid with trivalent chromium in chrome-plating; addition of iron sulfate in cement to transform chromate to Cr^{III}; and design of platinum compounds that are not sensitizing.

REFERENCES

Abbracchio MP, Evans RM, Heck JD, Cantoni O & Costa M (1982) The regulation of ionic nickel uptake and cytotoxicity by specific amino acids and serum components. Biol Trace Elem Res, **4**: 289–301.

ACGIH (1991) Documentation of the threshold limit values and biological exposure indices. Vol. 1. Cincinnati, Ohio, American Conference of Governmental Industrial Hygienists.

Ackley K & Caruso JA (2003) Liquid chromatography. In: Cornelis R, Crews H, Caruso J & Heumann KG eds. Handbook of elemental speciation I. Techniques and methodology. Chichester, John Wiley & Sons, pp 147–162.

Adriano DC (1986) Trace elements in the terrestrial environment. New York, Springer-Verlag.

Adriano DC (1992) Biogeochemistry of trace metals. Boca Raton, Florida, Lewis Publishers.

Ahsanullah M & Ying W (1995) Toxic effects of dissolved copper on *Penaeus merguiensis* and *Penaeus monodon*. Bull Environ Contam Toxicol, **55**(1): 81–88.

Aitio A & Jarvisalo Y (1986) Levels of welding fume components in tissue and body fluids. In: Stern RM, Berlin A, Fletcher AC & Jarvisalo J eds. Health hazards and biological effects of welding fumes and gases. Amsterdam, Elsevier, pp 169–179 (Excerpta Medica / International Congress Series 676).

Aitio A, Järvisalo J, Kiilunen M, Tossavainen A & Vaittinen P (1984) Urinary excretion of chromium as an indicator of exposure to trivalent chromium sulphate in leather tanning. Int Arch Occup Environ Health, **54**: 241–249.

Aiyar J, Berkovits J, Floyd RA & Wetterhahn KE (1991) Reaction of chromium(VI) with glutathione or with hydrogen peroxide: Identification of reactive intermediates and their role in chromium(VI)-induced DNA damage. Environ Health Perspect, **92**: 53–62.

Alajouanine T, Derobert L & Thieffry S (1958) Comprehensive clinical study of 210 cases of poisoning by organic salts of tin. Rev Neurol Paris, **98**: 85–96.

Alda JO & Garay R (1990) Chloride (or bicarbonate)-dependent copper uptake through the anion exchanger in human red blood cells. Am J Physiol, **259**: C570–576.

Aldenberg T & Slob W (1991) Confidence limits for hazardous concentrations based on logistically distributed NOEC toxicity data. Bilthoven, National Institute for Public Health and the Environment (RIVM).

Alexander J (1993) Toxicity versus essentiality of chromium. Scand J Work Environ Health, **19**: 126–127.

Alfrey AC (1985) Gastrointestinal absorption of aluminum. Clin Nephrol, **24**(suppl 1): 84–87.

Ali I & Jain CK (2004) Advances in arsenic speciation techniques. Int J Environ Anal Chem, **84**: 947–964.

Allen HE & Hansen DJ (1996) The importance of trace metal speciation to water quality criteria. Water Environ Res, **68**(1): 42–54.

Alsop DH & Wood CM (1999) Influence of waterborne cations on zinc uptake and toxicity in rainbow trout, Oncorhynchus mykiss. Can J Fish Aquat Sci, **56**: 2112–2119.

Alt F, Bambauer A, Hoppstock K, Mergler B & Tölg G (1993) Platinum traces in airborne particulate matter — determination of whole content, particle-size distribution and soluble platinum. Fresenius J Anal Chem, **346**: 693–696.

Alvarez-Llamas G, de la Campa MD & Sanz-Medel A (2005) ICP-MS for specific detection in capillary electrophoresis. Trends Anal Chem, **24**: 28–36.

Anard D, Kirsch-Volders M, Elhajouji A, Belpaeme K & Lison D (1997) In vitro genotoxic effects of hard metal particles assessed by alkaline single cell gel and elution assays. Carcinogenesis, **18**: 177–184.

Anderson RA (1986) Chromium metabolism and its role in disease processes in man. Clin Physiol Biochem, **4**: 31–41.

Anderson RA, Polansky MM, Bryden NA, Patterson, KY, Veillon C & Glinsman WH (1983) Effects of chromium supplementation on urinary Cr excretion of human subjects and correlation of Cr excretion with selected clinical parameters. J Nutr, **113**: 276–281.

Andre N, Paut O, Arditti J, Fabre P, Bremond V, Alhmana T, Bellus JF, Jouglard J & Camboulives J (1998) Severe potassium dichromate poisoning after accidental nasal introduction. Arch Pediatr, **5**: 145–148.

Ankley GT, Phipps GL, Leonard EN, Benoit DA, Mattson VR, Koslan PA, Cotter AM, Dierkes JR, Hansen DJ & Mahony JD (1991) Acid volatile sulfide as a factor mediating cadmium and nickel bioavailability in contaminated sediments. Environ Toxicol Chem, **10**: 1299–1308.

Antman KH (2001) Introduction: the history of arsenic trioxide in cancer therapy. Oncologist, **6**(suppl 2): 1–2.

Anttila A, Pukkala E, Aitio A, Rantanen T & Karjalainen S (1998) Update of cancer incidence among workers at a copper/nickel smelter and nickel refinery. Int Arch Occup Environ Health, **71**: 245–250.

Aoyagi S & Baker DH (1994) Copper–amino acid complexes are partially protected against inhibitory effects of L-cysteine and L-ascorbic acid on copper absorption in chicks. J Nutr, **124**: 388–395.

Aposhian HV, Zakharyan RA, Avram MD, Kopplin MJ & Wollenberg ML (2003) Oxidation and detoxification of trivalent arsenic species. Toxicol Appl Pharmacol, **193**: 1–8.

Apostoli P (1997) Element speciation in biological monitoring. Int Arch Occup Environ Health, **69**: 369–371.

Apostoli P (1999) The role of element speciation in environmental and occupational medicine. Fresenius J Anal Chem, **363**: 499–504.

Apostoli P, Romeo L, Buchet J-P & Alessio L (1997) Metabolism of arsenic after acute occupational arsine intoxication. J Toxicol Environ Health, **52**: 331–342.

Apostoli P, Bartoli D, Alessio L & Buchet JP (1999) Biological monitoring of occupational exposure to inorganic arsenic. Occup Environ Med, **56**: 1–7.

Apostoli P, Lucchini R & Alessio L (2000) Are current biomarkers suitable for the assessment of manganese exposure in individual workers? Am J Ind Med, **37**(3): 283–290.

Arakawa Y, Wada O & Yu TH (1981) Dealkylation and distribution of tin compounds. Toxicol Appl Pharmacol, **60**: 1–7.

Archibald FS & Tyree C (1987) Manganese poisoning and the attack of trivalent manganese upon catecholamines. Arch Biochem Biophys, **256**: 638–650.

Artik S, von Vultee C, Gleichmann E, Schwarz T & Griem P (1999) Nickel allergy in mice: enhanced sensitization capacity of nickel at higher oxidation states. J Immunol, **163**: 1143–1152.

Artiola JF (2005) Speciation of copper in the environment. In: Cornelis R, Crews H, Caruso J & Heumann KG eds. Handbook of elemental speciation II. Species in the environment, food, medicine and occupational health. Chichester, John Wiley & Sons, pp 174–186.

ATSDR (1999a) Toxicological profile for cadmium. Atlanta, Georgia, United States Department of Health and Human Services, Public Health Service, Agency for Toxic Substances and Disease Registry.

ATSDR (1999b) Toxicological profile for mercury. Atlanta, Georgia, United States Department of Health and Human Services, Public Health Service, Agency for Toxic Substances and Disease Registry.

ATSDR (2000) Toxicological profile for chromium. Atlanta, Georgia, United States Department of Health and Human Services, Public Health Service, Agency for Toxic Substances and Disease Registry.

ATSDR (2003a) Toxicological profile for selenium. Atlanta, Georgia, United States Department of Health and Human Services, Public Health Service, Agency for Toxic Substances and Disease Registry.

ATSDR (2003b) Draft toxicological profile for nickel. Atlanta, Georgia, United States Department of Health and Human Services, Public Health Service, Agency for Toxic Substances and Disease Registry.

ATSDR (2004) Toxicological profile for cobalt. Atlanta, Georgia, United States Department of Health and Human Services, Public Health Service, Agency for Toxic Substances and Disease Registry.

ATSDR (2005a) Toxicological profile for arsenic (draft for public comment). Atlanta, Georgia, United States Department of Health and Human Services, Public Health Service, Agency for Toxic Substances and Disease Registry.

ATSDR (2005b) Toxicological profile for lead. Atlanta, Georgia, United States Department of Health and Human Services, Public Health Service, Agency for Toxic Substances and Disease Registry.

Baes CF & Mesmer RE (1986) The hydrolysis of cations. Malabar, Florida, Robert E. Krieger Publishing.

Bagchi D, Stohs SJ, Downs BW, Bagchi M & Preuss HG (2002) Cytotoxicity and oxidative mechanisms of different forms of chromium. Toxicology, **180**: 5–22.

Baker D & Czarnecki-Maulden G (1987) Pharmacologic role of cysteine in ameliorating or exacerbating mineral toxicities. J Nutr, **117**: 1003–1010.

Baker DB, Gann PGH & Brooks SM (1990) Cross-sectional study of platinum salts sensitization among precious metals refinery workers. Am J Ind Med, **18**: 653–664.

Ballatori N (2002) Transport of toxic metals by molecular mimicry. Environ Health Perspect, **110**(suppl 5): 689–694.

Ballatori N & Clarkson TW (1982) Developmental changes in the biliary excretion of methylmercury and glutathione. Science, **216**: 61–63.

Balmes JR (1987) Respiratory effects of hard-metal dust exposure. Occup Med, **2**: 327–344.

Barats MS, Gonick HC, Rothenberg S, Balabanian M & Manton WI (2000) Severe lead-induced peripheral neuropathy in a dialysis patient. Am J Kidney Dis, **35**: 963–968.

Barceloux DG (1999) Cobalt. J Toxicol Clin Toxicol, **37**: 201–216.

Barlett RJ & James BR (1991) Skin permeation and cutaneous hypersensitivity as the basis for making risk assessments of chromium as a soil contaminant. Environ Health Perspect, **92**: 111–119.

Barltrop D & Meek F (1979) Effect of particle size on lead absorption from the gut. Arch Environ Health, **34**: 280–285.

Barrow L & Tanner MS (1988) Copper distribution among serum proteins in paediatric liver disorders and malignancies. Eur J Clin Invest, **18**: 555–560.

Bartsch H (2000) Studies on biomarkers in cancer etiology and prevention: a summary and challenge of 20 years interdisciplinary research. Mutat Res, **462**: 255–279.

Baselt R & Cravey R (1995) Disposition of toxic drugs and chemicals in man, 4th ed. Chicago, Illinois, Year Book Medical Publishers.

Basu N, Stamler CJ, Loua KM & Chan HM (2005) An interspecies comparison of mercury inhibition on muscarinic acetylcholine receptor binding in the cerebral cortex and cerebellum. Toxicol Appl Pharmacol, **205**: 71–76.

Baxter PJ, Adams PH, Aw T-C, Cockroft A & Harrington JM (2000) Hunter's diseases of occupations, 9th ed. London, Arnold.

Behne D & Kyriakopoulos A (2001) Mammalian selenium-containing proteins. Annu Rev Nutr, **21**: 453–473.

Beliles RP (1994) The metals. In: Clayton GD & Clayton FE eds. Patty's industrial hygiene and toxicology, 4th ed. Vol. II, Part C. New York, John Wiley & Sons, pp 1879–2352.

Bentley R & Chasteen TG (2002) Microbial methylation of metalloids: arsenic, antimony, and bismuth. Microbiol Mol Biol Rev, **66**: 250–271.

Bergdahl IA & Skerfving S (1997) Partition of circulating lead between plasma and red cells does not seem to be different for internal and external sources of lead. Am J Ind Med, **32**(3): 317–318.

Bergman HL & Dorward-King EJ (1997) Reassessment of metals criteria for aquatic life protection. Pensacola, Florida, SETAC Press.

Berlin M & Johansson LG (1964) Mercury in mouse brain after inhalation of mercury vapor and after intravenous injection of mercury salt. Nature, **204**: 85–86.

Berlin M & Ullberg S (1963) Accumulation and retention of mercury in the mouse. I. An autoradiographic study after a single intravenous injection of mercuric chloride. Arch Environ Health, **6**: 589–601.

Berlin M, Fazackerley J & Nordberg G (1969) The uptake of mercury in the brains of mammals exposed to mercury vapor and to mercuric salts. Arch Environ Health, **18**: 719–729.

Berlin MH, Nordberg GF & Serenius F (1986) On the site and mechanism of mercury vapor resorption in the lung. A study in the guinea pig using mercuric nitrate Hg 203. Arch Environ Health, **18**: 42–50.

Bernard A & Lauwerys R (1986) Effects of cadmium exposure in man. In: Foulkes EC ed. Handbook of experimental pharmacology. Vol. 80. Cadmium. Berlin, Springer-Verlag, pp 135–177.

Bernstam L, Lan CH, Lee J & Nriagu JO (2002) Effects of arsenic on human keratinocytes: morphological, physiological, and precursor incorporation studies. Environ Res, **89**(3): 220–235.

Bernstein IL, Chan-Yeung M, Malo J-L & Bernstein DI eds (1999) Asthma in the workplace, 2nd ed. New York, Marcel Dekker.

Besser JM, Ingersoll CG & Giesy JP (1996) Effects of spatial and temporal variation of acid-volatile sulfide on the bioavailability of copper and zinc in freshwater sediments. Environ Toxicol Chem, **15**(3): 286–293.

Besser R, Kramer G, Thumler R, Bohl J, Gutmann L & Hopf HC (1987) Acute trimethyltin limbic-cerebellar syndrome. Neurology, **37**: 945–950.

Bettley FR & O'Shea JA (1975) The absorption of arsenic and its relation to carcinoma. Br J Dermatol, **92**: 563–568.

B'Hymer C & Caruso JA (2004) Arsenic and its speciation analysis using high-performance liquid chromatography and inductively coupled plasma mass spectrometry. J Chromatogr A, **1045**: 1–13.

Block M & Glynn AW (1992) Influence of xanthates on the uptake of [109]Cd by Eurasian dace (*Phoxinus phoxinus*) and the rainbow trout (*Oncorhynchus mykiss*). Environ Toxicol Chem, **11**: 873–879.

Bluhm RE, Breyer JA, Bobbitt RG, Welch LW, Wood AJ & Branch RA (1992) Elemental mercury vapour toxicity, treatment, and prognosis after acute, intensive exposure in chloralkali plant workers. Part II: Hyperchloraemia and genitourinary symptoms. Hum Exp Toxicol, **11**: 211–215.

Booker DV, Chamberlain AC & Newton D (1969) Uptake of radio-active lead following inhalation and injection. Br J Radiol, **42**: 457–466.

Bouyssiere B, Szpunar J, Potin-Gautier M & Lobinski R (2003) Sample preparation techniques for elemental speciation studies. In: Cornelis R, Crews H, Caruso J & Heumann KG eds. Handbook of elemental speciation I. Techniques and methodology. Chichester, John Wiley & Sons, pp 95–118.

Brandi G, Pantaleo MA, Galli C, Falcone A, Antonuzzo A, Mordenti P, Di Marco MC & Biasco G (2003) Hypersensitivity reactions related to oxaliplatin (OHP). Br J Cancer, **89**: 477–481.

Brereton P, Macarthur R & Crews HM (2003) Food: Sampling with special reference to legislation, uncertainty and fitness for purpose. In: Cornelis R, Crews H, Caruso J & Heumann KG eds. Handbook of elemental speciation I. Techniques and methodology. Chichester, John Wiley & Sons, pp 47–58.

Bress WC & Bidanset JH (1991) Percutaneous in vivo and in vitro absorption of lead. Vet Hum Toxicol, **33**(3): 212–214.

Bruland KW (1989) Complexation of zinc by natural organic ligands in the central north Pacific. Limnol Oceanogr, **34**: 269–285.

Bucher JR, Hailey JR, Roycroft JR, Haseman JK, Sills RC, Grumbein SL, Mellick PW & Chou BJ (1999) Inhalation toxicity and carcinogenicity studies of cobalt sulfate. Toxicol Sci, **49**: 56–67.

Buchet JP (2005) Arsenic speciation in human tissues. In: Cornelis R, Caruso J, Crews H & Heumann KG eds. Handbook of elemental speciation II. Species in the environment, food, medicine and occupational health. Chichester, John Wiley & Sons, pp 86–93.

Buchet JP & Lauwerys R (1985) Study of inorganic arsenic methylation by rat liver in vitro: relevance for the interpretation of observations in man. Arch Toxicol, **57**: 125–129.

Buchet JP, Lauwerys R & Roels H (1981a) Urinary excretion of inorganic arsenic and its metabolites after repeated ingestion of sodium metaarsenite by volunteers. Int Arch Occup Environ Health, **48**: 111–118.

Buchet JP, Lauwerys R & Roels H (1981b) Comparison of the urinary excretion of arsenic metabolites after a single oral dose of sodium arsenite, monomethylarsonate, or dimethylarsinate in man. Int Arch Occup Environ Health, **48**: 71–79.

Buchet JP, Lauwerys R & Yager JW (1995) Lung retention and bio-availability of arsenic after single intratracheal administration of sodium arsenite, sodium arsenate, fly ash and copper smelter dust in the hamster. Environ Geochem Health, **17**: 182–188.

Budz-Jørgensen E, Grandjean P, Jørgensen PJ, Weihe P & Keiding N (2004) Association between mercury concentrations in blood and hair in methylmercury-exposed subjects at different ages. Environ Res, **95**: 385–393.

Bunker VW, Lawson MS, Delves HT & Clayton BE (1984) The uptake and excretion of chromium by the elderly. Am J Clin Nutr, **39**: 797–802.

Burgess WA (1995) Recognition of health hazards in industry. New York, Wiley.

Burns TM, Shneker BF & Juel VC (2001) Gasoline sniffing multifocal neuropathy. Pediatr Neurol, **25**: 419–421.

Burrows D ed. (1983) Chromium: metabolism and toxicity. Boca Raton, Florida, CRC Press, 172 pp.

Byard RW & Couper R (1998) Death after exposure to dimethylmercury. N Engl J Med, **339**: 1243.

Byrne RH, Kump LR & Cantrell KJ (1988) The influence of temperature and pH on trace metal speciation in seawater. Mar Chem, **25**: 163–181.

Cairney S, Maruff P, Burns C & Currie B (2002) The neurobehavioural consequences of petrol (gasoline) sniffing. Neurosci Biobehav Rev, **26**: 81–89.

Cairney S, Maruff P, Burns CB, Currie J & Currie BJ (2004) Neurological and cognitive impairment associated with leaded gasoline encephalopathy. Drug Alcohol Depend, **73**: 183–188.

Cairney S, Maruff P, Burns CB, Currie J & Currie BJ (2005) Neurological and cognitive recovery following abstinence from petrol sniffing. Neuropsychopharmacology, **30**(5): 1019–1027.

Cairo G & Pietrangelo A (2000) Iron regulatory proteins in pathobiology. Biochem J, **352**: 241–250.

Calne DB, Chu NS, Huang CC, Lu CS & Olanow W (1994) Manganism and idiopathic parkinsonism: similarities and differences. Neurology, **44**: 1583–1586.

Calverley AE, Rees D, Dowdeswell RJ, Linnett PJ & Kielkowski D (1995) Platinum salt sensitivity in refinery workers — incidence and effects of smoking and exposure. Occup Environ Med, **52**: 661–666.

Campbell D, Gonzales M & Sullivan JB (1992) Mercury. In: Sullivan JB Jr & Krieger GR eds. Hazardous materials toxicology: clinical principles of environmental health. Baltimore, Maryland, Williams and Wilkins, pp 824–833.

Canfield DE & Thamdrup B (1994) The production of ^{34}S-depleted sulfide during bacterial disproportionation of elemental sulfur. Science, **266**: 1973–1975.

Carlson-Lynch H, Beck BD & Boardman PD (1994) Arsenic risk assessment. Environ Health Perspect, **102**: 354–356.

Catterall WA (1995) Structure and function of voltage-gated ion channels. Annu Rev Biochem, **64**: 493–531.

Catterall WA (2000) Structure and regulation of voltage-gated Ca^{2+} channels. Annu Rev Cell Dev Biol, **16**: 521–555.

Cedar H & Razin A (1990) DNA methylation and development. Biochim Biophys Acta, **1049**: 1–8.

Centers for Disease Control and Prevention (2003) Barium toxicity after exposure to contaminated contrast solution — Goias State, Brazil. Morb Mortal Wkly Rep, **52**: 1047–1048.

Ceulemans M, Lobinski R, Dirkx WMR & Adams FC (1993) Rapid sensitive speciation analysis of butyltin and phenyltin compounds in water by capillary gas-chromatography atomic-emission spectrometry (GC-AES) after in-situ ethylation and in-liner preconcentration. Fresenius J Anal Chem, **347**: 256–262.

Chamberlain AC (1985) Prediction of response of blood lead to airborne and dietary lead from volunteer experiments with lead isotopes. Proc R Soc Lond B Biol Sci, **224**(1235): 149–182.

Chamberlain AC, Clough WS, Heard MJ, Newton D, Stott AN & Wells AC (1975) Uptake of lead by inhalation of motor exhaust. Proc R Soc Lond B Biol Sci, **192**(1106): 77–110.

Chaney RL (1988) Metal speciation and interaction among elements affect trace element transfer in agricultural and environmental food-chains. In: Kramer JR & Allen HE eds. Metal speciation: theory, analysis, and application. Boca Raton, Florida, Lewis Publishers, pp 219–259.

Charleston JS, Body RL, Bolender RP, Mottet NK, Vahter ME & Burbacher TM (1996) Changes in the number of astrocytes and microglia in the thalamus of the monkey *Macaca fascicularis* following long-term subclinical methylmercury exposure. Neurotoxicology, **17**: 127–138.

Chassaigne H (2003) Electrospray method for elemental analysis. In: Cornelis R, Crews H, Caruso J & Heumann KG eds. Handbook of elemental speciation I. Techniques and methodology. Chichester, John Wiley & Sons, pp 356–377.

Chassaigne H, Chéry CC, Bordin G, Vanhaecke F & Rodriguez AR (2004) 2-Dimensional gel electrophoresis technique for yeast selenium-containing proteins — sample preparation and MS approaches for processing 2-D gel protein spots. J Anal At Spectrom, **19**: 85–95.

Chen JY, Tsao GC, Zhao Q & Zheng W (2001) Differential cytotoxicity of Mn(II) and Mn(III): special reference to mitochondrial [Fe-S] containing enzymes. Toxicol Appl Pharmacol, **175**: 160–168.

Cherian MG & Chan HM (1993) Biological functions of metallothionein — a review. In: Suzuki T, Imura N & Kimura M eds. Metallothionein III: biological roles and medical implications. Basel, Birkhauser, pp 87–109.

Chéry CC (2003) Gel electrophoresis for speciation purposes. In: Cornelis R, Crews H, Caruso J & Heumann KG eds. Handbook of elemental speciation I. Techniques and methodology. Chichester, John Wiley & Sons, pp 224–239.

Chéry CC, Dumont E, Cornelis R & Moens L (2001) Two-dimensional gel electrophoresis of selenized yeast and autoradiography of Se-75-containing proteins. Fresenius J Anal Chem, **371**: 775–781.

Chéry CC, Chassaigne H, Verbeeck L, Cornelis R, Vanhaecke F & Moens L (2002) Detection and quantification of selenium in proteins by means of gel electrophoresis and electrothermal vaporization ICP-MS. J Anal At Spectrom, **17**: 576–580.

Chéry CC, Dumont E, Moens L, Vanhaecke F & Cornelis R (2005) Influence of reducing agents on the integrity of selenocompounds. Exploratory work for selenoproteome analysis. J Anal At Spectrom, **20**: 118–120.

Chia SE, Foo SC, Gan SL, Jeyaratnam J & Tian CS (1993) Neurobehavioral functions among workers exposed to manganese ore. Scand J Work Environ Health, **19**: 264–270.

Chiappino G (1994) Hard metal disease: clinical aspects. Sci Total Environ, **150**(1–3): 65–68.

Choudhury H, Harvey T, Thayer WC, Lockwood TF, Stiteler W, Goodrum PE, Hassett JM & Diamond G (2001) Urinary cadmium elimination as a biomarker of exposure for evaluating a cadmium dietary exposure — biokinetics model. J Toxicol Environ Health A, **63**(5): 321–350.

Christensen JM, Byrialsen K, Vercoutere K, Cornelis R & Quevauviller P (1999) Certification of Cr(VI) and total leachable Cr contents in welding dust loaded on a filter (CRM 545). Fresenius J Anal Chem, **363**: 28–32.

Chu CC, Huang CC, Ryu SJ & Wu TN (1998) Chronic inorganic mercury induced peripheral neuropathy. Acta Neurol Scand, **98**: 461–465.

Cinca I, Dumitrescu I, Onaca P, Serbanescu A & Nestorescu B (1980) Accidental ethyl mercury poisoning with nervous system, skeletal muscle, and myocardium injury. J Neurol Neurosurg Psychiatry, **43**: 143–149.

Clarkson T (1991) Methylmercury. Fundam Appl Toxicol, **16**: 20–21.

Clarkson TW (1979) Effects — General principles underlying the toxic action of metals. In: Friberg L, Nordberg GF & Vouk V eds. Handbook on the toxicology of metals. Vol. 1. Amsterdam, Elsevier/North-Holland Biomedical Press, pp 99–117.

Clarkson TW (1993) Molecular and ionic mimicry of toxic metals. Annu Rev Pharmacol Toxicol, **33**: 545–571.

Clarkson TW (1994) The toxicology of mercury and its compounds. In: Watras CJ & Huchabee JW eds. Mercury pollution: integration and synthesis. Boca Raton, Florida, Lewis Publishers, pp 631–643.

Clarkson TW (2002) The three modern faces of mercury. Environ Health Perspect, **110**(suppl 1): 11–23.

Clarkson TW, Magos L & Greenwood MR (1972) The transport of elemental mercury into fetal tissues. Biol Neonate, **21**: 239–244.

Clarkson TW, Hursh JB, Sager PR & Syversen TLM (1988) Mercury. In: Clarkson TW, Friberg L, Nordberg GF & Sager PR eds. Biological monitoring of toxic metals. New York, Plenum Press, pp 199–246.

Clary JJ (1975) Nickel chloride–induced metabolic changes in the rat and guinea pig. Toxicol Appl Pharmacol, **31**: 55–65.

Cleare MJ, Hughes EG, Jacoby B & Pepys J (1976) Immediate (type I) allergic responses to platinum compounds. Clin Allergy, **6**: 183–195.

Coale KH & Bruland KW (1988) Copper complexation in the northeast Pacific. Limnol Oceanogr, **33**: 1084–1101.

Coale KH & Bruland KW (1990) Spatial and temporal variability in copper complexation in the north Pacific. Deep Sea Res A, **37**: 317–336.

Cohen SM, Arnold LL, Uzvolgyi E, Cano M, St John M, Yamamoto S, Lu X & Le XC (2002) Possible role of dimethylarsinous acid in dimethylarsinic acid–induced urothelial toxicity and regeneration in the rat. Chem Res Toxicol, **15**: 1150–1157.

Cornelis R, Heinzow B, Herber RFM, Christensen JM, Paulsen OM, Sabbioni E, Templeton DM, Thomassen Y, Vahter M & Vesterberg O (1996) Sample collection guidelines for trace-elements in blood and urine. J Trace Elem Med Biol, **10**: 103–127.

Cornelis R, De Kimpe J & Zhang X (1998) Trace elements in clinical samples revisited — separation is knocking at the door. Sample preparation, separation of the species and measurement methods. Spectrochim Acta B, **53**: 187–196.

Cornelis R, Crews H, Donard OXF, Ebdon L & Quevauviller P (2001) Trends in certified reference materials for the speciation of trace elements. Fresenius J Anal Chem, **370**: 120–125.

Cornelis R, Crews H, Caruso J & Heumann KG eds (2003) Handbook of elemental speciation I. Techniques and methodology. Chichester, John Wiley & Sons.

Cornelis R, Crews H, Caruso J & Heumann K eds (2005) Handbook of elemental speciation II. Species in the environment, food, medicine and occupational health. Chichester, John Wiley & Sons.

Cossa P, Duplay, Fischgold, Arfel Capd, Lafon, Passouant, Minvielle & Radermecker J (1958) [Toxic brain diseases caused by stalinon; anatomo-clinical and electroencephalographic aspects.] Rev Neurol, **98**: 97–108 (in French).

Cossa P, Duplay, Arfel Capd, Lafon, Passouant, Minvielle & Radermecker J (1959) Toxic encephalopathy caused by stalinon; anatomoclinical & EEG aspects. Acta Neurol Psychiatr Belg, **59**: 281–303.

Counter SA, Buchanan LH & Ortega F (2005) Neurocognitive impairment in lead-exposed children of Andean lead-glazing workers. J Occup Environ Med, **47**: 306–312.

Couper J (1837) On the effects of black oxide of manganese when inhaled into the lungs. Br Ann Med Pharmacol, **1**: 41–42.

Crecelius EA (1977) Changes in the chemical speciation of arsenic following ingestion by man. Environ Health Perspect, **19**: 147–150.

Crews H (2005) Speciation of lead in food and wine. In: Cornelis R, Crews H, Caruso J & Heumann KG eds. Handbook of elemental speciation II. Species in the environment, food, medicine and occupational health. Chichester, John Wiley & Sons, pp 247–251.

Cristaudo A, Sera F, Severino V, De Rocco M, Di Lella E & Picardo M (2005) Occupational hypersensitivity to metal salts, including platinum, in the secondary industry. Allergy, **60**:159–164.

Croot PL, Karlson B, van Elteren JT & Kroon JJ (1999) Uptake of ^{64}Cu-oxine by marine phytoplankton. Environ Sci Technol, **33**: 3615–3621.

Crossgrove JS, Allen DD, Bukaveckas BL, Rhineheimer SS & Yokel RA (2003) Manganese distribution across the blood–brain barrier. I. Evidence for carrier-mediated influx of manganese citrate as well as manganese and manganese transferrin. Neurotoxicology, **24**: 3–13.

Cugell DW (1992) The hard metal diseases. Clin Chest Med, **13**: 269–279.

Czerczak S & Gromiec J (2001) Nickel, ruthenium, rhodium, palladium, osmium, and platinum. In: Bingham E, Cohrssen B & Powell CH eds. Patty's toxicology. Vol. 3. New York, John Wiley & Sons, pp 195–380.

Dabek-Zlotorzynska E & Keppel-Jones K (2003) Sampling: collection, storage — occupational health. In: Cornelis R, Crews H, Caruso J & Heumann KG eds. Handbook of elemental speciation I. Techniques and methodology. Chichester, John Wiley & Sons, pp 59–72.

Dabrio M, Rodriguez AR, Bordin G, Bebianno MJ, De Ley M, Šestáková I, Vašák M & Nordberg M (2002) Recent developments in quantification methods for metallothionein. J Inorg Biochem, **88**: 123–134.

Daenen M, Rogiers P, Van de Walle C, Rochette F, Demedts M & Nemery B (1999) Occupational asthma caused by palladium. Eur Respir J, **13**: 213–216.

Dagle GE, Cannon WC, Stevens DL & McShane JF (1983) Comparative disposition of inhaled ^{238}Pu and ^{239}Pu nitrates in beagles. Health Phys, **44**: 275–277.

Daintith J ed. (2004) A dictionary of chemistry. Oxford, Oxford University Press.

Dally H & Hartwig A (1997) Induction and repair inhibition of oxidative DNA damage by nickel(II) and cadmium(II) in mammalian cells. Carcinogenesis, **18**: 1021–1026.

Danielsson B, Hassoun E & Denker L (1982) Embryotoxicity of chromium: distribution in pregnant mice and effects on embryonic cells in vitro. Arch Toxicol, **51**: 233–245.

Danscher G (1981) Light and electron microscopic localization of silver in biological tissue. Histochemistry, **71**: 177–186.

Das KK & Dasgupta S (1997) Alteration of testicular biochemistry during protein restriction in nickel treated rats. Biol Trace Elem Res, **60**: 243–249.

Das KK & Dasgupta S (2000) Effect of nickel on testicular nucleic acid concentrations of rats on protein restriction. Biol Trace Elem Res, **73**: 175–180.

Das KK & Dasgupta S (2002) Effect of nickel sulfate on testicular steroidogenesis in rats during protein restriction. Environ Health Perspect, **110**: 923–926.

Davidson T, Kluz T, Burns F, Rossman T, Zhang Q, Uddin A, Nadas A & Costa M (2004) Exposure to chromium (VI) in the drinking water increases susceptibility to UV-induced skin tumors in hairless mice. Toxicol Appl Pharmacol, **196**: 431–437.

Davies JM, Easton DF & Bidstrup PL (1991) Mortality from respiratory cancer and other causes in United Kingdom chromate production workers. Br J Ind Med, **48**: 299–313.

Davis JM, Ruby MV & Bergstrom PD (1994) Factors controlling lead bio-availability in the Butte mining district, Montana, USA. Environ Geochem Health, **16**: 147–157.

De Boeck M, Lison D & Kirsch-Volders M (1998) Evaluation of the in vitro direct and indirect genotoxic effects of cobalt compounds using the alkaline comet assay. Influence of interdonor and interexperimental variability. Carcinogenesis, **19**: 2021–2029.

De Boeck M, Lombaert N, De Backer S, Finsy R, Lison D & Kirsch-Volders M (2003) In vitro genotoxic effects of different combinations of cobalt and metallic carbide particles. Mutagenesis, **18**: 177–186.

De Cremer K (2003) Sampling of clinical samples: collection and storage. In: Cornelis R, Crews H, Caruso J & Heumann KG eds. Handbook of elemental speciation I. Techniques and methodology. Chichester, John Wiley & Sons, pp 23–46.

De Flora S, Bagnasco M, Serra D & Zanacchi P (1990) Genotoxicity of chromium compounds. A review. Mutat Res, **238**: 99–172.

Deleu D, Hanssens Y, al Salmy HS & Hastie I (1998) Peripheral polyneuropathy due to chronic use of topical ammoniated mercury. J Toxicol Clin Toxicol, **36**: 233–237.

Demedts M, Gheysens B, Nagels J, Verbeken E, Lauweryns J, Van den Eeckhout A, Lahaye D & Gyselen A (1984) Cobalt lung in diamond polishers. Am Rev Respir Dis, **130**: 130–135.

De Schamphelaere KAC, Heijerick DG & Jannsen CR (2002) Refinement and field validation of a biotic ligand model predicting acute copper toxicity to *Daphnia magna*. Comp Biochem Physiol C Pharmacol Toxicol Endocrinol, **133**: 243–258.

Desilva PE (1981) Determination of lead in plasma and studies on its relationship to lead in erythrocytes. Br J Ind Med, **38**(3): 209–217.

De Vevey E, Bitton G, Rossel D, Ramos LD, Guerrero LM & Tarradellas J (1993) Concentration and bioavailability of heavy metals in sediments in Lake Yojoa (Honduras). Bull Environ Contam Toxicol, **50**(2): 253–259.

Diaz RS & Monreal J (1994) Thallium mediates a rapid chloride/hydroxyl ion exchange through myelin lipid bilayers. Mol Pharmacol, **46**: 1210–1216.

Di Toro DM, Mahoney JD, Hansen DJ, Scott KJ, Hicks MB, Mayr SM & Redmond MS (1990) Toxicity of cadmium in sediments: the role of acid volatile sulfide. Environ Toxicol Chem, **9**: 1487–1502.

Di Toro DM, Zarba CS, Hansen DJ, Berry WJ, Swarz RC, Cowan CE, Pavlou SP, Allen HE, Thomas NA & Paquin PR (1991) Technical basis for the equilibrium partitioning method for establishing sediment quality criteria. Environ Toxicol Chem, **10**: 1541–1584.

Di Toro DM, Allen HE, Bergman HL, Meyer JS, Paquin PR & Santore RC (2001) Biotic ligand model of the acute toxicity of metals. 1. Technical basis. Environ Toxicol Chem, **20**: 2383–2396.

Dizdaroglu M (1991) Chemical determination of free radical–induced damage to DNA. Free Radic Biol Med, **10**: 225–242.

Dizdaroglu M (1992) Oxidative damage to DNA in mammalian chromatin. Mutat Res, **275**: 331–342.

Dizdaroglu M, Rao G, Halliwell B & Gajewski E (1991) Damage to the DNA bases in mammalian chromatin by hydrogen peroxide in the presence of ferric and cupric ions. Arch Biochem Biophys, **285**: 317–324.

Doll R, Morgan LG & Speizer FE (1970) Cancers of the lung and nasal sinuses in nickel workers. Br J Cancer, **24**: 623–632.

Donaldson RM & Barreras RF (1966) Intestinal absorption of trace quantities of chromium. J Lab Clin Med, **68**: 484–493.

Donat JR & Bruland KW (1990) A comparison of two voltammetric techniques for determining zinc speciation in northeast Pacific Ocean waters. Mar Chem, **28**: 301–323.

Dorman DC, Struve MF, James RA, Marshall MW, Parkinson CU & Wong BA (2001a) Influence of particle solubility on the delivery of inhaled manganese to the rat brain: manganese sulfate and manganese tetroxide pharmacokinetics following repeated (14-day) exposure. Toxicol Appl Pharmacol, **170**: 79–87.

Dorman DC, Struve MF, James RA, McManus BE, Marshall MW & Wong BA (2001b) Influence of dietary manganese on the pharmacokinetics of inhaled manganese sulfate in male CD rats. Toxicol Sci, **60**: 242–251.

Dorman DC, Brenneman KA, McElveen AM, Lynch SE, Roberts KC & Wong BA (2002a) Olfactory transport: a direct route of delivery of inhaled manganese phosphate to the rat brain. J Toxicol Environ Health A, **65**: 1493–1511.

Dorman DC, Struve MF & Wong BA (2002b) Brain manganese concentrations in rats following manganese tetroxide inhalation are unaffected by dietary manganese intake. Neurotoxicology, **23**: 185–195.

Downs JC, Milling D & Nichols CA (1995) Suicidal ingestion of barium-sulfide-containing shaving powder. Am J Forensic Med Pathol, **16**: 56–61.

Draper MH (1997) A re-assessment of respiratory cancers at the Clydach nickel refinery: new evidence of causation. In: Duffus JH ed. Carcinogenicity of inorganic substances — risks from occupational exposure. Cambridge, Royal Society of Chemistry, p 181.

Driscoll KE, Carter JM, Howard BW & Hassenbein DG (1994) Mutagenesis in rat lung epithelial cells after in vivo silica exposure or ex vivo exposure to inflammatory cells. Am J Respir Crit Care Med, **149**: A553.

Duffus JH (1993) Glossary for chemists of terms used in toxicology (IUPAC recommendations 1993). Pure Appl Chem, **65**: 2003–2122.

Duffus JH (1996) Epidemiology and the identification of metals as human carcinogens. Sci Prog, **79**: 311–326.

Duffus JH (2001) Risk assessment and trace element speciation. In: Ebdon L, Pitts L, Cornelis R, Crews H, Donard OFX & Quevauviller P eds. Trace element speciation for environment, food and health. Cambridge, Royal Society of Chemistry, pp 354–372.

Dunn JD, Clarkson TW & Magos L (1981) Ethanol reveals novel mercury detoxification step in tissues. Science, **213**: 1123–1125.

Dunnick JK, Elwell MR, Radovsky AE, Benson JM, Hahn FF, Nikula KJ, Barr EB & Hobbs CH (1995) Comparative carcinogenic effects of nickel subsulfide, nickel oxide, or nickel sulfate hexahydrate chronic exposures in the lung. Cancer Res, **55**: 5251–5256.

Dyall-Smith DJ & Scurry JP (1990) Mercury pigmentation and high mercury levels from the use of a cosmetic cream. Med J Aust, **153**: 409–410, 414–415.

Dyg S, Cornelis R, Griepink B & Quevauviller P (1994) Development and interlaboratory testing of aqueous and lyophilized Cr(III) and Cr(VI) reference materials. Anal Chim Acta, **286**: 297–308.

Ebdon L, Pitts L, Cornelis R, Crews H, Donard OXF & Quevauviller P eds (2001) Trace element speciation for environment, food and health. Cambridge, Royal Society of Chemistry.

Elinder CG & Nordberg M (1985) Metallothionein. In: Friberg L, Elinder CG, Kjellström T & Nordberg GF eds. Cadmium and health. Vol. I. Boca Raton, Florida, CRC Press, pp 65–79.

Emons H (2003) Sampling: collection, processing and storage of environmental samples. In: Cornelis R, Crews H, Caruso J & Heumann KG eds. Handbook of elemental speciation I. Techniques and methodology. Chichester, John Wiley & Sons, pp 7–22.

Emteborg H, Sinemus HW, Radziuk B, Baxter DC & Frech W (1996) Gas chromatography coupled with atomic absorption spectrometry — A sensitive instrumentation for mercury speciation. Spectrochim Acta B At Spectrosc, **51**: 829–837.

Emtestam L, Caerlsson B, Marcussin AJ, Wallin J & Moeller E (1989) Specificity of HLA restricting elements for human nickel reactive T cell clones. Tissue Antigens, **33**: 531–541.

Esaki N, Nakamura T, Tanaka H & Soda K (1982) Selenocysteine lyase, a novel enzyme that specifically acts on selenocysteine. Mammalian distribution and purification and properties of pig liver enzyme. J Biol Chem, **257**: 4386–4391.

Feldman RG (1999) Occupational and environmental neurotoxicology. Philadelphia, Pennsylvania, Lippincott-Raven.

Feldmann J (1997) Summary of a calibration method for the determination of volatile metal(loid) compounds in environmental gas samples by using gas chromatography inductively coupled plasma mass spectrometry. J Anal At Spectrom, **12**: 1069–1076.

Fenoglio I, Martra G, Prandi L, Tomatis M, Coluccia S & Fubini B (2000) The role of mechanochemistry in the pulmonary toxicity caused by particulate minerals. J Mater Synth Process, **8**: 145–153.

Ferraz HB, Bertolucci PH, Pereira JS, Lima JG & Andrade LA (1988) Chronic exposure to the fungicide maneb may produce symptoms and signs of CNS manganese intoxication. Neurology, **38**: 550–553.

Finley BL, Kerger BD, Katona MW, Gargas ML, Corbett GC & Paustenbach DJ (1997) Human ingestion of chromium (VI) in drinking water: pharmacokinetics following repeated exposure. Toxicol Appl Pharmacol, **142**(1): 151–159.

Fishman BE, McGinley PA & Gianutsos G (1987) Neurotoxic effects of methylcyclopentadienyl manganese tricarbonyl (MMT) in the mouse: basis of MMT-induced seizure activity. Toxicology, **45**: 193–201.

Flanagan PR, McLellan JS, Haist J, Cherian G, Chamberlain MJ & Valberg LS (1978) Increased dietary cadmium absorption in mice and human subjects with iron deficiency. Gastroenterology, **74**: 841–846.

Forbes JR, Hsi G & Cox DW (1999) Role of the copper-binding domain in the copper transport function of ATP7B, the P-type ATPase defective in Wilson disease. J Biol Chem, **274**: 12408–12413.

Forgacs Z, Paksy K, Lazar P & Tatrai E (1998) Effect of Ni^{2+} on the testosterone production of mouse primary Leydig cell culture. J Toxicol Environ Health A, **55**: 213–224.

Fortemps E, Amand G, Bomboir A, Lauwerys R & Laterre EC (1978) Trimethyltin poisoning. Report of two cases. Int Arch Occup Environ Health, **41**: 1–6.

Foulkes E (2001) Mercury. In: Bingham E, Cohrssen B & Powell C eds. Patty's toxicology. Vol. 2. New York, John Wiley & Sons, pp 327–352.

Fragueiro S, Lavilla I & Bendicho C (2004) Direct coupling of solid phase microextraction and quartz tube–atomic absorption spectrometry for selective and sensitive determination of methylmercury in seafood: an assessment of chloride and hydride generation. J Anal At Spectrom, **19**: 250–254.

Francesconi KA & Pannier F (2004) Selenium metabolites in urine: a critical overview of past work and current status. Clin Chem, **50**: 2240–2253.

Franchini I, Magnani F & Mutti A (1983) Mortality experience among chromeplating workers. Initial findings. Scand J Work Environ Health, **9**: 247–252.

Frausto da Silva JJR & Williams RJP (1991) The biological chemistry of the elements, 1st ed. Oxford, Oxford University Press.

Frausto da Silva JJR & Williams RJP (2001) The biological chemistry of the elements, 2nd ed. Oxford, Oxford University Press.

Freeman GB, Dill JA, Johnson JD, Kurtz PJ, Parham F & Matthews HB (1996) Comparative absorption of lead from contaminated soil and lead salts by weanling Fischer 344 rats. Fundam Appl Toxicol, **33**: 109–119.

Friberg L & Elinder CG (1993) Biological monitoring of toxic metals. Scand J Work Environ Health, **19**: 7–10.

Friberg L & Nordberg G (1973) Inorganic mercury — a toxicological and epidemiological appraisal. In: Miller MW & Clarkson TW eds. Mercury, mercurials and mercaptans. Springfield, Illinois, Charles C. Thomas, pp 5–22.

Fullerton A, Andersen JR, Hoelgaard A & Menne T (1986) Permeation of nickel salts through human skin in vitro. Contact Dermatitis, **15**: 173–177.

Galimov EM (1981) The biological fractionation of isotopes. London, Academic Press.

Galvan-Arzate S & Rios C (1994) Thallium distribution in organs and brain regions of developing rats. Toxicology, **90**: 63–69.

Galvan-Arzate S, Martinez A, Medina E, Santamaria A & Rios C (2000) Subchronic administration of sublethal doses of thallium to rats: effects on distribution and lipid peroxidation in brain regions. Toxicol Lett, **116**: 37–43.

Gammelgaard B, Fullerton A, Avnstorp C & Menné T (1992) Permeation of chromium salts through human skin in vitro. Contact Dermatitis, **27**: 302–310.

Gao M, Binks SP, Chipman JK, Levy LS, Braithwaite RA & Brown SS (1992) Induction of DNA strand breaks in peripheral lymphocytes by soluble chromium compounds. Hum Exp Toxicol, **11**: 77–82.

García Alonso JI & Encinar JR (2003) Gas chromatography and other gas based methods. In: Cornelis R, Crews H, Caruso J & Heumann KG eds. Handbook of elemental speciation I. Techniques and methodology. Chichester, John Wiley & Sons, pp 162–200.

Gargas ML, Norton RL, Paustenbach DJ & Finley BL (1994) Urinary excretion of chromium by humans following ingestion of chromium picolinate: implications of biomonitoring. Drug Metab Dispos, **22**(4): 522–529.

Garvey JS & Chang CC (1981) Detection of circulating metallothionein in rats injected with zinc or cadmium. Science, **214**: 805–807.

Gelaude I, Dams R, Resano M, Vanhaecke F & Moens L (2002) Direct determination of methylmercury and inorganic mercury in biological materials by solid sampling–electro-thermal vaporization–inductively coupled plasma–isotope dilution–mass spectrometry. Anal Chem, **74**: 3833–3842.

Geubel AP, Mairlot MC, Buchet JP & Lauwerys R (1988) Abnormal methylation capacity in human liver cirrhosis. Int J Clin Pharmacol Res, **8**: 117–122.

Gheysens B, Auwerx J, Van den Eeckhout A & Demedts M (1985) Cobalt-induced bronchial asthma in diamond polishers. Chest, **88**: 740–744.

Gianutsos G & Murray MT (1982) Alterations in brain dopamine and GABA following inorganic or organic manganese administration. Neurotoxicology, **3**: 75–81.

Gibb HJ, Lees PS, Pinsky PF & Rooney BC (2000) Lung cancer among workers in chromium chemical production. Am J Ind Med, **38**: 606.

Gibbons RA, Dixon SN, Hallis K, Russel AM, Sansom BF & Symonds HW (1976) Manganese metabolism in cows and goats. Biochim Biophys Acta, **444**: 1–10.

Gilani SH & Marano M (1980) Congenital abnormalities in nickel poisoning in chick embryos. Arch Environ Contam Toxicol, **9**: 17–22.

Gledhill M & van den Berg CMG (1994) Determination of complexation of iron(III) with natural organic complexing ligands in seawater using cathodic stripping voltammetry. Mar Chem, **47**: 41–54.

Gordon T & Fine JM (1993) Metal fume fever. Occup Med, **8**(3): 504–517.

Gosselin R & Smith R (1984) Clinical toxicology of commercial products. Baltimore, Maryland, Williams & Wilkins.

Graf E, Mahoney JR, Bryant RG & Eaton JW (1984) Iron-catalyzed hydroxyl radical formation: Stringent requirement for free iron coordination site. J Biol Chem, **259**: 3620–3624.

Grandjean P, Andersen O & Nielsen GD (1988) Carcinogenicity of occupational nickel exposures: an evaluation of the epidemiological evidence. Am J Ind Med, **13**: 193–209.

Grasseschi R, Rajanna B, Ramaswamy B, Levine D, Klaassen D & Wesselius L (2003) Cadmium accumulation and detoxification by alveolar macrophages of cigarette smokers. Chest, **124**(5): 1927–1928.

Gray C, Sivaloganathan S & Simpkins KC (1989) Aspiration of high-density barium contrast medium causing acute pulmonary inflammation — report of two fatal cases in elderly women with disordered swallowing. Clin Radiol, **40**: 397–400.

Greger JL & Baier MJ (1983) Excretion and retention of low or moderate levels of aluminium by human subjects. Food Chem Toxicol, **21**: 473–477.

Grimsley EW & Adams-Mount L (1994) Occupational lead intoxication: report of four cases. South Med J, **87**: 689–691.

Grimsrud TK, Berge SR, Haldorsen T & Andersen A (2005) Can lung cancer risk among nickel refinery workers be explained by occupational exposures other than nickel? Epidemiology, **16**: 146–154.

Grobler SR, Rossouw RJ & Kotze D (1988) Effect of airborne lead on the blood lead levels of rats. In: Griffin TB & Knelson JG eds. Lead. Stuttgart, Georg Thieme, pp 212–240.

Groopman JD & Kensler TW (1999) The light at the end of the tunnel for chemical specific biomarkers: daylight or headlight? Carcinogenesis, **20**: 1–11.

Grootveld M, Bell JD, Halliwell B, Aruoma OI, Bomford A & Sadler PJ (1989) Non-transferrin-bound iron in plasma or serum from patients with idiopathic hemochromatosis. Characterization by high performance liquid chromatography and nuclear magnetic resonance spectroscopy. J Biol Chem, **264**: 4417–4422.

Gross PR, Katz SA & Samitz MH (1968) Sensitization of guinea pigs to chromium salts. J Invest Dermatol, **50**: 424–427.

Gross SB (1981) Human oral and inhalation exposures to lead: summary of Kehoe balance experiments. J Toxicol Environ Health, **8**(3): 333–377.

Guenther K & Kastenholz B (2005a) Speciation of cadmium in the environment. In: Cornelis R, Crews H, Caruso J & Heumann KG eds. Handbook of elemental speciation II. Species in the environment, food, medicine and occupational health. Chichester, John Wiley & Sons, pp 94–106.

Guenther K & Kastenholz B (2005b) Speciation of zinc. In: Cornelis R, Crews H, Caruso J & Heumann KG eds. Handbook of elemental speciation II. Species in the environment, food, medicine and occupational health. Chichester, John Wiley & Sons, pp 489–508.

Gunshin H & Hediger MA (2002) The divalent metal-ion transporter (DCT1/DMT1/Nramp2). In: Templeton DM ed. Molecular and cellular iron transport. New York, Marcel Dekker, pp 155–173.

Gunshin H, Mackenzie B, Berger UV, Gunshin Y, Romero MF, Boron WF, Nussberger S, Gollan JL & Hediger MA (1997) Cloning and characterization of a mammalian proton-coupled metal-ion transporter. Nature, **388**: 482–488.

Gutknecht J (1981) Inorganic mercury (Hg^{2+}) transport through lipid bilayer membranes. J Membr Biol, **61**: 61–66.

Haber LT, Erdreicht L, Diamond GL, Maier AM, Ratney R, Zhao Q & Dourson ML (2000) Hazard identification and dose response of inhaled nickel-soluble salts. Regul Toxicol Pharmacol, **31**: 210–230.

Halbach S, Ballatori N & Clarkson TW (1988) Mercury vapor uptake and hydrogen peroxide detoxification in human and mouse red blood cells. Toxicol Appl Pharmacol, **96**(3): 517–524.

Halliwell B & Gutteridge JMC (1990) Role of free radicals and catalytic metal ions in human disease: An overview. Methods Enzymol, **186**: 1–88.

Hansen MB, Johansen JD & Menne T (2003) Chromium allergy: significance of both Cr(III) and Cr(VI). Contact Dermatitis, **49**: 206–212.

Harada M, Nakachi S, Tasaka K, Sakashita S, Muta K, Yanagida K, Doi R, Kizaki T & Ohno H (2001) Wide use of skin-lightening soap may cause mercury poisoning in Kenya. Sci Total Environ, **269**: 183–187.

Hare L & Tessier A (1996) Predicting animal cadmium concentrations in lakes. Nature, **380**: 430–432.

Harrington CF (2000) The speciation of mercury and organomercury compounds by using high-performance liquid chromatography. Trends Anal Chem, **19**: 167–179.

Harrington CF, Eigendorf GK & Cullen WR (1996) The use of high-performance liquid chromatography for the speciation of organotin compounds. Appl Organomet Chem, **10**: 339–362.

Harris WR (2002) Iron chemistry. In: Templeton DM ed. Molecular and cellular iron transport. New York, Marcel Dekker, pp 1–40.

Harris WR & Chen Y (1994) Electron paramagnetic resonance and difference ultraviolet studies of Mn^{2+} binding to serum transferrin. J Inorg Biochem, **54**(1): 1–19.

Harrison GI & Morel FMM (1983) Antagonism between cadmium and iron in the marine diatom *Thalassiosira weissflogii*. J Phycol, **19**: 495–507.

Harrison PM & Arosio P (1996) Ferritins: molecular properties, iron storage function and cellular regulation. Biochim Biophys Acta, **1275**: 161–203.

Harry P, Mauras Y, Chennebault JM, Allain P & Alquier P (1984) [Acute renal failure following skin burns by chromic acid (chromium VI).] Presse Med, **13**: 2520 (in French).

Hart BA, Bertram PE & Scaife BD (1979) Cadmium transport by *Chlorella pyrenoidosa*. Environ Res, **18**: 327–335.

Hartmann M & Hartwig A (1998) Disturbance of DNA damage recognition after UV-irradiation by nickel(II) and cadmium(II) in mammalian cells. Carcinogenesis, **19**: 617–621.

Hartwig A (1994) Role of DNA repair inhibition in lead- and cadmium-induced genotoxicity: A review. Environ Health Perspect, **102**(suppl 3): 45–50.

Hartwig A, Snyder RD, Schlepegrell R & Beyersmann D (1991) Modulation by Co(II) of UV-induced DNA repair, mutagenesis and sister-chromatid exchanges in mammalian cells. Mutat Res, **248**: 177–185.

Hartwig A, Groblinghoff UD, Beyersmann D, Natarajan AT, Filon R & Mullenders LH (1997) Interaction of arsenic(III) with nucleotide excision repair in UV-irradiated human fibroblasts. Carcinogenesis, **18**: 399–405.

Hartwig A, Asmuss M, Ehleben I, Herzer U, Kostelac D, Pelzer A, Schwerdtle T & Burkle A (2002) Interference by toxic metal ions with DNA repair processes and cell cycle control: molecular mechanisms. Environ Health Perspect, **110**(suppl 5): 797–799.

Hay WJ, Rickards AG, McMenemey WH & Cumings JN (1963) Organic mercurial encephalopathy. J Neurol Neurosurg Psychiatry, **26**: 199–202.

Hayes KF & Traina SJ (1998) Metal ion speciation and its significance in ecosystem health. In: Huang PM ed. Soil chemistry and ecosystem health. Madison, Wisconsin, Soil Science Society of America, pp 46–83 (Special Publication No. 52).

Heijerick DG, de Schamphelaere KAC & Jannsen CR (2002) Biotic ligand model development predicting Zn toxicity to the alga *Pseudokirchneriella subcapitata*: possibilities and limitations. Comp Biochem Physiol C Pharmacol Toxicol Endocrinol, **133**: 207–218.

Heisterkamp M & Adams FC (1999) In situ propylation using sodium tetrapropylborate as a fast and simplified sample preparation for the speciation analysis of organolead compounds using GC-MIP-AES. J Anal At Spectrom, **14**: 1307–1311.

Hennecke J & Wiley DC (2001) T cell receptor–MHC interactions up close. Cell, **104**: 1–4.

Hesdorffer CS, Milne FJ, Terblanche J & Meyers AM (1986) Arsine gas poisoning: the importance of exchange transfusions in severe cases. Br J Ind Med, **43**: 353–355.

Heumann KG (2003) Calibration in elemental speciation analysis. In: Cornelis R, Crews H, Caruso J & Heumann KG eds. Handbook of elemental speciation I. Techniques and methodology. Chichester, John Wiley & Sons, pp 547–562.

Heumann KG (2004) Isotope-dilution ICP-MS for trace element determination and speciation: from a reference method to a routine method? Anal Bioanal Chem, **378**: 318–329.

Heumann KG (2005) Metal complexes of humic substances. In: Cornelis R, Crews H, Caruso J & Heumann KG eds. Handbook of elemental speciation II. Species in the environment, food, medicine and occupational health. Chichester, John Wiley & Sons, pp 621–637.

Hewitt CD, Herman MM, Lopes MB, Savory J & Wills MR (1991) Aluminium maltol-induced neurocytoskeletal changes in fetal rabbit midbrain in matrix culture. Neuropathol Applied Neurobiol, **17**: 47–60.

Hider RC (2002) Nature of nontransferrin-bound iron. Eur J Clin Invest, **32**(suppl 1): 50–54.

Hill S (2005) Environmental speciation of lead. In: Cornelis R, Crews H, Caruso J & Heumann KG eds. Handbook of elemental speciation II: Species in the environment, food, medicine and occupational health. Chichester, John Wiley & Sons, pp 239–246.

Hilmy MI, Rahim SA & Abbas AH (1976) Normal and lethal mercury levels in human beings. Toxicology, **6**: 155–159.

Hindmarsh JT & McCurdy RF (1986) Clinical and environmental aspects of arsenic toxicity. CRC Crit Rev Clin Lab Sci, **23**: 315–348.

Hirano S, Tsukamoto N & Suzuki KT (1990) Biochemical changes in the rat lung and liver following intratracheal instillation of cadmium oxide. Toxicol Lett, **50**: 97–105.

Hlavay J & Polyák K (2003) Sample preparation — fractionation (sediments, soil, aerosols, and fly ashes). In: Cornelis R, Crews H, Caruso J & Heumann KG eds. Handbook of elemental speciation I. Techniques and methodology. Chichester, John Wiley & Sons, pp 119–146.

Hoet P (2005a) Speciation of chromium in occupational exposure and clinical aspects. In: Cornelis R, Crews H, Caruso J & Heumann KG eds. Handbook of elemental speciation II. Species in the environment, food, medicine and occupational health. Chichester, John Wiley & Sons, pp 136–157.

Hoet P (2005b) Speciation of lead in occupational exposure and clinical aspects. In: Cornelis R, Crews H, Caruso J & Heumann KG eds. Handbook of elemental speciation II. Species in the environment, food, medicine and occupational health. Chichester, Wiley & Sons, pp 252–276.

Hoffman RS (2003) Thallium toxicity and the role of Prussian blue in therapy. Toxicol Rev, **22**: 29–40.

Hoffmann P (2005) Speciation of iron in the environment. In: Cornelis R, Crews H, Caruso J & Heumann KG eds. Handbook of elemental speciation II. Species in the environment, food, medicine and occupational health. Chichester, John Wiley & Sons, pp 200–217.

Hogstedt C & Alexandersson R (1987) Mortality among hard-metal workers in Sweden. Scand J Work Environ Health, **13**: 177–178.

Hong JS, Tilson HA, Hudson P, Ali SF, Wilson WE & Hunter V (1983) Correlation of neurochemical and behavioral effects of triethyl lead chloride in rats. Toxicol Appl Pharmacol, **69**: 471–479.

Hong S, Candelone J-P, Patterson CC & Boutron CF (1994) Greenland ice evidence of hemispheric lead pollution two millennia ago by Greek and Roman civilizations. Science, **265**: 1841–1843.

Horvat M & Byrne AR (1992) Preliminary study of the effects of some physical parameters on the stability of methylmercury in biological samples. Analyst, **117**: 665–668.

Horvat M & Gibičar D (2005) Speciation of mercury: environment, food, clinical and occupational health. In: Cornelis R, Crews H, Caruso J & Heumann KG eds. Handbook of elemental speciation II. Species in the environment, food, medicine and occupational health. Chichester, John Wiley & Sons, pp 281–304.

Hostynek JJ (2003) Factors determining percutaneous metal absorption. Food Chem Toxicol, **41**(3): 327–345.

Hostynek JJ, Dreher F, Nakada T, Schwindt D, Anigbogu A & Maibach HI (2001) Human stratum corneum adsorption of nickel salts: investigation of depth profiles by tape stripping in vivo. Acta Derm Venereol Suppl (Stockh), **212**: 11–18.

Houk RS (2003) Elemental speciation by inductively coupled plasma–mass spectrometry with high resolution instruments. In: Cornelis R, Crews H, Caruso J & Heumann KG eds. Handbook of elemental speciation I. Techniques and methodology. Chichester, John Wiley & Sons, pp 378–416.

Howarth RW, Marino R & Cole JJ (1988) Nitrogen fixation in freshwater, estuarine, and marine ecosystems. 2. Biogeochemical controls. Limnol Oceanogr, **33**: 688–701.

Hrudey SE, Weiping C & Rousseaux C (1996) Bio-availability in environmental risk assessment. Boca Raton, Florida, CRC Press.

Huang CC, Chu NS, Shih TS & Wu TN (1997) Occupational neurotoxic diseases in Taiwan: a review of the outbreaks and clinical features. Changgeng Yi Xue Za Zhi, **20**: 71–78.

Hudson RJM (1998) Which aqueous species control the rates of trace metal uptake by aquatic biota? Observations and predictions of non-equilibrium effects. Sci Total Environ, **219**: 95–115.

Hudson RJM & Morel FMM (1993) Trace metal transport by marine microorganisms: implications of metal coordination kinetics. Deep Sea Res, **40**: 129–150.

Hughes K, Meek ME, Newhook R & Chan P (1995) Speciation in health risk assessments of metals: evaluation of effects associated with forms present in the environment. Regul Toxic Pharmacol, **22**: 213–220.

Hughes MF (2002) Arsenic toxicity and potential mechanisms of action. Toxicol Lett, **133**: 1–16.

Hughes MF, Mitchell CT, Edwards BC & Rahman MS (1995) In vitro percutaneous absorption of dimethylarsinic acid in mice. J Toxicol Environ, **45**: 279–290.

Hughes MS & Birch NJ (1992) Isotopic differences in the lithium transport rate in human erythrocytes during simultaneous incubations with the stable isotopes ^{6}Li and ^{7}Li. C R Acad Sci III, **314**: 153–158.

Hurrell RF, Reddy MB, Juillerat MA & Cook JD (2003) Degradation of phytic acid in cereal porridges improves iron absorption by human subjects. Am J Clin Nutr, **77**: 1213–1219.

Hursh JB (1985) Partition coefficients of mercury (^{203}Hg) vapor between air and biological fluids. J Appl Toxicol, **5**: 327–332.

Hursh JB & Mercer TT (1970) Measurement of ^{212}Pb loss from human lungs. J Appl Physiol, **28**(3): 268–274.

Hursh JB, Sichak SP & Clarkson TW (1988) In vitro oxidation of mercury by the blood. Pharmacol Toxicol, **63**: 266–273.

Hursh JB, Clarkson TW, Miles EF & Goldsmith LA (1989) Percutaneous absorption of mercury vapor by man. Arch Environ Health, **44**(2): 120–127.

IARC (1980) Some metals and metallic compounds. Lyon, International Agency for Research on Cancer, 438 pp (IARC Monographs on the Evaluation of Carcinogenic Risks to Humans, Vol. 23).

IARC (1987) Arsenic and arsenic compounds. In: Overall evaluations of carcinogenicity: An updating of IARC monographs Volumes 1 to 42. Lyon, International Agency for Research on Cancer, pp 100–106 (IARC Monographs on the Evaluation of Carcinogenic Risks to Humans, Supplement 7).

IARC (1990) Chromium, nickel and welding. Lyon, International Agency for Research on Cancer, 677 pp (IARC Monographs on the Evaluation of Carcinogenic Risks to Humans, Vol. 49).

IARC (2004) Some drinking-water disinfectants and contaminants, including arsenic. Lyon, International Agency for Research on Cancer (IARC Monographs on the Evaluation of Carcinogenic Risks to Humans, Vol. 84).

IARC (2006) Cobalt in hard metals and cobalt sulfate, gallium arsenide, indium phosphide and vanadium pentoxide. Lyon, International Agency for Research on Cancer (IARC Monographs on the Evaluation of Carcinogenic Risks to Humans, Vol. 86).

Iida M, Terada K, Sambongi Y, Wakabayashi T, Miura N, Koyama K, Futai M & Sugiyama T (1998) Analysis of functional domains of Wilson disease protein (ATP7B) in *Saccharomyces cerevisiae*. FEBS Lett, **428**: 281–285.

International Committee on Nickel Carcinogenesis in Man (1990) Report of the International Committee on Nickel Carcinogenesis in Man. Scand J Work Environ Health, **16**: 1–82.

Iregren A (1990) Psychological test performance in foundry workers exposed to low levels of manganese. Neurotoxicol Teratol, **12**: 673–675.

Iserson KV, Banner W, Froede RC & Derrick MR (1983) Failure of dialysis therapy in potassium dichromate poisoning. J Emerg Med, **1**: 143–149.

Ishimatsu S, Kawamoto T, Matsuno K & Kodama Y (1995) Distribution of various nickel compounds in rat organs after oral administration. Biol Trace Elem Res, **49**(1): 43–52.

Itoh M & Suzuki KI (1997) Effects of dose on the methylation of selenium to mono-methylselenol and trimethylselenonium ion in rats. Arch Toxicol, **71**: 461–466.

Jacobs IA, Taddeo J, Kelly K & Valenziano C (2002) Poisoning as a result of barium styphnate explosion. Am J Ind Med, **41**: 285–288.

Jacquet P & Mayence A (1982) Application of the in vitro embryo culture to the study of the mutagenic effects of nickel in male germ cells. Toxicol Lett, **11**: 193–197.

James AC (1978) Lung deposition of sub-micron aerosols calculated as a function of age and breathing rate. London, HMSO, pp 71–75 (National Radiological Protection Board Report NRPB/R&D2).

Jansen LH & Berrens L (1968) Hypersensitivity of chromium compounds. Dermatologica, **137**: 1–16.

Jin T, Lu J & Nordberg M (1998) Toxicokinetics and biochemistry of cadmium with special emphasis on the role of metallothionein. Neurotoxicology,**19**: 529–536.

Johnson CH & VanTassell VJ (1991) Acute barium poisoning with respiratory failure and rhabdomyolysis. Ann Emerg Med, **20**: 1138–1142.

Jones PJH & Leatherdale ST (1991) Stable isotopes in clinical research: safety reaffirmed. Clin Sci, **80**: 277–280.

Juberg D & Hearne F (2001) Silver and gold. In: Bingham E, Cohrssen B & Powell C eds. Patty's toxicology. Vol. 2. New York, John Wiley & Sons, pp 123–175.

Jung GY, Kim YS & Lim HB (1997) Simultaneous determination of chromium(III) and chromium(VI) in aqueous solution by capillary electrophoresis with on-column UV–VIS detection. Anal Sci, **13**: 463–467.

Kägi JHR & Nordberg M eds (1979) Metallothionein. Basel/Boston/Stuttgart, Birkhauser Verlag.

Kakela R, Kakela A & Hyvarinen H (1999) Effects of nickel chloride on reproduction of the rat and possible antagonistic role of selenium. Comp Biochem Physiol C Pharmacol Toxicol Endocrinol, **123**: 27–37.

Kambe T, Yamaguchi-Iwai Y, Sasaki R & Nagao M (2004) Overview of mammalian zinc transporters. Cell Mol Life Sci, **61**: 49–68.

Karlson U & Frankenberger WT (1993) Biological alkylation of selenium and tellurium. In: Sigel H & Sigel A eds. Metal ions in biological systems. Vol. 29. Biological properties of metal alkyl derivatives. New York, Marcel Dekker, pp 185–227.

Kasprzak KS (1996) Oxidative DNA damage in metal-induced carcinogenesis. In: Chang LW, Magos L & Suzuki T eds. Toxicology of metals. Boca Raton, Florida, CRC Lewis Publishers, pp 299–320.

Kasprzak KS, Marchow L & Breborowicz J (1973) Pathological reactions in rat lungs following intratracheal injection of nickel subsulfide and 3,4-benzpyrene. Res Commun Chem Pathol Pharmacol, **6**: 237–245.

Kasprzak KS, Zastawny TH, North SL, Riggs CW, Diwan BA, Rice JM & Dizdaroglu M (1994) Oxidative DNA base damage in renal, hepatic, and pulmonary chromatin of rats after intraperitoneal injection of cobalt(II) acetate. Chem Res Toxicol, **7**: 329–335.

Kasten U, Mullenders LHF & Hartwig A (1997) Cobalt(II) inhibits the incision and the polymerization step of nucleotide excision repair in human fibroblasts. Mutat Res, **383**: 81–89.

Katz S & Salem H (1993) The toxicology of chromium with respect to its chemical speciation: a review. J Appl Toxicol, **13**: 217–224.

Katz SA & Salem H (1994) The biological and environmental chemistry of chromium. New York, VCH Publishers.

Kawanishi S, Inoue S & Yamamoto K (1994) Active oxygen species in DNA damage induced by carcinogenic metal compounds. Environ Health Perspect, **102**(suppl 3): 17–20.

Kelleher P, Pacheco K & Newman LS (2000) Inorganic dust pneumonias: the metal-related parenchymal disorders. Environ Health Perspect, **108**(suppl 4): 685–696.

Kenyon EM & Hughes MF (2001) A concise review of the toxicity and carcinogenicity of dimethylarsinic acid. Toxicology, **160**: 227–236.

Kerger BD, Finley BL, Corbett GC, Dodge DG & Paustenbach DJ (1997) Ingestion of chromium(VI) in drinking water by human volunteers: absorption, distribution, and excretion of single and repeated doses. J Toxicol Environ Health, **50**: 67–95.

Kern F, Roberts N, Ostlere L, Langtry J & Staughton RC (1991) Ammoniated mercury ointment as a cause of peripheral neuropathy. Dermatologica, **183**: 280–282.

Kerper LE, Ballatori N & Clarkson TW (1992) Methylmercury transport across the blood–brain barrier by an amino acid carrier. Am J Physiol, **262**: R761–R765.

Kerper LE, Mokrzan EM, Clarkson TW & Ballatori N (1996) Methylmercury efflux from brain capillary endothelial cells is modulated by intracellular glutathione but not ATP. Toxicol Appl Pharmacol, **141**: 526–531.

Kersten M, Förstner U, Krause P, Kriews M, Dannecker W, Garbe-Schönberg C-D, Höck M, Terzenbach U & Graßl H (1993) Pollution source reconnaissance using stable lead isotope ratios ($^{206/207}$Pb). In: Vernet J-P ed. Impact of heavy metals on the environment. Amsterdam, Elsevier, pp 311–325.

Khan A, Hill JM, Grater W, Loeb E, MacLellan A & Hill N (1975) Atopic hypersensitivity to *cis*-dichlorodiammineplatinum(II) and other platinum complexes. Cancer Res, **35**: 2766–2770.

Khayat A & Dencker L (1982) Fetal uptake and distribution of metallic mercury vapor in the mouse: influence of ethanol and aminotriazole. Int J Biol Res Pregnancy, **3**: 38–46.

Kiilunen M, Kivisto H, Ala-Laurila P, Tossavainen A & Aitio A (1983) Exceptional pharmacokinetics of trivalent chromium during occupational exposure to chromium lignosulfonate dust. Scand J Work Environ Health, **9**: 265–271.

Kjellstrom T & Nordberg GF (1978) A kinetic model of cadmium metabolism in the human being. Environ Res, **16**(1–3): 248–269.

Klaassen CD ed (1999) Metallothionein IV. Basel, Birkhäuser Verlag.

Klaassen CD (2001) Heavy metals and heavy-metal antagonists. In: Hardman JG, Limbird LE & Gilman AG eds. The pharmacological basis of therapeutics. New York, McGraw-Hill, pp 1851–1875.

Klein CB & Costa M (1997) DNA methylation, heterochromatin, and epigenetic carcinogens. Mutat Res, **386**: 163–180.

Klein CB, Conway K, Wang XW, Bhamra RK, Lin X, Cohen MD, Annab L, Barrett JC & Costa M (1991) Senescence of nickel-transformed cells by an X chromosome: possible epigenetic control. Science, **251**: 796–799.

Kligman AM (1966) The identification of contact allergens by human assay. III. The maximisation test: a procedure for screening and rating contact sensitizers. J Invest Dermatol, **47**: 393–408.

Koller LD (1998) Cadmium. In: Zelikoff JT & Thomas PT eds. Immunotoxicology of environmental and occupational metals. London, Taylor & Francis, pp 41–61.

Komura J & Sakamoto M (1991) Short-term oral administration of several manganese compounds in mice: physiological and behavioral alterations caused by different forms of manganese. Bull Environ Contam Toxicol, **46**: 921–928.

Komura J & Sakamoto M (1994) Chronic oral administration of methylcyclopentadienyl manganese tricarbonyl altered brain biogenic amines in the mouse: comparison with inorganic manganese. Toxicol Lett, **73**: 65–73.

Koplan JP, Wells AV, Diggory HJ, Baker EL & Liddle J (1977) Lead absorption in a community of potters in Barbados. Int J Epidemiol, 6(3): 225–230.

Korallus U, Ulm K & Steinmann-Steiner-Haldenstaett W (1993) Bronchial carcinoma mortality in the German chromate-producing industry: the effects of process modification. Int Arch Occup Environ Health, 65: 171–178.

Kreyberg S, Torvik A, Bjorneboe A, Wiik-Larsen W & Jacobsen D (1992) Trimethyltin poisoning: report of a case with postmortem examination. Clin Neuropathol, 11: 256–259.

Kruck TP & McLachlan DR (1989) Aluminum as a pathogenic factor in senile dementia of the Alzheimer type: ion specific chelation. Prog Clin Biol Res, 317: 1155–1167.

Krueger I, Mullenders LH & Hartwig A (1999) Nickel(II) increases the sensitivity of V79 Chinese hamster cells towards cisplatin and transplatin by interference with distinct steps of DNA repair. Carcinogenesis, 20: 1177–1184.

Kruszewski M (2003) Labile iron pool: the main determinant of cellular response to oxidative stress. Mutat Res, 531: 81–92.

Kurosaki K, Nakamura T, Mukai T & Endo T (1995) Unusual findings in a fatal case of poisoning with chromate compounds. Forensic Sci Int, 75: 57–65.

Kurta DL, Dean BS & Krenzelok EP (1993) Acute nickel carbonyl poisoning. Am J Emerg Med, 11: 64–66.

Kusaka Y, Iki M, Kumagai S & Goto S (1996) Epidemiological study of hard metal asthma. Occup Environ Med, 53: 188–193.

LaFleur PD (1973) Retention of mercury when freeze-drying biological materials. Anal Chem, 45: 1534–1536.

La Fontaine S, Firth SD, Lockhart PJ, Brooks H, Parton RG, Camakaris J & Mercer JFB (1998) Functional analysis and intracellular localization of the human Menkes protein (MNK) stably expressed from a cDNA construct in Chinese hamster ovary cells (CHO-K1). Hum Mol Genet, 7: 1293–1300.

Lahaye D, Demedts M, van den Oever R & Roosels D (1984) Lung diseases among diamond polishers due to cobalt? Lancet, 1(8369): 156–157.

Laitung JK & Earley M (1984) The role of surgery in chromic acid burns: our experience with two patients. Burns Incl Therm Inj, 10: 378–380.

Landolph JR, Dews PM, Ozbun L & Evans DP (1996) Metal-induced gene expression and neoplastic transformation. In: Chang LW ed. Toxicology of metals. Boca Raton, Florida, CRC Lewis Publishers, pp 321–329.

Langård S & Norseth T (1986) Chromium. In: Friberg L, Nordberg GF & Vouk V eds. Handbook on the toxicology of metals, 2nd ed. Amsterdam, Elsevier Science Publishers, pp 185–210.

Langford N & Ferner R (1999) Toxicity of mercury. J Hum Hypertens, 13: 651–659.

Lanphear BP, Dietrich K, Auinger P & Cox C (2000) Cognitive deficits associated with blood lead concentrations <10 microg/dL in US children and adolescents. Public Health Rep, **115**: 521–529.

Larese FL, Maina G, Adami G, Venifer M, Coceani N, Bussani R, Massiccio M, Barbieri P & Spinelli P (2004) In vitro percutaneous absorption of cobalt. Int Arch Environ Health, **77**: 85–95.

Lasfargues G, Lison D, Maldague P & Lauwerys R (1992) Comparative study of the acute lung toxicity of pure cobalt powder and cobalt–tungsten carbide mixture in rat. Toxicol Appl Pharmacol, **112**: 41–50.

Lasfargues G, Wild P, Moulin JJ, Hammon B, Rosmorduc B, Rondeau du Noyer C, Lavandier M & Moline J (1994) Lung cancer mortality in a French cohort of hard-metal workers. Am J Ind Med, **26**: 585–595.

Lasfargues G, Lardot C, Delos M, Lauwerys R & Lison D (1995) The delayed lung responses to single and repeated intratracheal administration of pure cobalt and hard metal powder in the rat. Environ Res, **69**: 108–121.

Lau TJ, Hackett RL & Sunderman FW (1972) The carcinogenicity of intravenous nickel carbonyl in rats. Cancer Res, **32**: 2253–2258.

Le SXC, Cullen WR & Reimer KJ (1994) Speciation of arsenic compounds in some marine organisms. Environ Sci Technol, **28**: 1598–1604.

Leach AM, McClenathan DM & Hieftje GM (2003) Plasma source time-of-flight mass spectrometry: a powerful tool for elemental speciation. In: Cornelis R, Crews H, Caruso J & Heumann KG eds. Handbook of elemental speciation I. Techniques and methodology. Chichester, John Wiley & Sons, pp 313–333.

Leblondel G & Allain P (1999) Manganese transport by Caco-2 cells. Biol Trace Elem Res, **67**(1): 13–28.

Lee AM & Fraumeni JF (1969) Arsenic and respiratory cancer in man: an occupational study. J Natl Cancer Inst, **42**: 1045–1052.

Lee J, Petris MJ &Thiele DJ (2002) Characterization of mouse embryonic cells deficient in the Ctr1 high affinity copper transporter. Identification of a Ctr1-independent copper transport system. J Biol Chem, **277**: 40253–40259.

Lee JG, Roberts SR & Morel FMM (1995) Cadmium: a nutrient for the marine diatom *Thalassiosira weissflogii*. Limnol Oceanogr, **40**: 1056–1063.

Lee YW, Klein CB, Kargacin B, Salnikow K, Kitahara J, Dowjat K, Zhitkovitch A, Christie NT & Costa M (1995) Carcinogenic nickel silences gene expression by chromatin condensation and DNA methylation: a new model for epigenetic carcinogens. Mol Cell Biol, **15**: 2547–2557.

Lee YW, Broday L & Costa M (1998) Effects of nickel on DNA methyltransferase activity and genomic DNA methylation levels. Mutat Res, **415**: 213–218.

Leffler PE, Jin T & Nordberg GF (2000) Differential calcium transport disturbances in renal membrane vesicles after cadmium–metallothionein injection in rats. Toxicology, **143**: 227–234.

Lerman SA, Clarkson TW & Gerson RJ (1983) Arsenic uptake and metabolism by liver cells is dependent on arsenic oxidation state. Chem Biol Interact, **45**: 401–406.

Lesko SA, Drocourt JL, Yang SU & Gajewski E (1982) Deoxyribonucleic acid–protein and deoxyribonucleic acid interstrand cross-links induced in isolated chromatin by hydrogen peroxide and ferrous ethylenediaminetetraacetate chelates. Biochemistry, **21**: 5010–5015.

Lewis BL, Luther GW, Lane H & Church TM (1995) Determination of metal–organic complexation in natural waters by SWASV with pseudopolarograms. Electroanalysis, **7**: 166–177.

Li JH & Rossman TG (1989) Inhibition of DNA ligase activity by arsenite: a possible mechanism of its comutagenesis. Mol Toxicol, **2**: 1–9.

Lin TS & Nriagu J (1998) Revised hydrolysis constants for thallium(I) and thallium(III) and the environmental implications. J Air Waste Manage Assoc, **48**: 151–156.

Lindemann T, Prange A, Dannecker W & Neidhart B (2000) Stability studies of arsenic, selenium, antimony and tellurium species in water, urine, fish and soil extracts using HPLC/ICP-MS. Fresenius J Anal Chem, **368**: 214–220.

Linna A, Oksa P, Palmroos P, Roto P, Laippala P & Uitti J (2003) Respiratory health of cobalt production workers. Am J Ind Med, **44**: 124–132.

Linnett PJ & Hughes EG (1999) 20 years of medical surveillance on exposure to allergenic and non-allergenic platinum compounds: the importance of chemical speciation. Occup Environ Med, **56**: 191–196.

Lison D (1996) Human toxicity of cobalt-containing dust and experimental studies on the mechanism of interstitial lung disease (hard metal disease). Crit Rev Toxicol, **26**: 585–616.

Lison D, Buchet JP, Swennen B, Molders J & Lauwerys R (1994) Biological monitoring of workers exposed to cobalt metal, salts, oxide and hard metal dust. Occup Environ Med, **51**: 447–450.

Lison D, Carbonnelle P, Mollo L, Lauwerys R & Fubini B (1995) Physicochemical mechanism of the interaction between cobalt metal and carbide particles to generate toxic activated oxygen species. Chem Res Toxicol, **8**: 600–606.

Lison D, De Boeck M, Verougstraete V & Kirsch-Volders M (2001) Update on the genotoxicity and carcinogenicity of cobalt compounds. Occup Environ Med, **58**: 619–625.

Liu J, Kershaw WC & Klaassen CD (1991) The protective effect of metallothionein on the toxicity of various metals in rat primary hepatocyte culture. Toxicol Appl Pharmacol, **107**(1): 27–34.

Lloyd DR & Phillips DH (1999) Oxidative DNA damage mediated by copper(II), iron(II) and nickel(II) Fenton reactions: evidence for site-specific mechanisms in the formation of double-strand breaks, 8-hydroxydeoxyguanosine and putative intrastrand cross-links. Mutat Res, **424**: 23–36.

Lloyd DR, Phillips DH & Carmichael PL (1997) Generation of putative intrastrand cross-links and strand breaks in DNA by transition metal ion-mediated oxygen radical attack. Chem Res Toxicol, **10**: 393–400.

Lloyd DR, Carmichael PL & Phillips DH (1998) Comparison of the formation of 8-hydroxy-2'-deoxyguanosine and single- and double-strand breaks in DNA mediated by Fenton reactions. Chem Res Toxicol, **11**: 420–427.

Lobinski R, Edmonds JS, Suzuki KT & Uden PC (2000) Species-selective determination of selenium compounds in biological materials. Pure Appl Chem, **72**: 447–461.

Lolin Y & O'Gorman P (1988) An intra-erythrocytic low molecular weight lead-binding protein in acute and chronic lead exposure and its possible protective role in lead toxicity. Ann Clin Biochem, **25**(6): 688–697.

Loubieres Y, de Lassence A, Bernier M, Vieillard-Baron A, Schmitt JM, Page B & Jardin F (1999) Acute, fatal, oral chromic acid poisoning. J Toxicol Clin Toxicol, **37**: 333–336.

Lu CC, Matsumoto N & Iijima S (1979) Teratogenic effects of nickel chloride on embryonic mice and its transfer to embryonic mice. Teratology, **19**: 137–142.

Lucchini R, Selis L, Folli D, Apostoli P, Mutti A, Vanoni O, Iregren A & Alessio L (1995) Neurobehavioral effects of manganese in workers from a ferroalloy plant after temporary cessation of exposure. Scand J Work Environ Health, **21**: 143–149.

Ludwig T & Oberleithner H (2004) Platinum complex toxicity in cultured renal epithelia. Cell Physiol Biochem, **14**: 431–440.

Lukanova A, Toniolo P, Zhitkovich A, Nikolova V, Panev T, Popov T, Taioli E & Costa M (1996) Occupational exposure to Cr(VI): comparison between chromium levels in lymphocytes, erythrocytes, and urine. Int Arch Occup Environ Health, **69**(1): 39–44.

Lustig S, De Kimpe J, Cornelis R, Schramel P & Michalke B (1999) Platinum speciation in clinical and environmental samples: scrutiny of data obtained by using gel electrophoresis techniques (flatbed and capillary). Electrophoresis, **20**: 1627–1633.

Lyman WJ (1995) Transport and transformation processes. In: Rand GM ed. Aquatic toxicology, 2nd ed. Washington, DC, Taylor & Francis.

Lynam DR, Pfeifer GD, Fort B & Gelbcke AA (1990) Environmental assessment of MMT fuel additive. Sci Total Environ, **93**: 107–114.

Mack DP & Dervan PB (1992) Sequence-specific oxidative cleavage of DNA by a designed metalloprotein, Ni(II).GGH(Hin139–190). Biochemistry, **31**: 9399–9405.

Mackay D (1982) Correlation of bioconcentration factors. Environ Sci Technol, **16**: 274–278.

Magos L (1968) Uptake of mercury by the brain. Br J Ind Med, **25**: 315–318.

Magos L (2001) Review on the toxicity of ethylmercury, including its presence as a preservative in biological and pharmaceutical products. J Appl Toxicol, **21**: 1–5.

Magos L (2003) Neurotoxic character of thimerosal and the allometric extrapolation of adult clearance half-time to infants. J Appl Toxicol, **23**: 263–269.

Magos L, Brown AW, Sparrow S, Bailey E, Snowden RT & Skipp WR (1985) The comparative toxicology of ethyl- and methylmercury. Arch Toxicol, **57**: 260–267.

Mancuso TF (1997) Chromium as an industrial carcinogen: Part I. Am J Ind Med, **31**: 129–139.

Mancuso TF & Hueper WC (1951) Occupational cancer and other health hazards in a chromate plant: a medical appraisal. I. Lung cancers in chromate workers. Ind Med Surg, **20**: 358–363.

Mann S, Droz PO & Vahter M (1996a) A physiologically based pharmacokinetic model for arsenic exposure. I. Development in hamsters and rabbits. Toxicol Appl Pharmacol, **137**: 8–22.

Mann S, Droz PO & Vahter M (1996b) A physiologically based pharmacokinetic model for arsenic exposure. II. Validation and application in humans. Toxicol Appl Pharmacol, **140**: 471–486.

Mao Y, Liu KJ, Jiang JJ & Shi X (1996) Generation of reactive oxygen species by Co(II) from H_2O_2 in the presence of chelators in relation to DNA damage and 2'- deoxy-guanosine hydroxylation. J Toxicol Environ Health, **47**: 61–75.

Mappes R (1977) [Experiments on excretion of arsenic in urine.] Int Arch Occup Environ Health, **40**: 267–272 (in German).

Marafante E & Vahter M (1987) Solubility, retention, and metabolism of intratracheally and orally administered inorganic arsenic compounds in the hamster. Environ Res, **42**(1): 72–82.

Marafante E, Vahter M, Norin H, Envall J, Sandstrom M, Christakopoulos A & Ryhage R (1987) Biotransformation of dimethylarsinic acid in mouse, hamster and man. J Appl Toxicol, **7**: 111–118.

Marcus RK (2003) Glow discharge plasmas as tunable sources for elemental speciation. In: Cornelis R, Crews H, Caruso J & Heumann KG eds. Handbook of elemental speciation I. Techniques and methodology. Chichester, John Wiley & Sons, pp 334–356.

Maring H, Settle DM, Buat-Ménard P, Dulac F & Patterson CC (1987) Stable lead isotope tracers of air mass trajectories in the Mediterranean region. Nature, **330**: 154–156.

Marino PE, Franzblau A, Lilis R & Landrigan PJ (1989) Acute lead poisoning in construction workers: the failure of current protective standards. Arch Environ Health, **44**: 140–145.

Martell AE & Motekaitis RJ (1992) The determination and use of stability constants. New York, VCH Publishers.

Martin RB (1986) The chemistry of aluminum as related to biology and medicine. Clin Chem, **32**: 1797–1805.

Martin RB, Savory J, Brown S, Bertholf RL & Wills MR (1987) Transferrin binding of Al^{3+} and Fe^{3+}. Clin Chem, **33**: 405–407.

Mason RP, Reinfelder RJ & Morel FMM (1996) Uptake, toxicity, and trophic transfer of mercury in a coastal diatom. Environ Sci Technol, **30**: 1835–1845.

Mass MJ, Tennant A, Roop BC, Cullen WR, Styblo M, Thomas DJ & Kligerman AD (2001) Methylated trivalent arsenic species are genotoxic. Chem Res Toxicol, **14**: 355–361.

Matey P, Allison KP, Sheehan TM & Gowar JP (2000) Chromic acid burns: early aggressive excision is the best method to prevent systemic toxicity. J Burn Care Rehabil, **21**: 241–245.

Mathur AK, Datta KK, Tandon SK & Dikshith TS (1977) Effect of nickel sulphate on male rats. Bull Environ Contam Toxicol, **17**: 241–248.

May P (1995) Modelling metal–ligand equilibria in blood plasma. In: Berthon G ed. Handbook of metal–ligand interactions in biological fluids: Bioinorganic chemistry. New York, Marcel Dekker, pp 1184–1194.

Maynard AD, Northage C & Hemingway M (1997) Measurement of short-term exposure to airborne soluble platinum in the platinum industry. Ann Occup Hyg, **41**: 77–94.

McArdle HJ, Gross SM, Danks DM & Wedd AG (1990) Role of albumin's copper binding site in copper uptake by mouse hepatocytes. Am J Physiol, **256**: G988–991.

McGeer JC, Playle RC, Wood CM & Galvez F (2000) A physiologically based acute toxicity model for predicting the effects of waterborne silver in rainbow trout in fresh waters. Environ Sci Technol, **34**: 4199–4207.

McGinley PA, Morris JB, Clay RJ & Gianutsos G (1987) Disposition and toxicity of methylcyclopentadienyl manganese tricarbonyl in the rat. Toxicol Lett, **36**: 137–145.

Meco G, Bonifati V, Vanacore N & Fabrizio E (1994) Parkinsonism after chronic exposure to the fungicide maneb (manganese ethylene-bis-dithiocarbamate). Scand J Work Environ Health, **20**: 301–305.

Mendelsohn AL, Dreyer BP, Fierman AH, Rosen CM, Legano LA, Kruger HA, Lim SW & Courtlandt CD (1998) Low-level lead exposure and behavior in early childhood. Pediatrics, **101**: E10.

Meplan C, Richard M-J & Hainaut P (2000) Metalloregulation of the tumor suppressor protein p53: zinc mediates the renaturation of p53 after exposure to metal chelators in vitro and in intact cells. Oncogene, **19**: 5227–5236.

Merget R, Kulzer R, Dierkes-Globish A, Breitstadt R, Gebler A, Kniffka A, Artelt S, Koenig HP, Alt F, Vormberg R, Baur X & Schultze-Werninghaus G (2000) Exposure–effects relationship of platinum salts allergy in a catalyst production plant: conclusion from a 5 years prospective cohort study. J Allergy Clin Immunol, **105**: 364–370.

Mergler D, Huel G, Bowler R, Iregren A, Belanger S, Baldwin M, Tardif R, Smargiassi A & Martin L (1994) Nervous system dysfunction among workers with long-term exposure to manganese. Environ Res, **64**: 151–180.

Mertz W, Roginski EE & Reba RC (1965) Biological activity and fate of trace quantities of intravenous chromium (3) in the rat. Am J Physiol, **209**: 489–494.

Mertz W, Roginski EE, Feldman FJ & Thurman DE (1969) Dependence of chromium transfer into the rat embryo on the chemical form. J Nutr, **99**: 363–367.

Metze D, Jakubowski N & Klockow D (2005) Speciation of chromium in environment and food. In: Cornelis R, Crews H, Caruso J & Heumann KG eds. Handbook of elemental speciation II. Species in the environment, food, medicine and occupational health. Chichester, John Wiley & Sons, pp 120–135.

Michalke B (2000) CE-ICP-MS advantages and improvements in selenium speciation. Spectroscopy, **15**: 30–39.

Michalke B (2003) Capillary electrophoresis in speciation analysis. In: Cornelis R, Crews H, Caruso J & Heumann KG eds. Handbook of elemental speciation I. Techniques and methodology. Chichester, John Wiley & Sons, pp 201–223.

Michalke B (2004) Selenium speciation in human serum of cystic fibrosis patients compared to serum from healthy persons. J Chromatogr A, **1058**: 203–208.

Milačič R (2005a) Speciation of aluminum in the environment. In: Cornelis R, Crews H, Caruso J & Heumann KG eds. Handbook of elemental speciation II. Species in the environment, food, medicine and occupational health. Chichester, John Wiley & Sons, pp 12–19.

Milačič R (2005b) Speciation of aluminum in food: sources, including potable water. In: Cornelis R, Crews H, Caruso J & Heumann KG eds. Handbook of elemental speciation II. Species in the environment, food, medicine and occupational health. Chichester, John Wiley & Sons, pp 20–26.

Milačič R (2005c) Speciation of aluminum in clinical aspects. In: Cornelis R, Crews H, Caruso J & Heumann KG eds. Handbook of elemental speciation II. Species in the environment, food, medicine and occupational health. Chichester, John Wiley & Sons, pp 27–39.

Miller WL, Lin K, King DW & Kester DR (1995) Photochemical redox cycling of iron in coastal seawater. Mar Chem, **50**: 63–77.

Mirimanoff N & Wilkinson KJ (2000) Regulation of zinc accumulation by a freshwater gram-positive bacterium (*Rhodococcus opacus*). Environ Sci Technol, **34**: 616–622.

Misra TK (1992) Bacterial resistance to inorganic mercury salts and organomercurials. Plasmid, **27**: 4–16.

Moffett JW (1995) Temporal and spatial variability of strong copper complexing ligands in the Sargasso Sea. Deep Sea Res, **42**(8): 1273–1295.

Moffett JW, Zika RG & Brand LE (1990) Distribution and potential sources and sinks of copper chelators in the Sargasso Sea. Deep Sea Res, **37**: 27–36.

Montes-Bayon M, DeNicola K & Caruso JA (2000) Liquid chromatography–inductively coupled plasma mass spectrometry. J Chromatogr A, **1000**: 457–476.

Morel FMM, Hudson RJM & Price NM (1991) Limitation of productivity by trace metals in the sea. Limnol Oceanogr, **36**(8): 1742–1755.

Morrow PE, Bates DV, Fish BR, Hatch TF & Mercer TT (1966) Deposition and retention models for internal dosimetry of the human respiratory tract. Health Phys, **12**: 173–207.

Morrow PE, Beiter H & Amato F (1980) Pulmonary retention of lead: an experimental study in man. Environ Res, **21**: 373–384.

Motsenbocker M & Tappel A (1982) Selenocysteine-containing selenium-transport protein in rat plasma. Biochim Biophys Acta, **719**: 147–153.

Moulin JJ, Portefaix P, Wild P, Mur JM, Smagghe G & Mantout B (1990) Mortality study among workers producing ferroalloys and stainless steel in France. Br J Ind Med, **47**: 537–543.

Moulin JJ, Wild P, Mur JM, Fournier Betz M & Mercier Gallay M (1993) A mortality study of cobalt production workers: an extension of the follow-up. Am J Ind Med, **23**: 281–288.

Moulin JJ, Wild P, Romazini S, Lasfargues G, Peltier A, Bozec C, Deguerry P, Pellet F & Perdrix A (1998) Lung cancer risk in hard-metal workers. Am J Epidemiol, **148**: 241–248.

Mukai H, Ambe Y, Muku T, Takeshite K & Fukuma T (1986) Seasonal variations in methylarsenic compounds in airborne particulate matter. Nature, **324**: 239–241.

Muller JG, Chen X, Dadis AC, Rokita SE & Burrows CJ (1992) Ligand effects associated with the intrinsic selectivity of DNA oxidation promoted by Ni(II) macrocyclic complexes. J Am Chem Soc, **114**: 6407–6411.

Muñoz-Olivas R & Cámara C (2003) Sample treatment for speciation analysis in biological samples. In: Cornelis R, Crews H, Caruso J & Heumann KG eds. Handbook of elemental speciation I. Techniques and methodology. Chichester, John Wiley & Sons, pp 95–118.

Murphy LS, Guillard RRL & Brown JF (1984) The effects of iron and manganese on copper sensitivity in diatoms: Differences in the responses of closely related neritic and oceanic species. Biol Oceanogr, **3**: 187–202.

Mutti A (1995) Use of intermediate end-points to prevent long-term outcomes. Toxicol Lett, **77**: 121–125.

Mutti A (1999) Biological monitoring in occupational and environmental toxicology. Toxicol Lett, **108**: 77–89.

Myers JE, Thompson ML, Ramushu S, Young T, Jeebhay MF, London L, Esswein E, Renton K, Spies A, Boulle A, Naik I, Iregren A & Rees DJ (2003) The nervous system effects of occupational exposure on workers in a South African manganese smelter. Neurotoxicology, **24**: 885–894.

Nackerdien Z, Kasprzak KS, Rao G, Halliwell B & Dizdaroglu M (1991) Nickel(II)- and cobalt(II)-dependent damage by hydrogen peroxide to the DNA bases in isolated human chromatin. Cancer Res, **51**: 5837–5842.

National Research Council (2003) Bioavailability of contaminants in soils and sediments: processes, tools, and applications. Washington, DC, National Academy Press.

Needleman HL, Riess JA, Tobin MJ, Biesecker GE & Greenhouse JB (1996) Bone lead levels and delinquent behavior. JAMA, **275**: 363–369.

Needleman HL, McFarland C, Ness RB, Fienberg SE & Tobin MJ (2002) Bone lead levels in adjudicated delinquents. A case control study. Neurotoxicol Teratol, **24**: 711–717.

Nesnow S, Roop BC, Lambert G, Kadiiska M, Mason RP, Cullen WR & Mass MJ (2002) DNA damage induced by methylated trivalent arsenicals is mediated by reactive oxygen species. Chem Res Toxicol, **15**: 1627–1634.

Neve J (1991) Method in determination of selenium states. J Trace Elem Electrolytes Health Dis, **5**: 1–6.

Nieboer E & Fletcher GG (1996) Determinants of reactivity in metal toxicology. In: Chang LW ed. Toxicology of metals. Boca Raton, Florida, CRC Lewis Publishers, pp 113–132.

Nieboer E, Fletcher GG & Thomassen Y (1999) Relevance of reactivity determinants to exposure assessment and biological monitoring of the elements. J Environ Monit, **1**: 1–14.

Nielands JB (1981) Iron absorption and transport in microorganisms. Annu Rev Nutr, **1**: 27–46.

Nielsen JB & Andersen O (1990) Disposition and retention of mercuric chloride in mice after oral and parenteral administration. J Toxicol Environ Health, **30**(3): 167–180.

Nierenberg DW, Nordgren RE, Chang MB, Siegler RW, Blayney MB, Hochberg F, Toribara TY, Cernichiari E & Clarkson T (1998) Delayed cerebellar disease and death after accidental exposure to dimethylmercury. N Engl J Med, **338**: 1672–1676.

Nohr D & Biesalski HK (2005) Speciation of copper in clinical and occupational aspects. In: Cornelis R, Crews H, Caruso J & Heumann KG eds. Handbook of elemental speciation II. Species in the environment, food, medicine and occupational health. Chichester, John Wiley & Sons, pp 187–199.

Nordberg GF, Piscator M & Nordberg M (1971) On the distribution of cadmium in blood. Acta Pharmacol Toxicol, **30**: 289–295.

Nordberg GF, Nordberg M, Piscator M & Vesterberg O (1972) Separation of two forms of rabbit metallothionein by isoelectric focusing. Biochem J, **126**: 491–498.

Nordberg GF, Goyer RA & Nordberg M (1975) Comparative toxicity of cadmium metallo-thionein and cadmium chloride on mouse kidney. Arch Pathol, **99**: 192–197.

Nordberg GF, Garvey JS & Chang CC (1982) Metallothionein in plasma and urine of cadmium workers. Environ Res, **28**: 179–182.

Nordberg M (1984) General aspect of cadmium: transport, uptake and metabolism by the kidney. Environ Health Perspect, **54**: 13–20.

Nordberg M (1998) Metallothioneins: historical review and state of knowledge. Talanta, **46**: 243–254.

Nordberg M & Nordberg GF (1987) On the role of metallothionein in cadmium induced renal toxicity. Experientia Suppl, **52**: 669–675.

Nordberg M & Nordberg GF (2000) Toxicological aspects of metallothionein. Cell Mol Biol, **46**(2): 451–463.

Nordberg M & Nordberg GF (2002) Cadmium. In: Sarkar B ed. Handbook of heavy metals in the environment. New York, Marcel Dekker, pp 231–269.

Nordberg M, Duffus JH & Templeton DM (2004) Glossary of terms used in toxicokinetics. Pure Appl Chem, **76**: 1033–1082.

Normandin L, Beaupré LA, Salehi F, St-Pierre A, Kennedy G, Mergler D, Butterworth RF, Philippe S & Zayed J (2004) Manganese distribution in the brain and neurobehavioral changes following inhalation exposure of rats to three chemical forms of manganese. Neurotoxicology, **25**(3): 433–441.

NTP (1994) National Toxicology Program technical report on the toxicology and carcino-genesis studies of nickel sulfate hexahydrate (CAS No. 10101-97-0) in F344/N rats and B6C3F1 mice (inhalation studies). Bethesda, Maryland, United States Department of Health and Human Services, Public Health Service, National Institutes of Health, National Toxicology Program (NIH Publication No. 94-3370).

NTP (2000) Toxicology and carcinogenesis studies of gallium arsenide (CAS No. 1303-00-0) in F344/N rats and B6C3F1 mice (inhalation studies). Bethesda, Maryland, United States Department of Health and Human Services, Public Health Service, National Institutes of Health, National Toxicology Program, pp 1–306 (Technical Report Series 492).

Nygren O & Lundgren C (1997) Determination of platinum in workroom air and in blood and in urine from nursing staff attending patients receiving cisplatin chemotherapy. Int Arch Occup Environ Health, **70**: 209–214.

Ogata M, Kenmotsu K, Hirota N, Meguro T & Aikoh H (1987) Reduction of mercuric ion and exhalation of mercury in acatalasemic and normal mice. Arch Environ Health, **42**(1): 26–30.

Ohsaki Y, Abe S, Kimura K, Tsuneta Y, Mikami H & Murao M (1978) Lung cancer in Japanese chromate workers. Thorax, **33**: 372–374.

Okubo T & Tsuchiya K (1977) An epidemiological study on lung cancer among chromium plating workers. Keio J Med, **26**: 171–177.

Oller AR, Costa M & Oberdörster G (1997) Carcinogenicity assessment of selected nickel compounds. Toxicol Appl Pharmacol, **143**: 152–166.

Oomen AG, Tolls J, Sips A & Groten JP (2003) Intestinal lead uptake and transport in relation to speciation: an in vitro study. Arch Environ Contam Toxicol, **44**(1): 116–124.

Ortner H (2003) Characterization of individual aerosol particles with special reference to speciation techniques. In: Cornelis R, Crews H, Caruso J & Heumann KG eds. Handbook of elemental speciation I. Techniques and methodology. Chichester, John Wiley & Sons, pp 505–525.

Ottaiano A, Tambaro R, Greggi S, Prato R, Di Maio M, Esposito G, Scala F, Barletta E, Losito S, De Vivo R, Iaffaioli VR & Pignata S (2003) Safety of cisplatin after severe hypersensitivity reactions to carboplatin in patients with recurrent ovarian carcinoma. Anticancer Res, **23**: 3465–3468.

Ozaki S, Ichimura T, Isobe T & Omata S (1993) Identification and partial characterization of a glycoprotein species with high affinity for methylmercury in peripheral nervous tissues of man and experimental animals. Arch Toxicol, **67**: 268–276.

Pagenkopf GK (1983) Gill surface interaction model for trace-metal toxicity to fishes: role of complexation, pH and water hardness. Environ Sci Technol, **17**: 342–347.

Pal PK, Samii A & Calne DB (1999) Manganese neurotoxicity: a review of clinical features, imaging and pathology. Neurotoxicology, **20**: 227–238.

Palecek E, Brazdova M, Cernocka H, Vlk D, Brazda V & Vojtesek B (1999) Effect of transition metals on binding of p53 protein to supercoiled DNA and to consensus sequence in DNA fragments. Oncogene, **18**: 3617–3625.

Pandey R & Singh SP (2001) Seminal toxicity of nickel sulfate in mice. Biol Trace Elem Res, **82**: 211–215.

Pandey R & Srivastava SP (2000) Spermatotoxic effects of nickel in mice. Bull Environ Contam Toxicol, **64**: 161–167.

Pandey R, Kumar R, Singh SP, Saxena DK & Srivastava SP (1999) Male reproductive effect of nickel sulphate in mice. Biometals, **12**: 339–346.

Paquin PR, Gorsuch JW, Apte S, Batley GE, Bowles KC, Campbell PG, Delos CG, Di Toro DM, Dwyer RL, Galvez F, Gensemer RW, Goss GG, Hostrand C, Janssen CR, McGeer JC, Naddy RB, Playle RC, Santore RC, Schneider U, Stubblefield WA, Wood CM & Wu KB (2002) The biotic ligand model: a historic overview. Comp Biochem Physiol C Pharmacol Toxicol Endocrinol, **133**: 3–35.

Park HS, Yu HJ & Jung K-S (1994) Occupational asthma caused by chromium. Clin Exp Allergy, **24**: 676–681.

Parkes JG & Templeton DM (2002) Transport of non-transferrin-bound iron by hepatocytes. In: Templeton DM ed. Molecular and cellular iron transport. New York, Marcel Dekker, pp 451–466.

Paustenbach DJ, Panko JM, Fredrick MM, Finley BL & Proctor DM (1997) Urinary chromium as a biological marker of environmental exposure: what are the limitations? Regul Toxicol Pharmacol, **26**: S23–34.

Paustenbach DJ, Finley BL, Mowat FS & Kerger BD (2003) Human health risk and exposure assessment of chromium (VI) in tap water. J Toxicol Environ Health A, **66**: 1295–1339.

Payne AS & Gitlin JD (1998) Functional expression of the Menkes disease protein reveals common biochemical mechanisms among the copper-transporting P-type ATPases. J Biol Chem, **273**: 3765–3770.

Pelissier-Alicot AL, Leonetti G, Champsaur P, Allain P, Mauras Y & Botta A (1999) Fatal poisoning due to intravasation after oral administration of barium sulfate for contrast radiography. Forensic Sci Int, **106**: 109–113.

Pershagen G, Lind B & Bjorklund NE (1982) Lung retention and toxicity of some inorganic arsenic compounds. Environ Res, **29**: 425–434.

Pershagen G, Nordberg G & Bjorklund NE (1984) Carcinomas of the respiratory tract in hamsters given arsenic trioxide and/or benzo[a]pyrene by the pulmonary route. Environ Res, **34**: 227–241.

Petersen R, Thomsen JF, Jorgensen NK & Mikkelsen S (2000) Half-life of chromium in serum and urine in a former plasma cutter of stainless steel. Occup Environ Med, **57**: 140–142.

Peterson EW & Cardoso ER (1983) The blood–brain barrier following experimental subarachnoid hemorrhage. Part 2: Response to mercuric chloride infusion. J Neurosurg, **58**: 345–351.

Petrilli F & Deflora A (1978) Metabolic deactivation of hexavalent chromium mutagenicity. Mutat Res, **54**: 137–147.

Petrucci F, Violante N, Senofonte O, Cristaudo A, Di Gregorio M, Forte G & Alimonti A (2005) Biomonitoring of a worker population exposed to latinum dust in a catalyst production plant. Occup Environ Health, **62**: 27–33.

Phinney JT & Bruland KW (1994) Uptake of lipophilic organic Cu, Cd, and Pb complexes in the coastal diatom, *Thalassiosira weissflogii*. Environ Sci Technol, **28**: 1781–1790.

Phoon WH, Chan MO, Goh CH, Edmondson RP, Kwek YK, Gan SL, Ngui SJ & Kwok SF (1984) Five cases of arsine poisoning. Ann Acad Med Singapore, **13**: 394–398.

Pinto SS & Bennett BM (1963) Effect of arsenic trioxide exposure on mortality. Arch Environ Health, **38**: 583–591.

Piotrowski JK, Szymanska JA, Skrzypinska-Gawrysiak M, Kotelo J & Sporny S (1992) Intestinal absorption of inorganic mercury in rat. Pharmacol Toxicol, **70**(1): 53–55.

Pippard EC, Acheson ED & Winter PD (1985) Mortality of tanners. Br J Ind Med, **42**: 285–287.

Playle RC (1998) Modelling metal interactions at fish gills. Sci Total Environ, **219**: 147–163.

Pollock CA & Ibels LS (1986) Lead intoxication in paint removal workers on the Sydney Harbour Bridge. Med J Aust, **145**: 635–639.

Pollock CA & Ibels LS (1988) Lead intoxication in Sydney Harbour Bridge workers. Aust N Z J Med, **18**: 46–52.

Pott EB, Henry PR, Ammerman CB, Merritt AM, Madison JB & Miles RD (1994) Relative bioavailability of copper in a copper–lysine complex for chicks and lambs. Anim Feed Sci Technol, **45**: 193–201.

Profrock D, Leonhard P & Prange A (2003) Determination of sulfur and selected trace elements in metallothionein-like proteins using capillary electrophoresis hyphenated to inductively coupled plasma mass spectrometry with an octopole reaction cell. Anal Bioanal Chem, **377**: 132–139.

Prohaska T & Stingeder G (2005) Arsenic and arsenic species in environment and human nutrition. In: Cornelis R, Crews H, Caruso J & Heumann KG eds. Handbook of elemental speciation II. Species in the environment, food, medicine and occupational health. Chichester, John Wiley & Sons, pp 69–85.

Qin H, Wang F & Guo J (2003) Structure and functions of ZRT and IRT-like protein. Wei Sheng Yan Jiu, **32**: 261–264.

Quevauviller P (2003) Reference materials. In: Cornelis R, Crews H, Caruso J & Heumann KG eds. Handbook of elemental speciation I. Techniques and methodology. Chichester, John Wiley & Sons, pp 563–590.

Rabinowitz MB (1987) Stable isotope mass spectrometry in childhood lead poisoning. Biol Trace Elem Res, **12**: 223–229.

Radabaugh TR & Aposhian HV (2000) Enzymatic reduction of arsenic compounds in mammalian systems: reduction of arsenate to arsenite by human liver arsenate reductase. Chem Res Toxicol, **13**: 26–30.

Rae CE, Bell CN Jr, Elliott CE & Shannon M (1991) Ten cases of acute lead intoxication among bridge workers in Louisiana. DICP, **25**: 932–937.

Raeburn D (1987) Calcium entry blocking drugs: their classification and sites of action in smooth muscle cells. Med Biol, **65**: 175–180.

Rahola T, Hattula T, Koralainen A & Miettinen JK (1973) Elimination of free and protein-bound ionic mercury (^{203}Hg^{2+}) in man. Ann Clin Res, **5**: 214–219.

Randell EW, Parkes JG, Olivieri NF & Templeton DM (1994) Uptake of non-transferrin-bound iron by both reductive and nonreductive processes is modulated by intracellular iron. J Biol Chem, **269**: 16046–16053.

Ravera O (2004) Importance and difficulties of research on metal speciation in the aquatic ecosystem: an ecologist's viewpoint. Ann Chim, **94**: 495–504.

Reaney SH, Kwik-Uribe CL & Smith DR (2002) Manganese oxidation state and its implications for toxicity. Chem Res Toxicol, **15**: 1119–1126.

Reinhard KJ & Ghazi AM (1992) Evaluation of lead concentrations in 18th-century Omaha Indian skeletons using ICP-MS. Am J Phys Anthropol, **89**: 183–195.

Remenda VH, Cherry JA & Edwards TD (1994) Isotopic composition of old ground water from Lake Agassiz: implications for late Pleistocene climate. Science, **266**: 1975–1978.

Rendall RE, Phillips JI & Renton KA (1994) Death following exposure to fine particulate nickel from a metal arc process. Ann Occup Hyg, **38**: 921–930.

Renshaw PF (1987) A diffusional contribution to lithium isotope effects. Biol Psychiatry, **22**: 73–78.

Rey C, Reinecke HJ & Besser R (1984) Methyltin intoxication in six men; toxicologic and clinical aspects. Vet Hum Toxicol, **26**: 121–122.

Riedel GF (1985) The relationship between chromium VI uptake, sulfate uptake, and chromium toxicity in the estuarine diatom *Thalassiosira pseudonana*. Aquat Toxicol, **7**: 191–204.

Riordan JR (1993) CFTR function. In: Dodge JA, Brock DJH & Widdicombe JH eds. Cystic fibrosis — Current topics. Vol. I. Chichester, John Wiley & Sons, pp 157–173.

Rios C, Galvan-Arzate S & Tapia R (1989) Brain regional thallium distribution in rats acutely intoxicated with Tl_2SO_4. Arch Toxicol, **63**: 34–37.

Robison SH, Cantoni O & Costa M (1982) Strand breakage and decreased molecular weight of DNA induced by specific metal compounds. Carcinogenesis, **3**: 657–662.

Roden DM & George AL (1996) The cardiac ion channels: relevance to management of arrhythmias. Annu Rev Med, **47**: 135–148.

Roels H, Lauwerys R, Buchet JP, Genet P, Sarhan MJ, Hanotiau I, de Fays M, Bernard A & Stanescu D (1987) Epidemiological survey among workers exposed to manganese: effects on lung, central nervous system, and some biological indices. Am J Ind Med, **11**: 307–327.

Roels HA, Ghyselen P, Buchet JP, Ceulemans E & Lauwerys RR (1992) Assessment of the permissible exposure level to manganese in workers exposed to manganese dioxide dust. Br J Ind Med, **49**: 25–34.

Roels H, Meiers G, Delos M, Ortega I, Lauwerys R, Buchet JP & Lison D (1997) Influence of the route of administration and the chemical form ($MnCl_2$, MnO_2) on the absorption and cerebral distribution of manganese in rats. Arch Toxicol, **71**: 223–230.

Roitz JS & Bruland KW (1997) Determination of dissolved manganese (II) in estuarine and coastal waters, by differential pulse cathodic stripping voltammetry. Anal Chim Acta, **344**: 175–180.

Romagnoli P, Labhardt AM & Sinigaglia F (1991) Selective interaction of Ni with an MHC-bound peptide. EMBO J, **10**: 1303–1306.

Romeo L, Apostoli P, Kovacic M, Martini S & Brugnone F (1997) Acute arsine intoxication as a consequence of metal burnishing operations. Am J Ind Med, **32**: 211–216.

Rosenberg E (2005) Speciation of tin. In: Cornelis R, Crews H, Caruso J & Heumann KG eds. Handbook of elemental speciation II. Species in the environment, food, medicine and occupational health. Chichester, John Wiley & Sons, pp 422–463.

Rosenman KD & Stanbury M (1996) Risk of lung cancer among former chromium smelter workers. Am J Ind Med, **29**: 491–500.

Rosman KJR, Chisholm W, Boutron CF, Candelone JP & Görlach U (1993) Isotopic evidence for the source of lead in Greenland snows since the late 1960s. Nature, **362**: 333–335.

Rosner MH & Carter DE (1987) Metabolism and excretion of gallium arsenide and arsenic oxides by hamsters following intratracheal instillation. Fundam Appl Toxicol, **9**: 730–737.

Rossman TG, Uddin AN & Burns FJ (2004) Evidence that arsenite acts as a cocarcinogen in skin cancer. Toxicol Appl Pharmacol, **198**: 394–404.

Roto P (1980) Asthma, symptoms of chronic bronchitis and ventilatory capacity among cobalt and zinc production workers. Scand J Work Environ Health, **6**(suppl 1): 1–49.

Rowbotham AL, Levy LS & Shuker LK (2000) Chromium in the environment: an evaluation of the exposure of the UK general population and possible adverse health effects. J Toxicol Environ Health B Crit Rev, **3**: 145–178.

Rowland I, Davies M & Grasso P (1978) Metabolism of methylmercuric chloride by the gastro-intestinal flora of the rat. Xenobiotica, **8**: 37–43.

Rubanyi G & Balogh I (1982) Effect of nickel on uterine contraction and ultrastructure in the rat. Am J Obstet Gynecol, **142**: 1016–1020.

Rue EL & Bruland KW (1995) Complexation of iron(III) by natural organic ligands in the central north Pacific as determined by a new competitive ligand equilibration/adsorptive cathodic stripping voltammetric method. Mar Chem, **50**: 117–138.

Rueter JG & Morel FMM (1982) The interaction between zinc deficiency and copper toxicity as it affects the silicic acid uptake mechanisms in *Thalassiosira pseudonana*. Limnol Oceanogr, **26**: 67–73.

Ruijten MW, Salle HJ, Verberk MM & Smink M (1994) Effect of chronic mixed pesticide exposure on peripheral and autonomic nerve function. Arch Environ Health, **49**: 188–195.

Ruiz E, Romero F & Besga G (1991) Selective solubilization of heavy metals in torrential river sediments. Toxicol Environ Chem, **33**: 1–6.

Saddique A & Peterson CD (1983) Thallium poisoning: a review. Vet Hum Toxicol, **25**: 16–22.

Sakurai H, Nishida M, Yoshimura T, Takada J & Koyama M (1985) Partition of divalent and total manganese in organs and subcellular organelles of $MnCl_2$-treated rats studied by ESR and neutron activation analysis. Biochim Biophys Acta, **841**: 208–214.

Samitz MH & Epstein E (1962) Experimental cutaneous chrome ulcers in guinea-pigs. Arch Environ Health, **5**: 463–468.

Samitz MH, Katz SA, Scheiner DM & Gross PR (1969) Chromium–protein interactions. Acta Derm Venereol, **49**: 142–146.

Sandborgh-Englund G, Elinder CG, Johanson G, Lind B, Skare I & Ekstrand J (1998) The absorption, blood levels, and excretion of mercury after a single dose of mercury vapor in humans. Toxicol Appl Pharmacol, **150**: 146–153.

Santore RC, Di Toro DM, Paquin PR, Allen HE & Meyer JS (2001) Biotic ligand model of the acute toxicity of metals. 2. Application to acute copper toxicity in freshwater fish and *Daphnia*. Environ Toxicol Chem, **20**: 2397–2402.

Santucci B, Cristaudo A, Cannistraci C & Picardo M (1995) Interaction of palladium ions with the skin. Exp Dermatol, **4**: 207–210.

Sarkar B (1995) Metal replacement in DNA-binding zinc finger proteins and its relevance to mutagenicity and carcinogenicity through free radical generation. Nutrition, **11**: 646–649.

Sartor FA, Rondia DJ, Claeys FD, Staessen JA, Lauwerys RR, Bernard AM, Buchet JP, Roels HA, Bruaux PJ & Ducoffre GM (1992) Impact of environmental cadmium pollution on cadmium exposure and body burden. Arch Environ Health, **47**: 347–353.

Sayato Y, Nakamuro K & Aando M (1980) Metabolic fate of chromium compounds. I. Comparative behavior of chromium in rat administered with $Na_2^{51}CrO_4$ and $^{51}CrCl_3$. J Pharmacobiodyn, **3**(1): 17–23.

Sbrana I, Caretto S, Lascialfari D, Rossi G, Marchi M & Loprieno N (1990) Chromosomal monitoring of chromium-exposed workers. Mutat Res, **242**: 305–312.

Scancar J & Milaćić R (2002) A novel approach for speciation of airborne chromium by convective-interaction media fast-monolithic chromatography with electrothermal atomic-absorption spectrometric detection. Analyst, **127**: 629–633.

Schaaper RM, Koplitz RM, Tkeshelashvili LK & Loeb LA (1987) Metal-induced lethality and mutagenesis: possible role of apurinic intermediates. Mutat Res, **177**: 179–188.

Schaumlöffel D (2005) Speciation of nickel. In: Cornelis R, Crews H, Caruso J & Heumann KG eds. Handbook of elemental speciation II. Species in the environment, food, medicine and occupational health. Chichester, John Wiley & Sons, pp 310–326.

Schiffl H, Weidmann P, Weiss M & Massry SG (1982) Dialysis treatment of acute chromium intoxication and comparative efficacy of peritoneal versus hemodialysis in chromium removal. Miner Electrolyte Metab, 7: 28–35.

Schneider W (1988) Iron hydrolysis and the biochemistry of iron — The interplay of hydroxide and biogenic ligands. Chimia (Aarau), 42: 9–20.

Schneider W & Schwyn B (1987) The hydrolysis of iron in synthetic, biological, and aquatic media. In: Stumm W ed. Aquatic surface chemistry: chemical processes at the particle–water interface. New York, John Wiley, pp 167–196.

Schorn TF, Olbricht C, Schuler A, Franz A, Wittek K, Balks HJ, Hausmann E & Wellhoener HH (1991) Barium carbonate intoxication. Intensive Care Med, 17: 60–62.

Schrauzer GN (2003) The nutritional significance, metabolism and toxicology of seleno-methionine. Adv Food Nutr Res, 47: 73–112.

SGOMSEC (2003) Special issue on methodologies for assessing exposures to metals: speciation, bioaccessibility, and bioavailability in the environment, food, and feed. Ecotoxicol Environ Saf, 56(1): 1–200.

Shi X, Chiu A, Chen CT, Halliwell B, Castranova V & Vallyathan V (1999a) Reduction of chromium(VI) and its relationship to carcinogenesis. J Toxicol Environ Health B Crit Rev, 2: 87–104.

Shi X, Ding M, Ye J, Wang S, Leonard SS, Zang L, Castranova V, Vallyathan V, Chiu A, Dalal N & Liu K (1999b) Cr(IV) causes activation of nuclear transcription factor-kappa B, DNA strand breaks and dG hydroxylation via free radical reactions. J Inorg Biochem, 75: 37–44.

Shi Z (1994) Nickel carbonyl: toxicity and human health. Sci Total Environ, 148: 293–298.

Shi ZC (1986) Acute nickel carbonyl poisoning: a report of 179 cases. Br J Ind Med, 43: 422–424.

Siegler RW, Nierenberg DW & Hickey WF (1999) Fatal poisoning from liquid dimethyl-mercury: a neuropathologic study. Hum Pathol, 30: 720–723.

Silbernagl S (1992) Renal physiology. In: Windhager EE ed. Handbook of physiology, 2nd ed. New York, Oxford University Press, p 1938.

Simkiss K & Taylor MG (1995) Transport of metals across membranes. In: Tessier A & Turner DR eds. Metal speciation and bio-availability in aquatic systems. New York, John Wiley & Sons, pp 1–44.

Simpson JR & Gibson RS (1992) Hair, serum and urine chromium concentrations in former employees of the leather tanning industry. Biol Trace Elem Res, 32: 155–159.

Sin YM, Lim YF & Wong MK (1983) Uptake and distribution of mercury in mice from ingesting soluble and insoluble mercury compounds. Bull Environ Contam Toxicol, **31**: 605–612.

Singh J & Snow ET (1998) Chromium(III) decreases the fidelity of human DNA polymerase beta. Biochemistry, **37**: 9371–9378.

Sinigaglia F (1994) The molecular basis of metal recognition by T cells. J Invest Dermatol, **102**: 398–401.

Sinigaglia F, Scheidegger D, Garotta G, Scherper R, Pletscher M & Lanzavecchia A (1985) Isolation and characterization of Ni-specific clones from patients with Ni-contact dermatitis. J Immunol, **135**: 3929–3932.

Skerfving S (1992) Biological monitoring of exposure to inorganic lead. In: Clarkson TW, Friberg L, Nordberg GF & Sager PR eds. Biological monitoring of toxic metals. New York, Plenum Press, pp 169–198.

Skoet R, Olsen J, Mathiesen B, Iversen L, Johansen DJ & Agner T (2004) A survey of occupational hand eczema in Denmark. Contact Dermatitis, **51**: 159–166.

Smith DR, Ilustre RP & Osterloh JD (1998) Methodological considerations for the accurate determination of lead in human plasma and serum. Am J Ind Med, **33**(5): 430–438.

Smith MK, George EL, Stober JA, Feng HA & Kimmel GL (1993) Perinatal toxicity associated with nickel chloride exposure. Environ Res, **61**: 200–211.

Smith SL (1997) An avoidable tragedy. Occup Hazards, **59**: 32.

Sorahan T & Harrington JM (2000) Lung cancer in Yorkshire chrome platers, 1972–97. Occup Environ Med, **57**: 385–389.

Sorahan T, Burges DC, Hamilton L & Harrington JM (1998) Lung cancer mortality in nickel/chromium platers, 1946–95. Occup Environ Med, **55**: 236–242.

Spedding M & Cavero I (1984) "Calcium antagonists": a class of drugs with a bright future. Part II. Determination of basic pharmacological properties. Life Sci, **35**: 575–587.

Speetjens JK, Collins RA, Vincent JB & Woski SA (1999) The nutritional supplement chromium(III) tris(picolinate) cleaves DNA. Chem Res Toxicol, **12**: 483–487.

Spini G, Profumo A, Riolo C, Beone GM & Zecca E (1994) Determination of hexavalent, trivalent and metallic chromium in welding fumes. Toxicol Environ Chem, **41**: 209–219.

Spuznar J (2000) Bio-inorganic speciation analysis by hyphenated techniques. Analyst, **125**: 963–988.

Squibb K & Fowler B (1984) Intracellular metabolism and effects of circulating cadmium–metallothionein in the kidney. Environ Health Perspect, **54**: 31–35.

Standeven AM & Wetterhahn KE (1991) Possible role of glutathione in chromium(VI) metabolism and toxicity in rats. Pharmacol Toxicol, **69**: 469–476.

Stauber JL & Florence TM (1987) Mechanisms of toxicity of ionic copper and copper complexes to algae. Mar Biol, **94**: 511–519.

Stern FB (2003) Mortality among chrome leather tannery workers: an update. Am J Ind Med, **44**: 197–206.

Stevens JT, Hall LL, Farmer JD, DiPasquale LC, Chernoff N & Durham WF (1977) Disposition of ^{14}C and/or ^{74}As-cacodylic acid in rats after intravenous, intratracheal, or peroral administration. Environ Health Perspect, **19**: 151–157.

Stewart DW & Hummel RP (1984) Acute poisoning by a barium chloride burn. J Trauma, **24**: 768–770.

Stift A, Friedl J, Langle F, Berlakovich G, Steininger R & Muhlbacher F (2000) Successful treatment of a patient suffering from severe acute potassium dichromate poisoning with liver transplantation. Transplantation, **69**: 2454–2455.

Stillman MJ, Shaw CF & Suzuki KT (1992) Metallothioneins: synthesis, structure and properties of metallothioneins, phytochelatins and metal-thiolate complexes. New York, VCH.

Stuhne-Sekalec L, Xu SX, Parkes JG, Olivieri NF & Templeton DM (1992) Speciation of tissue and cellular iron with on-line detection by inductively coupled plasma–mass spectrometry. Anal Biochem, **205**: 278–284.

Styblo M, Drobna Z, Jaspers I, Lin S & Thomas DJ (2002) The role of biomethylation in toxicity and carcinogenicity of arsenic: a research update. Environ Health Perspect, **110**(suppl 5): 767–771.

Sue YJ (1994) Mercury. In: Goldfrank LR, Flomenbaum NE, Howland MA, Hoffman RS & Weisman RS eds. Goldfrank's toxicologic emergencies, 5th ed. Norwalk, Connecticut, Appleton & Lange, pp 1051–1062.

Sun BG, Macka M & Haddad PR (2004) Speciation of arsenic and selenium by capillary electrophoresis. J Chromatogr A, **1039**: 201–208.

Sun XF, Ting BT & Janghorbani M (1987) Excretion of trimethylselenonium ion in human urine. Anal Biochem, **167**: 304–311.

Sunda WG & Hansen PJ (1979) Chemical speciation of copper in river water: effect of total copper, pH, carbonate, and dissolved organic matter. In: Jenne EA ed. Chemical modeling in aqueous systems: speciation, sorption, solubility and kinetics. Washington, DC, American Chemical Society.

Sunda WG & Huntsman SA (1983) Effect of competitive interactions between manganese and copper on cellular manganese and growth in estuarine and oceanic species of the diatom, *Thalassiosira*. Limnol Oceanogr, **28**: 924–934.

Sunda WG & Huntsman SA (1987) Microbial oxidation of manganese in a North Carolina estuary. Limnol Oceanogr, **32**: 552–564.

Sunda WG & Huntsman SA (1988) Effect of sunlight on redox cycles of manganese in the southwestern Sargasso Sea. Deep Sea Res, **35**(8): 1297–1317.

Sunda WG & Huntsman SA (1991) The use of chemiluminescence and ligand competition with EDTA to measure copper concentration and speciation in seawater. Mar Chem, **36**: 137–163.

Sunda WG & Huntsman SA (1992) Feedback interactions between zinc and phytoplankton in seawater. Limnol Oceanogr, **37**: 25–40.

Sunda WG & Huntsman SA (1995) Cobalt and zinc interreplacement in marine phytoplankton: biological and geochemical implications. Limnol Oceanogr, **40**: 1404–1417.

Sunda WG & Huntsman SA (1996) Antagonisms between cadmium and zinc toxicity and manganese limitation in a coastal diatom. Limnol Oceanogr, **41**: 373–387.

Sunda WG & Huntsman SA (1998a) Processes regulating cellular metal accumulation and physiological effects: Phytoplankton as model systems. Sci Total Environ, **219**: 165–181.

Sunda WG & Huntsman SA (1998b) Control of Cd concentrations in a coastal diatom by interactions among free ionic Cd, Zn and Mn in seawater. Environ Sci Technol, **32**: 2961–2968.

Sunda WG & Huntsman SA (1998c) Interactions among Cu^{2+}, Zn^{2+} and Mn^{2+} in controlling cellular Mn, Zn and growth rate in the coastal alga *Chlamydomonas*. Limnol Oceanogr, **43**: 1055–1064.

Sundberg J, Jonsson S, Karlsson MO, Hallen IP & Oskarsson A (1998) Kinetics of methylmercury and inorganic mercury in lactating and nonlactating mice. Toxicol Appl Pharmacol, **151**: 319–329.

Sunderman FW (1984) Nickel in the human environment. Lyon, International Agency for Research on Cancer (IARC Scientific Publications No. 53).

Sunderman FW (1989) Mechanisms of nickel carcinogenesis. Scand J Work Environ Health, **15**: 1–12.

Sunderman FW & Donnelly AJ (1965) Studies of nickel carcinogenesis metastasizing pulmonary tumors in rats induced by the inhalation of nickel carbonyl. Am J Pathol, **70**: 1027–1041.

Sunderman FW & Kincaid JF (1954) Nickel poisoning. II. Studies on patients suffering from acute exposure to vapors of nickel carbonyl. J Am Med Assoc, **155**: 889–894.

Sunderman FW, Shen SK, Mitchell JM, Allpass PR & Damjanov I (1978) Embryotoxicity and fetal toxicity of nickel in rats. Toxicol Appl Pharmacol, **43**: 381–390.

Sunderman FW, Allpass PR, Mitchell JM, Baselt RC & Albert DM (1979) Eye malformations in rats: induction by prenatal exposure to nickel carbonyl. Science, **203**: 550–553.

Sunderman FW, Shen SK, Reid MC & Allpass PR (1980) Teratogenicity and embryotoxicity of nickel carbonyl in Syrian hamsters. Teratog Carcinog Mutagen, **1**: 223–233.

Sunderman FW, Dingle B, Hopfer SM & Swift T (1988) Acute nickel toxicity in electroplating workers who accidently [sic] ingested a solution of nickel sulfate and nickel chloride. Am J Ind Med, **14**: 257–266.

Sunderman FW, Hopfer SM, Sweeney KR, Marcus AH, Most BM & Creason J (1989) Nickel absorption and kinetics in human volunteers. Proc Soc Exp Biol Med, **191**: 5–11.

Suzuki KT & Ogra Y (2002) Metabolic pathway for selenium in the body: speciation by HPLC-ICP-MS with enriched Se. Food Addit Contam, **19**: 974–983.

Swennen B, Buchet JP, Stanescu D, Lison D & Lauwerys R (1993) Epidemiological survey of workers exposed to cobalt oxides, cobalt salts, and cobalt metal. Br J Ind Med, **50**: 835–842.

Szpunar J, Schmitt VO, Lobinski R & Monod JL (1996) Rapid speciation of butyltin compounds in sediments and biomaterials by capillary gas chromatography – microwave-induced plasma atomic emission spectrometry after microwave-assisted leaching/digestion. J Anal At Spectrom, **11**: 193–199.

Takahashi M, Fukuda K, Ohkubo Y, Tokuhiro N, Tsuchiya R, Yoshie M & Hirai Y (2004) Nonfatal barium intravasation into the portal venous system during barium enema examination. Intern Med, **43**: 1145–1150.

Takahashi Y, Tsuruta S, Hasegawa J, Kameyama Y & Yoshida M (2001) Release of mercury from dental amalgam fillings in pregnant rats and distribution of mercury in maternal and fetal tissues. Toxicology, **163**: 115–126.

Takahashi Y, Tsuruta S, Arimoto M, Tanaka H & Yoshida M (2003) Placental transfer of mercury in pregnant rats which received dental amalgam restorations. Toxicology, **185**: 23–33.

Tam GKH, Charbonneau SM, Bryce F, Pomroy C & Sandi E (1979) Metabolism of inorganic arsenic (^{74}As) in humans following oral ingestion. Toxicol Appl Pharmacol, **50**: 319–322.

Taylor A, Branch S, Halls D, Patriarca M & White M (2005) Atomic spectrometry update. Clinical and biological materials, foods and beverages. J Anal At Spectrom, **20**: 323–369.

Taylor D (1962) The absorption of cobalt from the gastro-intestinal tract of the rat. Phys Med Biol, **6**: 445–451.

Taylor GA, Ferrier IN, McLoughlin IJ, Fairbairn AF, McKeith IG, Lett D & Edwardson JA (1992) Gastrointestinal absorption of aluminium in Alzheimer's disease: response to aluminium citrate. Age Ageing, **21**: 81–90.

Teitelbaum DT & Kier LC (1969) Arsine poisoning. Report of five cases in the petroleum industry and a discussion of the indications for exchange transfusion and hemodialysis. Arch Environ Health, **19**: 133–143.

Templeton DM (1990) Cadmium uptake by cells of renal origin. J Biol Chem, **265**: 21764–21770.

Templeton DM (1995) Therapeutic use of chelating agents in iron overload. In: Goyer RA & Cherian MG eds. Handbook of experimental pharmacology. Vol. 115. Toxicology of metals — biochemical aspects. Berlin, Springer-Verlag, pp 303–331.

Templeton DM (2003) The importance of trace element speciation in biomedical science. Anal Bioanal Chem, **375**: 1062–1066.

Templeton DM (2004) Mechanisms of immunosensitization to metals. Pure Appl Chem, **76**: 1255–1268.

Templeton DM (2005) Selected examples of important metal–protein species. In: Cornelis R, Crews H, Caruso J & Heumann KG eds. Handbook of elemental speciation II. Species in the environment, food, medicine and occupational health. Chichester, John Wiley & Sons, pp 638–650.

Templeton DM & Cherian MG (1991) Toxicological significance of metallothionein. Methods Enzymol, **205**: 11–24.

Templeton DM, Ariese F, Cornelis R, Danielsson L-G, Muntau H, van Leeuwen H & Lobinski L (2000) Guidelines for terms related to chemical speciation and fractionation of elements: definitions, structural aspects, and methodological approaches. Pure Appl Chem, **72**: 1453–1470.

Tenenbein M (1997) Leaded gasoline abuse: the role of tetraethyl lead. Hum Exp Toxicol, **16**: 217–222.

Terrill PJ & Gowar JP (1990) Chromic acid burns; beware, be aggressive, be watchful. Br J Plast Surg, **43**: 699–701.

Thayer JS (1993) Global bioalkylation of the heavy elements. In: Sigel H & Sigel A eds. Metal ions in biological systems. Vol. 29. Biological properties of metal alkyl derivatives. New York, Marcel Dekker, pp 1–36.

Thévenod F (2003) Nephrotoxicity and the proximal tubule. Insights from cadmium. Nephron Physiol, **93**: 87–93.

Thier R & Bolt HM (2001) European aspects of standard setting in occupational hygiene and medicine. Rev Environ Health, **16**: 81–86.

Thomas M, Bowie D & Walker R (1998) Acute barium intoxication following ingestion of ceramic glaze. Postgrad Med J, **74**: 545–546.

Thomson C (1998) Selenium speciation in human body fluids. Analyst, **123**: 827–831.

Thomson C, Robinson M, Campbell D & Rea H (1982) Effect of prolonged supplementation with daily supplements of selenomethionine and sodium selenite on glutathione peroxidase activity in blood of New Zealand residents. Am J Clin Nutr, **36**: 24–29.

Tilson HA, Mactutus CF, McLamb RL & Burne TA (1982) Characterization of triethyl lead chloride neurotoxicity in adult rats. Neurobehav Toxicol Teratol, **4**: 671–681.

Tjalve H & Henriksson J (1999) Uptake of metals in the brain via olfactory pathways. Neurotoxicology, **20**(2–3): 181–195.

Toll LL & Hurlbut KM eds (2002) 13. Arzneikompendium der Schweiz 2001. POISINDEX® System. Greenwood Village, Colorado, Micromedex.

Toribara TY, Clarkson TW & Nierenberg DW (1997) Chemical safety: more on working with dimethylmercury. Chem Eng News, **75**: 6.

Town RM, Emons H & Buffle J (2003) Speciation analysis by electrochemical methods. In: Cornelis R, Crews H, Caruso J & Heumann KG eds. Handbook of elemental speciation I. Techniques and methodology. Chichester, John Wiley & Sons, pp 427–460.

Trinder D, Oates PS, Thomas C, Sadleir J & Morgan EH (2000) Localisation of divalent metal transporter 1 (DMT1) to the microvillus membrane of rat duodenal enterocytes in iron deficiency, but to hepatocytes in iron overload. Gut, **46**: 270–276.

Trull AK, Demers LM, Holt DW, Johnston A, Tredger JM & Price CP (2002) Biomarkers of disease. Cambridge, Cambridge University Press.

Turner DR, Whitfield M & Dickson AG (1981) The equilibrium speciation of dissolved components in freshwater and seawater at 25°C and 1 atm pressure. Geochim Cosmochim Acta, **45**: 855–881.

Turner M, Smith J & Kilkpper R (1975) Absorption of natural methylmercury (MeHg) from fish. Clin Res, **23**: 2–7.

Uden PC (2005) Speciation of selenium. In: Cornelis R, Crews H, Caruso J & Heumann KG eds. Handbook of elemental speciation II. Species in the environment, food, medicine and occupational health. Chichester, John Wiley & Sons, pp 346–365.

Uehara T, Watanabe H, Itoh F, Inoue S, Koshida H, Nakamura M, Yamate J & Maruyama T (2005) Nephrotoxicity of a novel antineoplastic platinum complex, neda-platin: a comparative study with cisplatinum in rats. Arch Toxicol, **79**: 451–460.

Umemura T, Sai K, Takagi A, Hasegawa R & Kurokawa Y (1990a) Oxidative DNA damage, lipid peroxidation and nephrotoxicity induced in the rat kidney after ferric nitrilotriacetate administration. Cancer Lett, **54**: 95–100.

Umemura T, Sai K, Takagi A, Hasegawa R & Kurokawa Y (1990b) Formation of 8-hydroxydeoxyguanosine (8-OH-dG) in rat kidney DNA after intraperitoneal administration of ferric nitrilotriacetate (Fe-NTA). Carcinogenesis, **11**: 345–347.

USEPA (1984) Health assessment document for chromium. Research Triangle Park, North Carolina, United States Environmental Protection Agency (Final Report No. EPA600/8-83-014F).

USEPA (1986) Air quality criteria for lead. Research Triangle Park, North Carolina, United States Environmental Protection Agency, Office of Research and Development, Office of Health and Environmental Assessment, Environmental Criteria and Assessment Office (Report No. EPA 600/8-83-028F).

USEPA (1997) Study report to Congress. Washington, DC, United States Environmental Protection Agency (EPA-452/R-97-003).

USEPA (2005) Procedures for the derivation of equilibrium partitioning sediment benchmarks (ESBs) for the protection of benthic organisms: metal mixtures (cadmium, copper, lead, nickel, silver and zinc). Washington, DC, United States Environmental Protection Agency, Office of Research and Development (Report No. EPA-600-R-02-011).

USFDA (1983) Mercury toxicity in ear irrigation. United States Food and Drug Administration. FDA Drug Bull, **13**: 5–6.

Vaglenov A, Nosko M, Georgieva R, Carbonell E, Creus A & Marcos R (1999) Genotoxicity and radioresistance in electroplating workers exposed to chromium. Mutat Res, **446**: 23–34.

Vahter M (1999) Methylation of inorganic arsenic in different mammalian species and population groups. Sci Prog, **82**: 69–88.

Vahter M (2002) Mechanisms of arsenic biotransformation. Toxicology, **181–182**: 211–217.

Vahter M & Norin H (1980) Metabolism of ^{74}As-labelled trivalent and pentavalent inorganic arsenic in mice. Environ Res, **21**: 446–457.

Vahter M, Concha G, Nermell B, Nilsson R, Dulout F & Natarajan N (1995) A unique metabolism of inorganic arsenic in native Andean women. Eur J Pharmacol Environ Toxicol Pharmacol, **293**: 455–462.

Valkonen S & Riikimäki V (2005) Speciation of aluminum in occupational health. In: Cornelis R, Crews H, Caruso J & Heumann KG eds. Handbook of elemental speciation II. Species in the environment, food, medicine and occupational health. Chichester, John Wiley & Sons, pp 40–46.

Van Assche F, Van Tilborg W & Waeterschoot H (1996) Environmental risk assessment for essential elements — case study zinc. In: Report of the international workshop on risk assessment of metals and their inorganic compounds, Angers, France, 13–15 November 1996. Ottawa, Ontario, The International Council on Metals and the Environment, pp 171–180.

van den Berg CMG, Merks AGA & Dursma EK (1987) Organic complexation and its control of the dissolved concentrations of copper and zinc in the Scheldt estuary. Estuarine Coastal Shelf Sci, **24**: 785–797.

Van Goethem F, Lison D & Kirsch-Volders M (1997) Comparative evaluation of the in vitro micronucleus test and the alkaline single cell gel electrophoresis assay for the detection of DNA damaging agents: genotoxic effects of cobalt powder, tungsten carbide and cobalt–tungsten carbide. Mutat Res, **392**(1–2): 31–43.

Vanhaecke F & Köllensperger G (2003) Detection by ICP–mass spectrometry. In: Cornelis R, Crews H, Caruso J & Heumann KG eds. Handbook of elemental speciation I. Techniques and methodology. Chichester, John Wiley & Sons, pp 281–312.

Varma PP, Jha V, Ghosh AK, Joshi K & Sakhuja V (1994) Acute renal failure in a case of fatal chromic acid poisoning. Ren Fail, **16**: 653–657.

Verity MA, Sarafian TS, Guerra W, Ettinger A & Sharp J (1990) Ionic modulation of triethyllead neurotoxicity in cerebellar granule cell culture. Neurotoxicology, **11**: 415–426.

Verougstraete V (2005) Speciation of cadmium in health and disease. In: Cornelis R, Crews H, Caruso J & Heumann KG eds. Handbook of elemental speciation II. Species in the environment, food, medicine and occupational health. Chichester, John Wiley & Sons, pp 107–119.

Versieck J & Cornelis R (1989) Trace elements in human plasma or serum. Boca Raton, Florida, CRC Press.

Versieck J, Barbier F, Cornelis R & Hoste J (1982) Sample contamination as a source of error in trace-element analysis of biological samples. Talanta, **29**: 973–984.

Villaverde MS & Verstraeten SV (2003) Effects of thallium(I) and thallium(III) on liposome membrane physical properties. Arch Biochem Biophys, **417**: 235–243.

Vincent JB (1999) Mechanisms of chromium action: low-molecular-weight chromium-binding substance. J Am Coll Nutr, **18**: 6–12.

Vuopala U, Huhti E, Takkunen J & Huikko M (1970) Nickel carbonyl poisoning. Report of 25 cases. Ann Clin Res, **2**: 214–222.

Walczyk T (2005) Iron speciation in biomedicine. In: Cornelis R, Crews H, Caruso J & Heumann KG eds. Handbook of elemental speciation II. Species in the environment, food, medicine and occupational health. Chichester, John Wiley & Sons, pp 219–238.

Walsh C (1979) Enzymatic reaction mechanisms. San Francisco, California, W.H. Freeman.

Walsh CT, Distefano MD, Moore MJ, Shewchuk LM & Verdine GL (1988) Molecular basis of bacterial resistance to organomercurial and inorganic mercuric salts. FASEB J, **2**: 124–138.

Walsh TJ, Schulz DW, Tilson HA & Dehaven DL (1986) Acute exposure to triethyl lead enhances the behavioral effects of dopaminergic agonists: involvement of brain dopamine in organolead neurotoxicity. Brain Res, **363**: 222–229.

Wapnir RA (1998) Copper absorption and bioavailability. Am J Clin Nutr, **67**: 1054–1060.

Wapnir RA & Stiel L (1986) Zinc intestinal absorption in rats: specificity of amino acids as ligands. J Nutr, **116**: 2171–2179.

Ward JM, Joung DM & Fauvie KA (1976) Comparative nephrotoxicity of platinum cancer therapeutic agents. Cancer Treat Rep, **60**: 1675–1678.

Warfvinge K, Hua J & Logdberg B (1994) Mercury distribution in cortical areas and fiber systems of the neonatal and maternal adult cerebrum after exposure of pregnant squirrel monkeys to mercury vapor. Environ Res, **67**: 196–208.

Webb DR, Sipes IG & Carter DE (1984) In vitro solubility and in vivo toxicity of gallium arsenide. Toxicol Appl Pharmacol, **76**: 96–104.

Wei M, Wanibuchi H, Morimura K, Iwai S, Yoshida K, Endo G, Nakae D & Fukushima S (2002) Carcinogenicity of dimethylarsinic acid in male F344 rats and genetic alterations in induced urinary bladder tumors. Carcinogenesis, **23**: 1387–1397.

Weiler RR (1987) Panel discussion: mechanism and health effects of chromium. Environ Health Perspect, **92**: 87–89.

Weinshilboum RM, Otterness DM & Szumlanski CL (1999) Methylation pharmacogenet-ics: catecol O-methyltransferase, thiopurine methyltransferase, and histamine N-methyl-transferase. Annu Rev Pharmacol Toxicol, **39**: 19–52.

Welter E (2003) Direct speciation of solids: X-ray absorption fine structure spectroscopy for species analysis in solid samples. In: Cornelis R, Crews H, Caruso J & Heumann KG eds. Handbook of elemental speciation I. Techniques and methodology. Chichester, John Wiley & Sons, pp 526–545.

Wetterhahn KE & Hamilton JW (1989) Molecular basis of hexavalent chromium carcino-genicity: effect and expression. Sci Total Environ, **86**: 113–129.

Whanger PD (2002) Selenocompounds in plants and animals and their biological significance. J Am Coll Nutr, **21**: 223–232.

Whanger PD, Xia Y & Thomson CD (1994) Protein technics for selenium speciation. J Trace Elem Electrolytes Health Dis, **8**: 1–7.

Whitlam JB & Brown KF (1981) Ultrafiltration in serum-protein binding determinations. J Pharm Sci, **70**: 146–150.

Whittaker P, Ali SF, Imam SZ & Dunkel VC (2002) Acute toxicity of carbonyl iron and sodium iron EDTA compared with ferrous sulfate in young rats. Regul Toxicol Pharmacol, **36**: 280–286.

WHO (1979) Mercury. Geneva, World Health Organization, International Programme on Chemical Safety (Environmental Health Criteria 1).

WHO (1980) Tin and organotin compounds. Geneva, World Health Organization, International Programme on Chemical Safety (Environmental Health Criteria 15).

WHO (1981) Manganese. Geneva, World Health Organization, International Programme on Chemical Safety (Environmental Health Criteria 17).

WHO (1988) Chromium. Geneva, World Health Organization, International Programme on Chemical Safety (Environmental Health Criteria 61).

WHO (1990a) Methylmercury. Geneva, World Health Organization, International Programme on Chemical Safety, pp 1–197 (Environmental Health Criteria 101).

WHO (1990b) Barium. Geneva, World Health Organization, International Programme on Chemical Safety (Environmental Health Criteria 107).

WHO (1991a) Nickel. Geneva, World Health Organization, International Programme on Chemical Safety (Environmental Health Criteria 108).

WHO (1991b) Inorganic mercury. Geneva, World Health Organization, International Programme on Chemical Safety (Environmental Health Criteria 118).

WHO (1992) Cadmium. Geneva, World Health Organization, International Programme on Chemical Safety (Environmental Health Criteria 134).

WHO (1994) Organic lead. Geneva, World Health Organization, International Programme on Chemical Safety (Poison Information Monograph 302).

WHO (1995) Inorganic lead. Geneva, World Health Organization, International Programme on Chemical Safety (Environmental Health Criteria 165).

WHO (1996a) Thallium. Geneva, World Health Organization, International Programme on Chemical Safety (Environmental Health Criteria 182).

WHO (1996b) Biological monitoring of chemical exposure in the workplace. Vol. 1. Geneva, World Health Organization, 300 pp.

WHO (1997) Triethyltin. Geneva, World Health Organization, International Programme on Chemical Safety (Poison Information Monograph 588).

WHO (1999a) Manganese and its compounds. Geneva, World Health Organization, International Programme on Chemical Safety (Concise International Chemical Assessment Document 12).

WHO (1999b) Trimethyltin compounds. Geneva, World Health Organization, International Programme on Chemical Safety (Poison Information Monograph; Group PIM G019).

WHO (2000a) Copper. Geneva, World Health Organization, International Programme on Chemical Safety (Environmental Health Criteria 200).

WHO (2000b) *Statement on thiomersal.* Geneva, World Health Organization, Global Advisory Committee on Vaccine Safety (http://www.who.int/vaccine_safety/topics/thiomersal/statement200308/en/index.html).

WHO (2001) Arsenic and arsenic compounds. Geneva, World Health Organization, International Programme on Chemical Safety (Environmental Health Criteria 224).

WHO (2003) Elemental mercury and inorganic mercury compounds: human health aspects. Geneva, World Health Organization, International Programme on Chemical Safety (Concise International Chemical Assessment Document 50).

WHO (2005) Tin and inorganic tin compounds. Geneva, World Health Organization, International Programme on Chemical Safety (Concise International Chemical Assessment Document 65).

Wild P, Perdrix A, Romazini S, Moulin JJ & Pellet F (2001) Lung cancer mortality in a site producing hard metals. Occup Environ Med, **57**: 568–573.

Wilhelm SW & Trick CG (1994) Iron-limited growth of cyanobacteria: Multiple siderophore production is a common response. Limnol Oceanogr, **39**(8): 1979–1984.

Williams RJP (1981) Physico-chemical aspects of inorganic element transfer through membranes. Phil Trans R Soc Lond B, **294**: 57–74.

Williams RJP (1985) The symbiosis of metal and protein functions. Eur J Biochem, **150**: 231–248.

Windisch W (2002) Interaction of chemical species with biological regulation of the metabolism of essential trace elements. Anal Bioanal Chem, **372**: 421–425.

Windisch WM, Gotterbarm GG & Roth FX (2001) Effect of potassium diformate in combination with different amounts and sources of excessive dietary copper on production performance in weaning piglets. Arch Anim Nutr, **54**(2): 87–100.

Wirth PL & Linder MC (1985) Distribution of copper among components of human serum. J Natl Cancer Inst, **75**: 277–283.

Wrobel K, Wrobel K, Kannamkumarath SS & Caruso JA (2003) Identification of selenium species in urine by ion-pairing HPLC-ICP-MS using laboratory-synthesized standards. Anal Bioanal Chem, **377**: 670–674.

Wu FY, Wu WY, Kuo HW, Liu CS, Wang RY & Lai JS (2001) Effect of genotoxic exposure to chromium among electroplating workers in Taiwan. Sci Total Environ, **279**: 21–28.

Wu J & Luther GW (1995) Complexation of iron(III) by natural organic ligands in the northwest Atlantic Ocean by a competitive ligand equilibration method and a kinetic approach. Mar Chem, **50**: 159–177.

Xie H, Holmes AL, Wise SS, Gordon N & Wise JP Sr (2004) Lead chromate–induced chromosome damage requires extracellular dissolution to liberate chromium ions but does not require particle internalization or intracellular dissolution. Chem Res Toxicol, **17**: 1362–1367.

Xue H & Sunda WG (1997) Comparison of $[Cu^{2+}]$ measurements in lake water determined by ligand exchange and cathodic stripping voltammetry and by ion-selective electrode. Environ Sci Technol, **31**: 1902–1909.

Xue H, Kistler D & Sigg L (1995) Competition of copper and zinc for strong ligands in a eutrophic lake. Limnol Oceanogr, **40**: 1142–1152.

Xue H, Oestreich A, Kistler D & Sigg L (1996) Free cupric ion concentrations and Cu complexation in selected Swiss lakes and rivers. Aqua Sci, **58**: 69–87.

Yager JW, Hicks JB & Fabianova E (1997) Airborne arsenic and urine excretion of arsenic metabolites during boiler cleaning operations in a Slovak coal-fired power plant. Environ Health Perspect, **105**: 836–842.

Yagminas AP, Little PB, Rousseaux CG, Franklin CA & Villeneuve DC (1992) Neuropathologic findings in young male rats in a subchronic oral toxicity study using triethyl lead. Fundam Appl Toxicol, **19**: 380–387.

Yamamoto S, Konishi Y, Matsuda T, Murai T, Shibata MA, Matsui Yuasa I, Otani S, Kuroda K, Endo G & Fukushima S (1995) Cancer induction by an organic arsenic compound, dimethylarsinic acid (cacodylic acid), in F344/DuCrj rats after pretreatment with five carcinogens. Cancer Res, **55**: 1271–1276.

Yamauchi H & Yamamura Y (1984) Metabolism and excretion of orally administered dimethylarsinic acid in the hamster. Toxicol Appl Pharmacol, **74**: 134–140.

Yamauchi H, Yamato N & Yamamura Y (1988) Metabolism and excretion of orally and intraperitoneally administered methylarsenic acid in the hamster. Bull Environ Contam Toxicol, **40**: 280–286.

Yamauchi H, Takahashi K, Yamamura Y & Kaise T (1989) Metabolism and excretion of orally and intraperitoneally administered trimethylarsine oxide in the hamster. Toxicol Environ Chem, **22**: 69–76.

Yamauchi H, Kaise T, Takahashi K & Yamamura Y (1990) Toxicity and metabolism of trimethylarsine in mice and hamster. Fundam Appl Toxicol, **14**: 399–407.

Yang JM, Jiang XZ, Chen QY, Li PJ, Zhou YF & Wang YL (1996) The distribution of $HgCl_2$ in rat body and its effects on fetus. Biomed Environ Sci, **9**: 437–442.

Yannai S & Sachs KM (1993) Absorption and accumulation of cadmium, lead and mercury from foods by rats. Food Chem Toxicol, **31**(5): 351–355.

Yokel RA, Lasley SM & Dorman DC (2006) The speciation of metals in mammals influences their toxicokinetics and toxicodynamics and therefore human health risk assessment. J Toxicol Environ Health B Crit Rev, **9**(1): 63–85.

Yoshida M, Yamamura Y & Satoh H (1986) Distribution of mercury in guinea pig offspring after in utero exposure to mercury vapor during late gestation. Arch Toxicol, **58**: 225–228.

Yoshida M, Aoyama H, Satoh H & Yamamura Y (1987) Binding of mercury to metallothionein-like protein in fetal liver of the guinea pig following in utero exposure to mercury vapor. Toxicol Lett, **37**: 1–6.

Yoshida M, Satoh M, Shimada A, Yamamoto E, Yasutake A & Tohyama C (2002) Maternal-to-fetus transfer of mercury in metallothionein-null pregnant mice after exposure to mercury vapor. Toxicology, **175**: 215–222.

Yoshida M, Watanabe C, Horie K, Satoh M, Sawada M & Shimada A (2005) Neurobehavioral changes in metallothionein-null mice prenatally exposed to mercury vapor. Toxicol Lett, **155**: 361–368.

Zanetti G & Fubini B (1997) Surface interaction between metallic cobalt and tungsten carbide particles as a primary cause of hard metal lung disease. J Mater Chem, **7**: 1647–1654.

Zelikoff JT & Thomas PT (1998) Immunotoxicology of environmental and occupational metals. London, Taylor & Francis.

Zhang J (1984) Clinical observations in ethyl mercury chloride poisoning. Am J Ind Med, **5**: 251–258.

Zhang X & Zhang C (2003) Atomic absorption and atomic emission spectrometry. In: Cornelis R, Crews H, Caruso J & Heumann KG eds. Handbook of elemental speciation I. Techniques and methodology. Chichester, John Wiley & Sons, pp 241–260.

Zhang X, Cornelis R, DeKimpe J & Mees L (1996) Arsenic speciation in serum of uraemic patients based on liquid chromatography with hydride generation atomic absorption spectrometry and on-line UV photo-oxidation digestion. Anal Chim Acta, **319**: 177–185.

Zhang XR, Cornelis R, De Kimpe J, Mees L & Lameire N (1998) Study of arsenic–protein binding in serum of patients on continuous ambulatory peritoneal dialysis. Clin Chem, **44**: 141–147.

Zheng W, Aschner M & Ghersi-Egea JF (2003) Brain barrier systems: a new frontier in metal neurotoxicological research. Toxicol Appl Pharmacol, **192**: 1–11.

Zhitkovich A, Quievryn G, Messer J & Motylevich Z (2002) Reductive activation with cysteine represents a chromium(III)-dependent pathway in the induction of genotoxicity by carcinogenic chromium(VI). Environ Health Perspect, **110**(suppl 5): 729–731.

RESUME

1. Thème et objet du document

Le présent document a pour objet, d'une part d'examiner et d'apprécier le rôle de la spéciation des éléments et de son analyse dans l'évaluation des dangers et des risques et d'autre part de fournir un certain nombre d'orientations à cet égard, plutôt que de passer en revue chaque élément et sa spéciation. Les effets sur l'environnement n'y sont pas pris en considération car ils figurent à l'ordre du jour d'une récente conférence ainsi que dans la documentation correspondante (SGOMSEC, 2003). Toutefois, le document traite de l'exposition de la population humaine dans l'environnement.

Ce document vise à rappeler aux experts en évaluation du risque ainsi qu'aux organismes de surveillance qu'il est important pour eux de prendre en compte la question de la spéciation dans leurs réflexions. Jusqu'ici, cet aspect des choses n'a pas été envisagé dans la plupart des évaluations portant sur les dangers et les risques. Il s'agit aussi, en préconisant le recours à l'analyse de la spéciation, de préciser comment elle peut influencer le mode d'action des divers éléments et de mieux comprendre leurs effets sur la santé.

Le document n'est pas axé sur les besoins nutritionnels mais sur la toxicité des différents éléments pour l'Homme. Par ailleurs, il n'est pas seulement question de l'exposition des consommateurs et de la population en général mais aussi de l'exposition professionnelle.

2. Définitions

On entend par « espèce chimique » la forme particulière sous laquelle se trouve un élément et qui est définie par sa composition isotopique, son état électronique, son degré d'oxydation ou sa structure complexe ou moléculaire. On peut définir la spéciation comme la distribution, à l'intérieur d'un système donné, d'un élément sous un certain nombre de formes chimiques déterminées et l'analyse de la spéciation comme l'identification et le dosage de la ou des espèces chimiques présentes dans l'échantillon.

Résumé

3. Aspects structuraux de la spéciation

Dans la définition de l'espèce chimique et de la spéciation sont pris en compte différents niveaux de structure atomique ou moléculaire auxquels se manifestent précisément des différences spécifiques. Dans le cas présent, les différences qui sont prises en compte résultent 1) de la composition isotopique, 2) de l'état électronique ou du degré d'oxydation, 3) de la forme, organique ou minérale du composé ou du complexe, 4) du fait qu'il s'agit d'un dérivé organométallique, 5) du fait qu'il s'agit d'un composé ou d'un complexe macromoléculaire. Certains de ces niveaux de structure sont plus importants que d'autres en ce qui concerne l'évaluation du risque. Par exemple, la stabilité de la composition isotopique, si elle est importante du point de vue théorique ou en chimie physique ou environnementale, n'est généralement que d'une importance minime en ce qui concerne l'évaluation du risque pour la santé humaine. De même, on connaît l'importance biologique de la spéciation des éléments au niveau macromoléculaire en physiologie, biochimie et nutrition mais on sait moins bien ce qu'elle représente du point de vue du risque de toxicité sur le lieu de travail ou dans l'environnement. La complexation par des composés organiques est d'importance moyenne; comme la plupart des chélates sont labiles comparativement aux complexes covalents, ils ont une influence sur la biodisponibilité et le captage par les cellules. Cela étant, ils se forment et s'échangent en fonction des ligands qui sont présents dans l'environnement local et leurs mouvements en direction des cibles cellulaires est à peu près imprévisible. En revanche, une spéciation selon les différents états de valence ou sous la forme de composés minéraux ou organométalliques covalents conditionne en grande partie la toxicité des métaux et les éléments semi-métalliques.

4. Techniques et méthodes d'analyse

Au cours des 20 dernières années, l'efficacité des méthodes d'analyse de la spéciation des éléments a fait de remarquables progrès. Il est désormais possible d'analyser la spéciation de presque tous les éléments, mais pas encore pour toutes les espèces chimiques de chacun d'entre eux. On a également appris à recueillir et à conserver les échantillons selon des modalités qui permettent d'éviter leur contamination et de maintenir en l'état les espèces chimiques qu'ils contiennent. On sait aussi préparer les échantillons de liquides biologiques, de tissus, d'eau ou de poussières aéroportées de manière à identifier et doser les espèces chimiques qu'ils contiennent. Cette préparation peut comporter une étape supplémentaire de purification, la mise en œuvre de diverses techniques d'extraction ou encore la concentration préalable ou la formation de dérivés des espèces en cause avant leur séparation. Les techniques de séparation les plus couramment utilisées sont la chromatographie en phase liquide ou gazeuse, l'électrophorèse capillaire et l'électrophorèse en gel. Si les espèces sont trop complexes, on peut les isoler par groupes en procédant par extractions successives. C'est la technique la plus utilisée pour le fractionnement des sédiments, des sols, des aérosols et des cendres volantes. Généralement, ces méthodes permettent l'identification de l'élément, mais la détection des molécules progresse, notamment en biologie clinique et en analyse bromatologique. Les méthodes d'analyse couramment utilisées pour la recherche des éléments sont la spectrométrie d'absorption atomique, la spectrométrie de fluorescence atomique, la spectrométrie d'émission atomique et la spectrométrie de masse avec source de plasma à couplage inductif. On peut en outre utiliser la spectrométrie de masse à temps de vol et les plasmas produits par décharge luminescente comme sources accordables pour la spéciation des éléments. La spectrométrie de masse en mode électrospray et la spectrométrie de masse avec désorption au laser d'une matrice sont des techniques idéales pour obtenir des informations sur la structure des espèces moléculaires. Les méthodes électrochimiques sont également de puissants outils pour l'analyse de la spéciation.

Dans l'analyse de la spéciation des éléments, l'étalonnage pose encore des problèmes, notamment dans le cas d'espèces chimiques inconnues. Le choix des substances de référence pour l'analyse de la spéciation est encore limité mais le nombre de celles qui sont homologuées est en augmentation.

L'analyse directe de la spéciation des éléments présents dans des particules est d'un grand intérêt dans l'évaluation des dangers pour la santé qui sont liés à l'environnement. Elle fournit de précieux renseignements sur les espèces chimiques présentes dans les couches superficielles de ces particules et permet d'en tirer un certain nombre de conclusions au sujet de leur origine, de leur formation, de leur transport et des réactions chimiques qui s'y produisent. Dans la plupart des cas, ces analyses nécessitent un appareillage de pointe.

5. Bioaccessibilité et biodisponibilité

Avant d'être biodisponibles pour l'être humain, les substances chimiques doivent être bioaccessibles. Une substance est dite bio-accessible s'il lui est possible d'entrer en contact avec un organisme vivant susceptible de l'absorber. La bioaccessibilité est un facteur de première importance dans le cas des particules, du fait que les substances présentes à l'intérieur de ces dernières peuvent ne jamais être bioaccessibles. Les espèces chimiques d'un élément qui sont accessible à la surface des particules ou qui sont présentes en solution peuvent devenir biodisponibles s'il existe des mécanismes qui en permettent le captage par les cellules. La vitesse d'absorption d'une substance par les cellules dépend généralement de la concentration extracellulaire de cette substance, qui se peut se trouver sous la forme d'ions libres dotés de propriétés appropriées ou d'espèces minérales cinétiquement labiles (ions libres plus complexes minéraux). La complexation par des ligands organiques et la sorption par les particules ont souvent pour effet de réduire la vitesse d'absorption d'un élément, du fait qu'elle diminue la concentration des ions libres et des complexes minéraux labiles. Il arrive toutefois dans certains cas que la formation de complexes organiques d'un élément en facilite l'absorption par les cellules. Par ailleurs, le site où les particules sont en contact prolongé avec les tissus – l'épithélium des alvéoles pulmonaires par exemple – peut constituer un foyer d'exposition chronique et de toxicité. Les systèmes d'absorption cellulaire ne sont jamais totalement spécifiques d'un élément donné et il font l'objet d'une compétition entre espèces chimiques analogues de différents éléments, ce qui peut conduire à une inhibition de l'absorption d'éléments essentiels au profit d'éléments potentiellement toxiques. En raison de ces interactions compétitives, c'est souvent le rapport des concentrations ioniques qui détermine l'absorption cellulaire des éléments toxiques ou nutritifs. Les relations naturelles entre toxicité et nutrition peuvent également être la conséquence de ces interactions. Il est donc important de bien définir les interactions entre espèces chimiques avant de procéder à une évaluation du risque en raison des profonds effets qu'elles exercent sur la biodisponibilité et la toxicité.

6. Toxicocinétique et surveillance biologique

6.1 Toxicocinétique

Pour étudier l'absorption, les mécanismes de fixation aux protéines, la distribution, le stockage, le métabolisme, l'excrétion, la réactivité, l'activité toxique des éléments métalliques eux-mêmes il faut prendre en considération les divers aspects de leur spéciation (présence sous forme inchangée, mécanismes biologiques qui modifient la spéciation, états de valence, présence sous forme de complexes métal-ligand).

L'absorption au niveau des voies respiratoires est déterminée par la taille, la solubilité et la réactivité chimique des espèces chimiques inhalées sous forme de particules. Au niveau des voies digestives, l'absorption de ces espèces varie en fonction de leur solubilité dans l'eau et les sucs gastro-intestinaux, de leurs propriétés physiques et chimiques, de la présence d'autres espèces réactives et du moment de l'ingestion (à jeun par exemple). Le passage transcutané constitue également une importante voie d'absorption pour quelques espèces chimiques d'un certain nombre d'éléments.

Après absorption, les espèces chimiques d'un élément peuvent former des complexes avec des protéines, et notamment avec des enzymes, et c'est par exemple le cas des éléments essentiels associés à la ferritine (fer, cuivre, zinc), à l'α-amylase (cuivre), à l'alcool-déshydrogénase (zinc) et à l'anhydrase carbonique (cuivre, zinc).

D'une façon générale, le fait d'enlever ou d'ajouter des électrons à un atome influe sur l'activité chimique de l'élément correspondant et par conséquent sur l'aptitude d'un métal à interagir avec sa cible tissulaire (ligand). L'influence de la charge sur le franchissement des barrières lipidiques est illustrée par le passage des couples chromate/bichromate, Fe^{2+}/Fe^{3+} et Hg^{+}/Hg^{0}.

Parmi les autres transformations métaboliques, la plus importante est la bioalkylation que le mercure, l'étain et le plomb, par exemple, sont susceptibles de subir chez les microorganismes, l'arsenic et le sélénium pouvant de leur côté, également subir une bioalkylation lors de leur métabolisation par les organismes supérieurs. L'alkylation augmente le degré d'hydrophobicité, ce qui conduit à une augmentation de la biodisponibilité et facilite la pénétration intracellulaire ainsi que l'accumulation dans les tissus graisseux. Pour certains métaux, l'importance de la bioalkylation tient au fait qu'une fois alkylée, l'espèce chimique sous laquelle se trouve le métal interagit également avec l'ADN. Les espèces métalliques alkylées franchissent plus facilement la barrière hémato-encéphalique et c'est pourquoi ces espèces alkylées sont d'importants neurotoxiques.

Les éléments métalliques peuvent être stockés dans les tissus ou les organes sous la forme d'espèces minérales – des sels par exemple – ou sous la forme de chélates, ou encore être séquestrés par fixation aux protéines ou à d'autres composés organiques.

L'excrétion d'un élément dépend de sa spéciation, de sa voie d'absorption et des diverses phases toxicocinétiques. Il est excrété sous la forme d'une espèce minérale ou organique, souvent à son degré d'oxydation le plus bas. Les éléments qui sont ingérés avec les aliments ou l'eau de boisson sont excrétés dans la bile et les matières fécales et il existe aussi des voies d'excrétion mineures telles que l'haleine, le lait, la sueur, le système pileux ou les ongles. L'excrétion des éléments essentiels est constamment régulée par des mécanismes homéostatiques qui dépendent de la nature de l'élément.

6.2   *Surveillance biologique*

La surveillance biologique a principalement pour but de mesurer la dose interne – c'est-à-dire la quantité de la substance chimique résultant de son absorption systémique. Dans la surveillance biologique, la spéciation peut s'envisager à trois niveaux : 1) la recherche et le dosage de l'espèce chimique en cause (arsenic, par ex.); 2) le fractionnement par les diverses techniques de la chimie analytique en espèces organiques et minérales ou 3) la prise en compte, dans l'analyse, des informations que l'on possède sur la distribution des différentes espèces de l'élément en cause (le mercure dans le plasma, les éléments figurés du sang et l'urine; le chrome dans les érythrocytes et le plasma).

Ce qui fait le grand intérêt de la surveillance biologique, c'est que cette méthode prend en compte la totalité des sources d'exposition et des voies de pénétration. Le dosage de la quantité totale d'un élément présente dans l'organisme est particulièrement important dans le cas des espèces métalliques car les métaux ont tendance à s'accumuler. Le rapport de la concentration des espèces toxicologiquement actives au niveau de l'organe cible à la concentration totale de l'élément que l'on mesure par la surveillance biologique varie selon l'espèce chimique en cause.

7. Les mécanismes moléculaires et cellulaires de la toxicité des métaux

Les métaux et les éléments semi-métalliques ont, sur les processus biologiques, de multiples effets qu'on peut, dans une large mesure, rationaliser une fois décrites leurs interactions avec les différents types de molécules biologiques. Ces interactions sont très dépendantes de la nature des espèces en cause. C'est par la description, au niveau cellulaire et moléculaire, de ses effets sur les structures et les processus biochimiques que l'on parvient le mieux à comprendre l'action qu'un élément exerce sur les systèmes biologiques. Dans ce domaine en particulier, on observe une combinaison d'effets caractéristiques de l'espèce chimique en cause. L'approche traditionnelle consiste à examiner les interactions des éléments métalliques avec les principaux types de molécules biologiques, comme les protéines, les lipides, les glucides et les acides nucléiques. Cette démarche présente encore un certain intérêt, mais devient plus intéressante lorsqu'elle est replacée dans un contexte donné.

La production, par catalyse métallique, d'espèces oxygénées réactives peut endommager les molécules biologiques : la spéciation détermine la réactivité – catalytique ou autre – avec l'oxygène. Lorsque des ions métalliques tels que Hg^{2+} ou Cd^{2+} se lient directement aux protéines, ils peuvent inhiber leur activité enzymatique, leur capacité d'assemblage en structures déterminées ou encore nombre d'autres fonctions. En pareil cas, c'est l'état de valence de l'élément dans l'espèce en cause ou la présence de ligands qui détermine la capacité de liaison aux biomolécules et par conséquent, le type de toxicité. La peroxydation des lipides catalysée par des éléments métalliques sous forme ionique ou de complexes dotés d'activité rédox détruit les barrières protectrices des cellules et des organites infracellulaires. La liaison des ions métalliques aux glucides est complexe tant par les structures qui en résultent que par ses conséquences biologiques, mais il est clair qu'elle influe sur des processus tels que l'assemblage des glycoprotéines sous la forme d'une matrice extracellulaire fonctionnelle. Les réactions d'échanges de ligands avec les restes glucidiques dépendent de la nature des espèces en cause. La liaison aux acides nucléiques perturbe la régulation du génome à de nombreux niveaux, par exemple en rendant l'ADN plus vulnérable aux lésions et en inhibant sa réparation.

L'action des éléments métalliques sur le système immunitaire est un autre aspect de leur toxicité. Nombre d'entre eux sont capables de provoquer une immunodépression, mais on sait peu de choses sur le rôle des différentes espèces de ces éléments. Certaines d'entre elles et notamment celles du nickel, du cobalt et du chrome ont une action sensibilisatrice sur la peau et sur le système respiratoire. On connaît toutefois dans une certaine mesure le rôle joué par la spéciation, et les sels d'or utilisés en thérapeutique, de même que certaines espèces du cobalt et du nickel, en sont des exemples intéressants qui commencent à nous permettre de faire la lumière sur les mécanismes en cause.

8. Effets sur la santé

La toxicité peut varier dans d'importantes proportions en fonction d'un certain nombre de facteurs : degré d'oxydation de l'élément, formation de complexes ou biotransformation de l'espèce en cause. Dans le chapitre consacré aux effets sur la santé, sont donnés les exemples les plus significatifs (par ordre de numéro atomique) de cas où l'importance de la spéciation sur le plan des effets sanitaires chez l'Homme a été démontrée. Il s'agit notamment des effets toxiques aigus (chrome, nickel, arsenic, étain, baryum, mercure, plomb), des effets allergiques (chrome, nickel, palladium, platine), de la toxicité pulmonaire (cobalt), de la neurotoxicité (manganèse, étain, mercure, thallium, plomb), de la néphrotoxicité (cadmium), des effets toxiques sur la reproduction (nickel, mercure), de la génotoxicité (chrome, cobalt) et de la cancérogénicité (chrome, cobalt, nickel, arsenic). Une étude générale des données montre que, lorsqu'elle est possible, la prise en compte de la spéciation permet de mieux cerner les mécanismes qui sont à la base de la toxicité d'un élément donné et d'affiner l'évaluation du risque en faisant porter sur l'espèce principalement en cause l'examen des conséquences de l'exposition à l'élément étudié.

RESUMEN

1. Ámbito y finalidad del documento

El presente documento tiene por objeto evaluar y ofrecer orientación sobre la función de la especiación elemental y su análisis en la evaluación del peligro y del riesgo, más que presentar un examen de cada elemento y su especiación. No se examinan los efectos en el medio ambiente, puesto que éste ha sido el tema de una conferencia reciente y de la documentación asociada (SGOMSEC, 2003). Sin embargo, se examina la exposición de la población humana por vías ambientales.

Este documento está orientado a los evaluadores del riesgo y los encargados de la reglamentación, para subrayar la importancia del examen de la especiación en sus deliberaciones. Hasta ahora, esta cuestión no se ha incluido en la mayor parte de las evaluaciones del peligro y del riesgo. Además, uno de los objetivos del documento es alentar el análisis de la especiación de los elementos para mejorar los conocimientos sobre sus efectos en el mecanismo de acción y comprender sus repercusiones en la salud.

La atención no se concentra en las necesidades nutricionales, sino en la toxicidad de los elementos para las personas. No sólo se hace un examen de la exposición del consumidor/general, sino también de la exposición profesional.

2. Definiciones

Una "especie" química es la "forma específica de un elemento definida por su composición isotópica, su estado electrónico o de oxidación y/o su estructura compleja o molecular". La "especiación" se puede definir como la distribución de un elemento entre especies químicas definidas en un sistema, y el "análisis de la especiación" como las actividades analíticas de identificación y/o medición de las cantidades de una o más especies químicas determinadas en una muestra.

3. Aspectos estructurales de la especiación

Las definiciones de especie y especiación de elementos se basan en varios niveles diferentes de estructura atómica y molecular en los que se manifiestan diferencias entre las especies. Aquí examinamos las diferencias en los niveles de: 1) composición isotópica, 2) estado electrónico o de oxidación, 3) compuestos y complejos inorgánicos y orgánicos, 4) especies organometálicas y 5) compuestos y complejos macromoleculares. Algunos de estos niveles estructurales son más importantes que otros para la evaluación del riesgo. Así pues, si bien la composición de los isótopos estables es importante tanto desde el punto de vista teórico como de la química física y del medio ambiente, tiene en general una importancia mínima en la evaluación del riesgo relativo a la salud humana. Al mismo tiempo, la especiación elemental a nivel macromolecular tiene importancia biológica en la fisiología, la bioquímica y la nutrición, pero se conoce mucho menos su importancia en relación con las toxicidad profesional o ambiental. La formación de complejos orgánicos tiene una importancia intermedia; dado que la mayor parte de los quelatos son lábiles en relación con los complejos covalentes, influyen en la biodisponibilidad y la absorción celular. Sin embargo, su formación y su intercambio guardan relación con la disponibilidad de ligandos en el entorno local y su tránsito hasta objetivos celulares no es del todo previsible. Por otra parte, su valencia y la especiación organometálica inorgánica y covalente tienen una gran importancia para la determinación de la toxicidad de los metales y los semimetales.

4. Técnicas analíticas y metodología

Durante los 20 últimos años se han conseguido progresos notables en la realización de análisis de la especiación elemental. Ya se puede realizar un análisis de la especiación para casi todos los elementos, pero no para todas las especies de cada elemento. Se han mejorado los conocimientos acerca de la recogida y el almacenamiento de las muestras, a fin de evitar la contaminación y conservar las especies intactas. Los conocimientos disponibles permiten preparar las muestras para identificar y cuantificar las especies presentes en los fluidos biológicos, los tejidos, el agua y el polvo suspendido en el aire. La preparación de las muestras puede incluir una fase de limpieza adicional, procedimientos de extracción o la concentración previa y la derivación de las especies antes de su separación. Las técnicas de separación de uso más general son la cromatografía líquida, la cromatografía de gases, la electroforesis capilar y la electroforesis en gel. Si las especies son demasiado complejas, se pueden aislar grupos de especies aplicando métodos de extracción secuencial. Éste es el sistema más utilizado en el fraccionamiento de sedimentos, suelos, aerosoles y cenizas volátiles. La detección suele ser la del elemento, aunque la detección molecular está ganando terreno, especialmente en el análisis clínico y bromatológico. Los métodos de detección elemental más utilizados son la espectrometría de absorción atómica, la espectrometría de fluorescencia atómica, la espectrometría de emisión atómica y la espectrometría de emisión atómica de plasma con acoplamiento inductivo. Además, se pueden utilizar como fuentes sintonizables para la especiación elemental la espectrometría de masas por tiempo de vuelo con fuentes de plasma y los plasmas de descarga luminiscente. Para obtener información estructural acerca de las especies moleculares son ideales la espectrometría de masas por electropulverización y la espectrometría de masas de ionización por desorción de láser asistida por matriz. Los métodos electroquímicos son también instrumentos importantes para el análisis de la especiación.

En el análisis de la especiación elemental, la calibración sigue siendo un problema, sobre todo en el caso de especies desconocidas. Hay un número limitado de materiales de referencia para la especiación elemental y cada vez son más los que están certificados.

El análisis de la especiación directa de elementos en partículas tiene de gran interés en la evaluación de los riesgos para la salud relacionados con el medio ambiente. Proporciona una información valiosa sobre las especies elementales que se encuentran en las capas superficiales de las partículas, permitiendo realizar deducciones acerca del origen, la formación, el transporte y las reacciones químicas. En la mayoría de los casos se necesitan aparatos muy complejos.

5. Bioaccesibilidad y biodisponibilidad

Las sustancias deben ser bioaccesibles antes de que puedan convertirse en biodisponibles para las personas. Una sustancia se define como bioaccesible si existe la posibilidad de que entre en contacto con un organismo vivo, que luego puede absorberla. La bioaccesibilidad es un aspecto importante que se ha de considerar en relación con las partículas, dado que las especies de su interior pueden no llegar a ser nunca bioaccesibles. Las especies elementales que son accesibles sobre la superficie de las partículas o en solución pueden estar biodisponibles si existen mecanismos para su absorción por las células vivas. La velocidad de su absorción por las células suele estar en relación con la concentración externa de iones libres con propiedades adecuadas o bien con especies inorgánicas cinéticamente lábiles (iones libres más complejos inorgánicos). La formación de complejos orgánicos y la unión de partículas con frecuencia reducen las tasas de absorción de elementos, al disminuir las concentraciones de iones libres y complejos inorgánicos lábiles. Sin embargo, en determinadas circunstancias los complejos orgánicos de un elemento pueden facilitar su absorción. Además, el lugar en el que las partículas tienen un contacto prolongado con los tejidos, como el epitelio alveolar de los pulmones, se puede convertir en un foco de exposición y toxicidad crónicas. Los sistemas de absorción no son nunca totalmente específicos de un solo elemento y en ellos se produce a menudo competencia entre especies químicas semejantes de elementos diferentes, con el resultado de la inhibición de la absorción de elementos esenciales y la absorción de elementos competidores potencialmente tóxicos. Debido a estas interacciones competitivas, las proporciones de iones controlan con frecuencia la absorción celular de elementos tóxicos y nutrientes. Antes de realizar una evaluación del riesgo hay que definir con claridad las interacciones de las especies químicas, debido a sus importantes repercusiones en la disponibilidad y la toxicidad.

6. Toxicocinética y biovigilancia

6.1 Toxicocinética

Al evaluar la absorción, los mecanismos de unión a proteínas, la distribución, el almacenamiento, el metabolismo, la excreción, la reactividad y la actividad tóxica de los propios elementos metálicos se deben tener en cuenta diversos aspectos de la especiación de los elementos (por ejemplo, las formas inalteradas, los mecanismos biológicos que modifican las especies, los diferentes estados de valencia y los complejos metal-ligando).

La absorción a través del tracto respiratorio depende del tamaño, la solubilidad y la reactividad química de las especies elementales inhaladas como partículas. La absorción de especies elementales en el tracto gastrointestinal varía en función de su solubilidad en agua y en los fluidos gastrointestinales, sus características químicas y físicas, la presencia de otros compuestos reactivos y el período de ingestión (por ejemplo en ayunas). La piel también puede ser una vía de absorción importante para algunas especies elementales.

Tras la absorción, las especies elementales pueden formar complejos con proteínas, incluidas las enzimas, por ejemplo los elementos esenciales asociados con la ferritina (hierro, cobre, zinc), la α-amilasa (cobre), la alcohol deshidrogenasa (zinc) y la anhidrasa carbónica (cobre, zinc).

En general, la eliminación de electrones de los átomos o su adición a ellos influye en la actividad química y, por consiguiente, en la capacidad de interacción de los elementos metálicos con determinados tejidos (ligandos). Son ejemplos de la importancia de la carga en relación con el tránsito a través de las barreras lipídicas los pasos de cromato/dicromato, Fe^{2+}/Fe^{3+} y Hg^+/Hg^0.

Entre las otras transformaciones metabólicas, la más importante es la bioalquilación que, por ejemplo, experimentan el mercurio, el estaño y el plomo en los microorganismos, mientras que el arsénico y el selenio sufren una bioalquilación adicional como parte de sus vías metabólicas en organismos superiores. La alquilación produce especies en un nivel hidrofóbico más elevado, dando lugar a un aumento de la biodisponibilidad, la penetración celular y la acumulación en tejidos grasos. La bioalquilación es importante para algunos metales, puesto que las especies metálicas alquiladas también interaccionan con el ADN. Dichas especies atraviesan la barrera hematoencefálica con más facilidad y por este motivo son sustancias neurotóxicas importantes.

En los tejidos/órganos se pueden almacenar elementos metálicos como especies inorgánicas o sales y como especies queladas o fijadas a proteínas y a otros compuestos orgánicos.

La excreción depende de la especiación, la vía de absorción y otras fases toxicocinéticas. Las especies excretadas son inorgánicas u orgánicas y con frecuencia están en el estado de oxidación más bajo. Los elementos ingeridos con los alimentos o el agua se excretan por medio de la bilis y las heces; son vías secundarias de excreción la respiración, la leche, el sudor, el pelo y las uñas. La excreción de elementos esenciales, en función del que se trate, está bajo el control constante de mecanismos homeostáticos eficaces.

6.2   *Biovigilancia*

El principal objetivo de la vigilancia biológica es la medición de la dosis interna, es decir, la cantidad de sustancia química que se absorbe de manera sistemática. La especiación en la vigilancia biológica se puede abordar en tres niveles diferentes: 1) el análisis de especies de elementos específicos (por ejemplo, el arsénico), 2) el fraccionamiento por medios analíticos químicos para obtener especies orgánicas e inorgánicas (por ejemplo, el mercurio, el plomo) o 3) la aplicación al análisis de la información sobre las diferencias en la distribución de las distintas especies de un elemento (el mercurio en el plasma, los eritrocitos, la orina; el plomo en los eritrocitos/plasma).

La vigilancia biológica tiene un valor especial porque el método integra la exposición a partir de todas las fuentes y por todas las vías de entrada. La medición de la carga corporal interna reviste una importancia particular para las especies de metales, debido a su tendencia a la acumulación. La proporción entre la concentración de especies importantes desde el punto de vista toxicológico en el lugar destinatario y la concentración elemental total medida en la biovigilancia es diferente para las distintas especies.

7.   Mecanismos moleculares y celulares de la toxicidad de los metales

Los metales y semimetales tienen efectos múltiples en los procesos biológicos, que se pueden racionalizar en gran medida después de describir las interacciones con las diversas clases de biomoléculas. Tales interacciones dependen fundamentalmente de las especies. Como mejor se comprenden los efectos de los distintos elementos en los sistemas biológicos es mediante los efectos de los elementos en las estructuras y los procesos bioquímicos, descritos a nivel celular y molecular. Sobre todo en este sector, es evidente una combinación de efectos característicos de una especie concreta. Tradicionalmente se han examinado las interacciones de los elementos metálicos con los principales tipos de biomoléculas, es decir, proteínas, lípidos, carbohidratos y ácidos nucleicos. Este método todavía tiene algún valor, pero aumenta su importancia cuando se pone en un contexto.

La generación catalítica mediante metales de especies reactivas de oxígeno puede dañar todas las biomoléculas: la especiación determina la reactividad – catalítica o de otro tipo – con el oxígeno. La unión directa a proteínas de iones como el Hg^{2+} y el Cd^{2+} puede inhibir las actividades enzimáticas, los ensamblajes estructurales y otras muchas funciones de las proteínas. Aquí, el estado de valencia y/o los ligandos asociados determinan la disponibilidad para la unión, y en consecuencia, la modalidad de la toxicidad. La peroxidación de los lípidos catalizada por elementos metálicos en su forma iónica y en complejos con actividad redox destruye las barreras protectoras de los orgánulos celulares y subcelulares. La unión de iones metálicos a carbohidratos se ve complicada tanto por la química estructural como por las consecuencias biológicas, pero afecta sin duda a procesos como el ensamblaje de las glucoproteínas en la matriz extracelular funcional. Las reacciones de intercambio de ligandos con grupos de azúcares dependen de la especie. La unión a ácidos nucleicos interfiere con la regulación del genoma en muchos niveles. Esto significa que facilita tanto la producción de daños en el ADN como la inhibición de su reparación.

Otra dimensión de la toxicidad de los metales está en los efectos de los distintos elementos en el sistema inmunitario. Si bien hay muchos elementos que pueden producir inmunosupresión, es poco lo que se conoce acerca de la función de las distintas especies elementales. Algunas de ellas, por ejemplo las del níquel, el cobalto y el cromo, son sensibilizadores cutáneos y del sistema respiratorio. Se conoce en cierto grado la función de la especiación, siendo las sales de oro, las especies de cadmio y las especies de níquel con actividad terapéutica ejemplos interesantes que comienzan a arrojar luz sobre los mecanismos.

8.   Efectos en la salud

La toxicidad puede variar de manera significativa en función del estado de oxidación del elemento, la formación de complejos y/o la transformación de las especies elementales. En el capítulo sobre los efectos en la salud, se ofrece una selección de los ejemplos más significativos (por orden de número atómico) en los que se ha demostrado la importancia de la especiación en relación con los efectos en la salud humana, con inclusión de la toxicidad aguda (cromo, níquel, arsénico, estaño, bario, mercurio, plomo), la alergia (cromo, níquel, paladio, platino), la toxicidad pulmonar (cobalto), la neurotoxicidad (manganeso, estaño, mercurio, talio, plomo), la nefrotoxicidad (cadmio), la toxicidad reproductiva (níquel, mercurio), la genotoxicidad (cromo, cobalto) y la carcinogenicidad (cromo, cobalto, níquel, arsénico). Una evaluación global de los datos indica que, cuando es posible, el examen de la especiación permite conocer mejor los mecanismos de la toxicidad de un elemento y perfeccionar la evaluación del riesgo, al concentrar la evaluación de las consecuencias de la exposición en las especies de mayor interés.

INDEX OF ELEMENTS

Aluminium (Al), 21, 24, 50, 57
  analysis, 46
  bioavailability, 16, 17, 53, 57, 58, 60
  biomonitoring, 110
Antimony (Sb), 13, 36
  analysis, 26, 40, 41, 43
  biomonitoring, 110
  biotransformation, 18
Arsenic (As), 13, 14, 20, 21, 24, 36
  absorption, 78–80
  acute toxicity, 7, 124–126
  analysis, 25, 26, 34–37, 40, 41, 43, 45, 46
  bioaccessibility, 49
  bioavailability, 14, 59
  biomonitoring, 5, 105, 107–110
  biotransformation, 5, 18, 19, 51, 97–102
  carcinogenicity, 7, 158–161
  detoxification, 19, 20
  distribution, 90, 91
  excretion, 91
  exposure, 60, 104, 105
  mode of action, 14, 113
Barium (Ba), 7, 57, 127, 128
Beryllium (Be), 58, 60, 120, 130
Bismuth (Bi), 36
Boron (B), 61
Cadmium (Cd), 7, 14, 57, 60, 86, 104
  absorption, 81
  analysis, 37, 46
  bioaccessibility, 49, 51
  bioavailability, 17, 53, 54, 56, 60, 61, 66, 67
  biomonitoring, 110
  distribution, 92
  excretion, 92, 93
  immunosuppression, 121

  mode of action, 6, 56, 113, 115, 117
  nephrotoxicity, 7, 21, 144, 145
Chromium (Cr), 4, 12, 13, 24, 57, 162, 163
  absorption, 73, 74
  acute toxicity, 7, 122, 123
  analysis, 27, 28, 30, 37, 41, 43, 45, 46
  bioaccessibility, 49
  bioavailability, 12, 13, 53, 54, 57–60, 67
  biomonitoring, 5, 106, 107, 109, 110
  biotransformation, 98
  carcinogenicity, 7, 12, 153, 154
  distribution, 86, 87
  excretion, 87, 88
  exposure, 60, 104, 105, 112
  genotoxicity, 7, 12, 148–150
  mode of action, 112, 119, 120
  sensitization, 6, 7, 120, 130–132
Cobalt (Co), 13, 14, 23, 57, 60, 63
  absorption, 76
  analysis, 30
  bioavailability, 53, 54, 60, 66, 67
  biomonitoring, 107
  biotransformation, 18
  carcinogenicity, 7, 154, 155
  genotoxicity, 7, 150–152
  lung toxicity, 7, 134, 135
  mode of action, 111, 113, 119, 120
  sensitization, 6, 120, 130
Copper (Cu), 4, 13, 14, 24, 50, 57, 60, 63, 85, 86
  absorption, 78

analysis, 34, 37, 38, 46
bioaccessibility, 51
bioavailability, 53, 56, 59–
    61, 66, 67
biomonitoring, 110
distribution, 89, 90
mode of action, 111, 112,
    115, 117–120
sensitization, 120
Germanium (Ge), 18
Gold (Au), 7, 57, 120
Iron (Fe), 4, 13–15, 17, 21, 24,
    50, 57, 63, 85, 97
absorption, 76
analysis, 43
bioaccessibility, 51
bioavailability, 53–56, 58,
    60, 62, 67
mode of action, 111, 112,
    115–117, 119
Lead (Pb), 11, 13, 14, 18, 20,
    21, 36, 57, 60
absorption, 83–85
acute toxicity, 7, 129, 130
analysis, 34, 45, 47
bioaccessibility, 49, 51
bioavailability, 53, 54, 60,
    61
biomonitoring, 5, 24, 105–
    107, 110
biotransformation, 5, 18, 20,
    51, 97
distribution, 96, 97
mode of action, 56, 113
neurotoxicity, 7, 142–144
Manganese (Mn), 13, 14, 50, 57,
    60, 63
absorption, 74–76
analysis, 30, 43
bioaccessibility, 51
bioavailability, 53, 54, 60,
    66, 67
biomonitoring, 108, 109
biotransformation, 98
distribution, 88
excretion, 88, 89

lung toxicity, 54, 60
mode of action, 14
neurotoxicity, 7, 136, 137
Mercury (Hg), 4, 13, 15, 18, 21,
    36, 57, 162
absorption, 81–83
acute toxicity, 7, 128, 129
analysis, 34, 36, 40–42, 45,
    47
bioaccessibility, 49
bioavailability, 52–55, 60,
    61
biomonitoring, 5, 24, 105,
    106, 109, 110
biotransformation, 5, 18, 20,
    51, 97, 102–104
distribution, 93–95
excretion, 95, 96
mode of action, 6, 56, 117,
    120
neurotoxicity, 7, 138–141
reproductive toxicity, 7,
    146–148
sensitization, 120
Molybdenum (Mo), 13, 50
bioavailability, 59, 61, 64,
    65, 67
Nickel (Ni), 7, 13, 14, 16
absorption, 77, 78
acute toxicity, 7, 123, 124
analysis, 30, 46
bioaccessibility, 49, 51
bioavailability, 17, 53, 54,
    57, 60
carcinogenicity, 7, 15, 156–
    158
exposure, 15, 60, 104, 105
mode of action, 111–114,
    119–121
reproductive toxicity, 7, 145,
    146
sensitization, 6, 7, 120, 121,
    130, 132
Palladium (Pd), 13, 57
sensitization, 7, 120, 130,
    132, 133

Platinum (Pt), 13, 57
   acute toxicity, 109
   analysis, 27, 38
   biomonitoring, 109, 110
   nephrotoxicity, 109
   reproductive toxicity, 109
   sensitization, 7, 109, 120,
     130, 133, 134
Plutonium (Pu), 12, 13
Selenium (Se), 13, 36, 60
   absorption, 80
   analysis, 26, 33–37, 40, 41,
     43, 46
   bioavailability, 59, 64
   biomonitoring, 110
   biotransformation, 5, 18, 19,
     97, 102
   detoxification, 19
   distribution, 91
   excretion, 91
   mode of action, 116, 118,
     119
Silicon (Si), 61
Silver (Ag), 13, 38, 57
   bioavailability, 53, 54, 60,
     61
   biomonitoring, 110
   distribution, 91, 92
   mode of action, 117
Tellurium (Te), 13, 26
Thallium (Tl), 13, 57
   analysis, 43
   mode of action, 56
   neurotoxicity, 7, 141, 142
Tin (Sn), 13, 20, 36, 57, 162
   acute toxicity, 7, 126, 127
   analysis, 34, 35, 42, 43, 45,
     46
   bioavailability, 54
   biotransformation, 5, 18, 97
   neurotoxicity, 7, 137, 138
Uranium (U), 11, 13
Vanadium (V), 13, 14, 57
   bioavailability, 59, 64, 65
   biomonitoring, 110

Zinc (Zn), 4, 13, 14, 50, 56, 57,
   63, 85, 86
   analysis, 34, 37
   bioaccessibility, 51
   bioavailability, 53, 54, 59,
     60, 62, 66, 67
   biomonitoring, 110
   distribution, 90
   exposure, 60
   mode of action, 114, 115,
     117

www.ingramcontent.com/pod-product-compliance
Lightning Source LLC
Chambersburg PA
CBHW061207220326
41597CB00015BA/1552